Contents

List of contributors

F. Ian Atkinson BSc(Hons), PhD, RGN, RMN, Senior Lecturer, School of Health, University of Teesside, Middlesbrough, TS1 3BA, England.

David C. Benton RGN, RMN, BSc, MPhil, Chief Executive, National Board for Nursing, Midwifery and Health Visiting for Scotland, 22 Queen Street, Edinburgh EH2 1NT, Scotland.

Senga Bond PhD, RN, FRCN, Professor of Nursing Research, Centre for Health Services Research, School of Health Sciences, University of Newcastle upon Tyne, 21 Claremont Place, Newcastle upon Tyne NE2 4AA, England.

Diana E. Carter BA, MSc, RGN, RM, RNT, Senior Lecturer, Nursing & Midwifery School, University of Glasgow, 68 Oakfield Avenue, Glasgow G12 8LS, Scotland.

Jennifer E. Clark MSc in Public Sector Management, CertEd, RN, RM, RHV, Senior Lecturer, School of Health Sciences Nursing, University of Birmingham, The Medical School, Edgbaston, Birmingham B15 2TT, England.

Desmond F.S. Cormack RNN, RGN, DipNurs, MPhil, DipEd, PhD, formerly Honorary Reader in Health and Nursing, Department of Health and Nursing, Queen Margaret University College, Clerwood Terrace, Edinburgh EH8 8TS, Scotland

Peter T. Donnan DCR, BA, BSc(Hons), MSc, PhD, Senior Research Fellow, Medicines Monitoring Unit, University of Dundee, Ninewells Hospital and Medical School, Dundee DD1 8SY, Scotland.

Robert J. Edelmann BSc, MPhil, PhD, FBPsS, CPsychol, Honorary Visiting Professor, Faculty of Social and Life Sciences, School of Psychology and Counselling, Roehampton Institute London, Whitelands College, West Hill, London SW15 3SN, England.

Paul Fulbrook MSc, BSc(Hons), PGDE, RGN, DPSN, Senior Lecturer in Research, Institute of Health and Community Studies, Bournemouth University, Royal London House, Christchurch Road, Bournemouth, Dorset BH1 3LT, England.

Lisbeth Hockey OBE, SRN, SCM, HV, QNCert, RNT, RFCN, BSc(Econ), PhD, Visiting Professor, Buckinghamshire Chilterns University College; and Honorary Reader in Health and Nursing, Department of Health and Nursing, Queen Margaret University College, Clerwood Terrace, Edinburgh EH12 8TS, Scotland.

Hazel E. McHaffie SRN, RM, PhD, Research Fellow, Medical Ethics, Department of Medicine, University of Edinburgh; and Deputy Director of Research, Institute of Medical Ethics, Department of Medicine, University of Edinburgh, Royal Infirmary, Lauriston Place, Edinburgh EH3 9YW, Scotland.

Tricia Murphy-Black RM, RGN, RCNT, MSc, PhD, Professor of Midwifery, Department of Nursing and Midwifery, University of Stirling, Stirling FK9 4LA, Scotland.

David Pontin RN, RSCN, RHV, PhD, Senior Lecturer, Institute of Health Studies (Somerset Centre), University of Plymouth, Taunton, Somerset TA1 5YD, England.

Sam Porter RN, DipNurs, BSSc, PhD, Senior Lecturer in Sociology, Department of Sociology and Social Policy, The Queen's University of Belfast, Belfast BT7 1NN, Northern Ireland.

Anne Marie Rafferty DPhil(Oxon), RGN, DN, Director, Centre for Policy in Nursing Research, London School of Hygiene and Tropical Medicine, Keppel Street, London WC1E 7HT, England.

Preface

The general inspiration for this book came from the now widely accepted sense of the need for *all* nurses, midwives and related groups to become aware of, and knowledgeable about, the application of the research process to their specialist areas – this applying equally to clinicians, educators and managers. All the teachers and colleagues from whom I have learned research skills are recognized as having sown the seeds of this work. These individuals, some of whom contributed to this book, have made a unique contribution to the development of research.

Students to whom I taught the subject and whose research I have supervised, also contributed to this work. It might be argued that one of the best means of extending one's knowledge of a subject is to teach it – research is no exception.

Not all will carry out research work, although the potential for all professionals to do so exists. Many will choose to remain consumers of the research undertaken by others, but a thorough understanding of the research process, as outlined in this book, is essential to both researchers and consumers of research. Thus, all individuals in the professions for whom this book was written require an understanding of the research process and this text offers one means of doing so. It has been prepared and designed to enable it to be used to introduce the subject either during or after training.

Although the title and much of the terminology used in this text may imply that it relates mainly to nurses and nursing, this is not so. The term *nurse* should be taken as 'shorthand' to also encompass other staff groups who are part of, or are in close relationship with, the nursing profession. Examples are midwives, health visitors, district nurses, occupational health nurses, and community mental health nurses. Indeed, because the research process is the same irrespective of the discipline being studied, other health care groups such as occupational therapists, psychologists, social workers, pharmacologists, and chiropodists may find this book of value.

Although the contribution to research by men *and* women in nursing, midwifery and so on is firmly recognized, they and researchers will be referred to as 'she' throughout this text. Where the subject of the research is referred to – for example, the patient or client – the term 'he' will be used, with the obvious exception of groups who are exclusively female, such as expectant mothers. Thus, the repeated use of the clumsy alternative 'he/she' or 'she or he' will be avoided.

Since the publication of the third edition of this book in 1996, the terms *evidence-based nursing/midwifery* have become commonly used. For readers who understand *evidence-based nursing/midwifery* to be synonymous with *research-based nursing/midwifery*, this text will contribute to that understanding. For readers who understand *evidence-based nursing/midwifery* to include, rather than to be synonymous with, *research-based nursing/midwifery*, this text will contribute to an understanding of the research element of the former term.

Finally, those who contributed to this book have done so recognizing that no single text or experience can, of itself, provide all the answers relating to the research process or any of its parts. This book should be used as part of a planned programme of study for one of two purposes. First, by those who wish to read and understand research findings, examples of this group are all trained nurses and midwives and those in training. Second, as part of a programme of study which will enable reading and understanding of research, and which will then underpin further reading and *supervised* research being undertaken by some individuals.

Desmond F.S. Cormack

Introduction to the research process

The purpose of Part I is to put the subsequent discussion of the research process into context and to 'set the scene' for the more detailed material which follows. The introduction is presented in the firm belief that this must precede a consideration of the detailed phases of the research process. Only with the initial, more general, introduction, will readers be able to optimize their understanding of research and their potential contribution to the development of a research-based profession. Chapter 1 presents a clear description of what research is and why it is of importance. Not all readers will have a prior belief in the value of research; this chapter provides a persuasive argument which will reinforce the views of the converted, and convert the sceptic.

The use of specialist research terms may inhibit the use of published research and frustrate attempts to understand what the research process is, and how to make use of it. The selected common terms and concepts discussed in Chapter 2 are intended to introduce readers to the specialist language of research. Although over-use of technical terms or 'jargon' is to be strongly condemned, a number of terms and concepts must be understood by the reader of research reports. The purpose of this chapter is not to present a comprehensive list of such terms, rather it is intended to demonstrate the need to understand the terms and the relative ease with which their meaning can be understood.

Because of the central importance of *validity and reliability* to the research process, an entire chapter has now been dedicated solely to these concepts (see Chapter 3).

Chapter 4 is intended to reduce the potential isolation which many aspiring researchers experience or fear because they are unaware of the many and varied agencies which are available to give support. Some of these agencies may be unknown; some may be known but thought of as being only for the use of 'others'.

A full consideration of ethical issues pervades all aspects of research, particularly those that deal with human subjects, as is often the case in health care. Chapter 5 considers these issues and offers guidelines which will direct both those who do and those who consume research.

Finally, Chapter 6 presents a sequential description of the research process and the interrelationship of each of its phases, while recognizing that there is no single *blueprint* for this process. This general overview of the research process should be seen as an introduction to the more detailed discussion of the steps in the process which are presented in Part II.

CHAPTER 1

The nature and purpose of research

Lisbeth Hockey

Since 1984, when the first edition of this book was published, research has been included, directly or indirectly, in most nursing curricula. The topic is gaining ever-increasing prominence in health care related conferences, study days, workshops and other professional activities within continuing professional education. Research has become a commonly used term in the professional vocabulary and it is incumbent on all nurses* to cultivate some familiarity with research and its appropriate use. From being 'urgent', as referred to in the first chapter of the third edition, 1996, research has become unavoidable and necessary.

The nature of research

What is research?

The essential nature of research lies in its intent to create new knowledge in whatever field. It does this through a process of systematic enquiry governed by scientific principles, as outlined in Chapter 6. The principles vary according to the specific science or discipline in which the research is undertaken. Although the term *research* is now commonplace, it still does not seem to be given its correct meaning by some people, both lay and professional. Definitions of research remain sparse, probably because authors of research texts continue to assume that the meaning of the term is self-evident. In my view this is an unwarranted assumption and misconceptions remain. In fact, it seems that increasing use of the term goes hand in hand with increasing misuse and abuse. There are still many people in all walks of life who believe that research connotes the kind of advanced scientific activity which is only undertaken by scientists in an academic setting, probably in a laboratory. While such activity is likely to be research, the inter-

---

* In this chapter, in line with the remainder of the book, the term *nurse* should be taken as 'shorthand' to also encompass other staff groups who are part of, or are in close relationship with, the nursing profession. Examples are midwives, health visitors, district nurses, occupational health nurses, and community mental health nurses.

pretation is narrow and does not include many other types of endeavour which are not necessarily undertaken by academic scientists in a laboratory. For others, it means little more than common sense, which is also a misguided belief. Common sense is extremely useful but not adequate. The essential characteristic of research is its scientific nature; research is a process which has to be undertaken according to certain scientific rules – the research process.

The research process can be learned and applied by people who are not necessarily academic scientists and it need not be confined to a laboratory. The research process consists of a sequence of steps which includes mental activities that are designed to increase the sum of what is known about certain phenomena in all types of disciplines.

Defining research

A definition, or rather an explanation of research, was offered by Macleod Clark & Hockey (1989) as

> 'an attempt to increase the sum of what is known, usually referred to as "a body of knowledge", by the discovery of new facts or relationships through a process of systematic scientific enquiry, the research process.'

It is important to recognize that it is not only the discovery of new facts which adds to available knowledge, but also that of new relationships.

The variations in the research process between the various disciplines are due to their own specific modes of thought and their own paradigms and theories. Thus, the physical scientist's approach to the exploration of new knowledge will be different from that of the historian or the behaviourist. The basic principles of the systematic process will be observed by all.

The main types of research are fully explained in Chapters 12–22 inclusive. It remains here merely to draw attention to the differences which stem from the basic scientific roots of the discipline in which the research is undertaken. Nursing provides an ideal way of illustrating this point and also demonstrates the need for nurses to familiarize themselves with the sciences underlying nursing.

Nursing research

What is nursing research? Is it different from other research and, if so, in what way? Many different definitions of nursing research have been advanced and there cannot be a totally right or wrong answer to the questions about its nature. Because nursing encompasses a wide range of activities, because it is interpreted differently in different parts of the world, and because it changes over time, a definition of the term 'nursing research' and an explanation of its nature should make provision for these variations.

Nursing research is defined here as research into those aspects of professional activity which are predominantly and appropriately the concern and responsibility of nurses. Where nurses have little or no appropriate or predominant responsibility, nursing research makes little sense. Where nurses have responsibility for nursing education, for the administration of nursing services, and for all aspects of nursing practice, nursing research encompasses all these areas. At the time when nurses were not the appropriate personnel to monitor patients' vital signs – for example, blood pressure – nursing research would not have included studies of such monitoring procedures. Similarly, in countries where nurses are not in control of nursing education, research in the field of nursing education would lie outside the scope of nursing research and the same is true for nursing administration.

In terms of the research process – the series of logical steps which have to be undertaken to develop further the available knowledge – nursing research is no different from any other. The same rules of the scientific method apply and, just as in any other research, the specific type, design and method of the research must be appropriate for the problems or questions to be investigated. Nursing represents a unique mix of several disciplines and any of the disciplines underlying nursing might be appropriate for research in nursing; for example, patients' anxiety can be viewed and studied from a psychological perspective, in which case psychological knowledge will be applied and psychological measurements might be utilized. Patients' anxiety can also be viewed and studied from a physiological perspective, in which case the biological sciences will be invoked to provide the necessary scientific guidelines. In time, nursing will develop more of its own nursing perspectives and nursing measures. It may be of interest to some to explore the development of nursing, which can be retrieved from documentary sources through systematic historical enquiry. Such historical research will also attempt to disentangle the events of the time, to explore primary and secondary sources in the hope of offering plausible explanations of events, and to throw new light on those events by the discovery of relationships.

The science of physiology has provided new knowledge about the relationship between skin integrity and pressure. However, it is possible that other variables, such as the action of certain drugs or mental state, may also play a part in causing skin sores.

In order to discover effective treatments, experimental research – that is, the collection of data in rigorously controlled situations – will be appropriate. Organizational change might best be explored through action research (see Chapter 16) which deliberately rules out any control of the situation.

Nursing research is also explained by Montgomery Robinson et al. (1991) in a self-learning module. Clamp (1994) describes research in nursing as 'providing a link between practice, education and theory, thereby making it essential for all nurses to become knowledgeable consumers or, for the minority research, doers'. It is important to recognize, therefore, that questions initiating research can and should originate in any field of nursing. Research must begin with a question and it invariably generates further questions. It is in this way that the knowledge underlying nursing grows like a spiral. There can be no end point as the universe will never be totally mastered (Fig. 1.1). It is this continuous never-ending potential to create and use further knowledge, the opportunity for ongoing learning, that not only enables nursing to develop its all-important body of knowledge but also makes life exciting and worth while for us all.

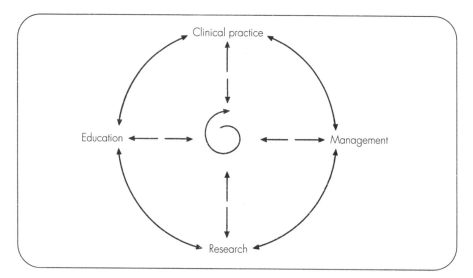

Fig. 1.1   The spiral of knowledge.

The purpose of nursing research

Deductive and inductive research

Nursing research may set out to test theories developed in other settings: for example, organizational theories developed in industry have been tested in nursing. It may set out to test theories or models developed by other researchers in nursing. Research which is designed to test general theories in particular situations is referred to as deductive research. It is also possible to study nursing inductively. Here, the particular situation would be the starting point for study. Inductive research, which also has its own scientific rules, might result in the identification of certain patterns, eventually leading to the formulation of hypotheses or the advancement of general theories which can then be tested deductively.

As suggested by the definitions of research given above, its purpose is to increase the body of knowledge, the sum of what is known. The purpose of research in nursing is, therefore, to increase the sum of what is known about the professional activity of nurses, which may be nursing education, administration or practice in its many forms and settings. Nursing research is relatively new and a great deal of what nurses do and teach is based on tradition, convention, intuition and beliefs rather than on evidence. Nursing research attempts to change this situation and to provide the professional discipline of nursing with a base which can be defended on grounds of scientifically established knowledge.

Nursing research begins with questions about nursing. Questions may be generated by an intelligent curiosity or by a wish to find out more about the respective activity; they may also be generated by an urgent need to identify more effective and, probably, less costly methods of providing nursing care, of educating nurses or of providing an effective administrative structure.

There are many unanswered questions in nursing and there are many more questions which have not yet been asked. The main purposes of nursing research may be summarized as:

1. To establish scientifically defensible reasons for nursing activities.
2. To provide nurses with an increased repertoire of scientifically defensible nursing intervention options.
3. To find ways of increasing the cost-effectiveness of nursing activities.
4. To provide a basis for standard setting and quality assurance.
5. To provide evidence of weaknesses and strengths in nursing.
6. To provide evidence in support of demands for resources in nursing.
7. To give the term *evidence-based practice* scientific credence.
8. To satisfy the academic curiosity of thinking nurses.
9. To facilitate interdisciplinary collaboration in nursing and nursing research.
10. To earn and defend a professional status for nursing.

At the first International Conference on Community Health Nursing Research in 1993, the purposes of community health nursing research embedded in 436 abstracts were distilled, as shown in Fig. 1.2. At the same conference the overall purposes of community health nursing were stated as:

'... an attempt to find means by which potential patients can be prevented from becoming actual patients and means by which the health and well-being of both groups in the community can be promoted.' (King *et al.*, 1993)

This mode of thought concerning community health nursing research can easily be adapted to embrace nursing research in general.

Although the main purpose of nursing research in the current business-oriented health service tends to be seen in terms of a direct pay-off for patient care, it is important not to lose sight of the other stated purposes.

The necessity of nursing research

In the opening paragraph of this chapter, the necessity of nursing research was stressed. This section is intended to support this statement. As early as 1972, the

---

Purposes

- Targeting of services
- Curriculum content
- Instrument construction/testing
- Theory construction/testing
- Client assessment
- Direct care provision
- Others

Overall purpose – explicit/implicit

'Better' understanding of self and others

'Better' quality of:

- service
- care
- education

Fig. 1.2 Purposes of community health nursing research (King *et al.*, 1993).

Committee on Nursing (1972) stressed the need to give nursing a research base, stating: '...a sense of the need for research should become part of the mental equipment of every practising nurse or midwife'.

Evidence-based nursing

The term *evidence-based nursing* is being used with increasing frequency and in many different contexts. It is to some extent influenced by one's understanding of 'evidence' (Kendall, 1997). Some readers are likely to consider the term synonymous with *research-based nursing*. Others may interpret it as part of research-based nursing while some seem to subordinate the research base to the evidence base. Whatever the reader's individual stance in relation to the two terms, this text should contribute to a clearer understanding.

Cormack (1979) suggested that the nursing profession will be recognized as being 'research based' when the above situation is achieved and when research becomes an integral part of nursing practice. From a paper by English (1994) it seems that the desired situation has not yet been achieved. He makes the point that

'in spite of an escalation of nursing research in the last 22 years, it has generally failed to influence clinical practice. Also, in spite of a considerable increase in nursing theory, nursing still cannot claim to be a research based profession.'

Other authoritative statements point to the urgent need for nursing research.

The International Council of Nurses

In 1985, the International Council of Nurses published *Guidelines for Nursing Research Development*. The introduction states the commitment of the ICN to the development of nursing research world wide (ICN, 1985):

'The International Council of Nurses is convinced of the importance of nursing research as a major contribution to meeting the health and welfare needs of people. The continuous and rapid scientific developments in a changing world highlight the need for research as a means of identifying new knowledge, improving professional education and practice, and effectively utilizing resources.

'The ICN believes that nursing research should be socially relevant. It should look towards the future while drawing on the past and being concerned with the present.'

and

'Nursing research should include what relates to a total research plan and what may be undertaken independently. In nursing research, available resources of different levels of sophistication should be utilized and research should comply with accepted ethical standards. Research findings should be widely disseminated and their utilization and implementation encouraged when appropriate.'

and

'ICN is aware that nursing research is at various stages of development in different countries ... but efforts to promote it are made elsewhere.'

British nursing education

The reforms of nursing education in the United Kingdom support the move into higher education with its research ethos. This is true from the first level of education to the level of a registered practitioner, as stated in *Project 2000* (UKCC, 1986) and especially for post-registration education as set out in detail by the United Kingdom Central Council for Nursing, Midwifery and Health Visiting in *The Future of Professional Practice: The Council's Standards for Education and Practice following Registration* (UKCC, 1994).

Professional accountability for nurses is high on the agenda in all countries where nursing is moving towards true professional status. It is embedded in the *Code of Professional Conduct* (UKCC, 1984). The document states:

'Each registered nurse, midwife and health visitor shall act, at all times, in such a manner as to justify public trust and confidence, to uphold and enhance the good standing and reputation of the profession, to serve the interests of society and above all to safeguard the interests of individual patients and clients.'

and 'Each registered nurse, midwife and health visitor is accountable for his or her practice....'

Research awareness is implicit in the above document. A nurse who is oblivious of the latest available knowledge relevant to his or her area of practice, and uses redundant methods, cannot expect public trust and confidence and such a nurse will not enhance the good standing and reputation of the profession. The interests of society will not be served and interests of individual patients and clients will not be safeguarded. Bassett (1992) suggested that nursing care should be based on a body of knowledge which gives an 'objective basis to justify nursing actions'. It is becoming increasingly obvious that nursing needs a scientifically defensible body of knowledge, that it must acknowledge and develop science rather than shy away from it (Closs, 1994, 1997).

Research involvement

Because nursing research is at different stages of development, the involvement of nurses must take different forms. First, there must be a research awareness, a recognition that questions can and should be asked, that reading of research articles and research-based texts is essential, and that research findings should be assessed in terms of their usefulness, their relevance, and their potential for implementation. Research awareness must be cultivated by all nurses in all spheres of activity and at all levels. Such awareness should be inculcated early in the professional preparation of nurses and kept alive throughout it. Existing professional and academic education must continue to strengthen and refine research awareness and its application to nursing.

The systematic collection of information, in which most nurses are involved in one way or another, is another form of research involvement. For example, community nurses who keep records for their employing authority should be keenly aware of the purpose of the information they collect and record, and of its ultimate use in the formulation of policy.

Many nurses, knowingly – or sometimes unknowingly – become research assistants for their medical colleagues; they may collect specimens, for example, as part of medical research, or help in some other way. Such involvement can be helpful as a learning experience but it should be part of an official and fully understood contract. The nurse's part of the contract should be the contribution of the nursing dimension to the research in return for which she should be initiated into the scientific aspects of the research process and should be encouraged to participate as a colleague in the preparation of research papers.

An increasing number of nurses, especially those in first-level management and teaching positions, find themselves with a research component as part of their job description. This aspect of their job should be clarified as soon as possible and jealously guarded. It is a precious jewel which gives opportunity for stimulating innovative activity. It should also provide legitimate time for thinking. Sometimes, nurses feel insecure in this research role and attempt to evade it by creating other 'more urgent' demands on their time. Although it is easy to do that, it may prove to be a retrograde step in the long-term. There are opportunities for nurses to obtain advice and help with the research component of their role and they should strive to develop confidence in it. It is almost bound to add to job satisfaction, providing, of course, that the thinking process is deemed to be both desirable and satisfying!

The research component of nursing may take many different forms: it may consist of initiating others in facilitating the creation of a research-oriented environment, or it may consist of direct personal involvement. Finally, research may be undertaken by the nurse on a full-time basis as a member of a research team or as an individual. Several opportunities for such research exist.

In spite of the many positive aspects of research involvement and its acknowledged defensible and urgent purposes and aims, there are still many arguments in favour of leaving research in nursing well alone. Some of these arguments stress the urgency of other nursing activities at a time of scarce resources. It is considered that research activity cannot be defended when finance and manpower are not adequate to provide the necessary care and essential professional preparation for the basic licence to practise nursing. Managers with limited budgets feel reluctant to support research, the results of which are often unpredictable, when they could use the money for other, seemingly more urgent and certainly more easily defensible purposes. Their views and hesitations must be respected and they must not be accused out of hand of being 'unprogressive'. Research does not always realize results that can be utilized and, therefore, the type of research to be undertaken must be considered carefully.

However, some importance must be attached to the beneficial effects of continuing research within an organization, the dynamism it ensures, and the interest it generates. A recognition of possible long-term benefits rather than immediate results may change the outlook of understandably careful managers. In the long term, it may be possible to save either time or money, or both on redundant equipment or practices by investing some of these resources in research in the short term.

Many members of the nursing profession fail to see, or do not wish to see, the importance of research and only perseverance and demonstration of its worth can be expected to change their attitude. Sometimes their lack of interest or enthusiasm is at least partially the fault of researchers who fail to communicate appropriately with their peer groups. The communication of research is as important as the research itself. This is discussed in Chapter 35.

There is also a body of opinion that holds that nursing research should be the concern of trained researchers and that it should not infiltrate the profession as a whole. Some reasons for this view are worthy of thought; poor research by incompetent people can do a great deal of harm and so can thoughtless implementation of findings. More urgent attention must therefore be devoted to the appropriate education of nursing personnel for different levels of research involvement. An evasion of that responsibility can be expected to reverse any progress which has been made in advancing the sum of what is known in and about nursing.

Summary and speculation for the future

It is recognized that a substantial part of the professional activity of nurses at all levels and in all spheres is based on convention rather than substantive knowledge. The need to extend that knowledge cannot be denied and the responsibility for research support cannot be evaded.

Research activity requires knowledge of the scientific method; the research process consists of a series of steps which is subject to scientific rules. Knowledge of the scientific method can be acquired and need not be the province of individuals who work in academic settings. All nurses must develop an awareness of research and recognize its relevance to nursing.

More direct involvement in research at different levels should be encouraged and valued. Uncertainty should be overcome by seeking help rather than by escapism and avoidance. Qualified researchers can help a great deal by teaching, explaining and communicating intelligibly. The reservations about the investment of manpower and finance in research must be viewed sympathetically and the long-term benefits, as well as the immediate gains, of a research-oriented environment should be allowed to enter into the debate quite apart from the possibility of usable research results. The need for research is clearly indicated in the official documents relating to the future of professional practice following registration as a qualified nurse (UKCC, 1994). This authoritative publication refers not merely to specific research training but also to the need for nurses to identify, apply and disseminate research findings relating to clinical practice development. Health Service users are becoming increasingly aware of their rights and encouraged to ask questions about their care. Patient expectations have been raised through the media and also by the introduction of the Patient's Charter Department of Health, 1993a).

The National Board for Nursing, Midwifery and Health Visiting for Scotland (NBS, 1994) also commits itself to the provision of leadership and liaison for research in education and practice. The future of nursing depends to no small extent on the development of nursing research. It is no coincidence that the terms 'research' and 'development' have been linked in official documents.

Another key concept, which is gaining momentum, is 'clinical governance' with the implied need to demonstrate clinical effectiveness. Newell (1997) referred to the challenge and opportunity for the nursing profession of pursuing means to establish clinical effectiveness. Research is necessary to achieve this. It is through the process of systematic enquiry by scientific principles that policy in health care should be influenced. The government department responsible for such policy in the UK supports this stance, as demonstrated in a policy statement by the Department of Health (1997). The research strategy for Scotland was revised in 1998 (The Scottish Office Department of Health, 1998); in its Foreword, the Minister for Health stated: 'There is need to integrate research more fully into the agenda of Health Boards and Trusts and to encourage research activity and usage.' That the need for research to inform health care policy is by no means confined to the UK is clearly evident from the profuse international literature.

The report of the taskforce convened to consider the future of research in nursing points to the way forward (Department of Health, 1993b) in recognizing the contribution of the nursing profession to research and development (R&D) in the NHS as a whole. A strategy for nursing research is being pursued and augurs well for the future. In *Research for Health* such a strategy for England and Wales is described (Department of Health, 1991); its declared primary objective is to see that R&D becomes an integral part of health care. Though not specifically addressed to the nursing profession, it clearly opens up new avenues for nursing involvement.

A clear indication of the UK government's resolution to support research is given:

> 'Good information for policy making and for the public means that we will continue to need high quality research and development and a way to ensure that research findings are widely disseminated and acted on. The Government will work across all departments and with other funders to ensure that research to support "our Healthier Nation" is put into place.' (Department of Health, 1998)

The Scottish Office has published its own strategy document (Chief Scientist Office, 1993) in which emphasis is given to better targeting of R&D in terms of value for money. The crunch point seems to lie in attempts to identify the impact of nursing research on health care, which is also stressed by Mulhall (1995).

In Scotland, a multi-disciplinary conference, held in 1992 and reported by Watt (1993), identified current problems in translating research findings into policy and practice. Although health care research in general was the focus of discussion at that time, nursing research, being an integral part of it, must consider itself included. Referring particularly to nursing research, Closs & Cheater (1994) stress the importance but also the complexity of appropriate utilization of nursing research and make a case for the development of a research culture in nursing which, as yet, has not been attained.

The challenges for nursing research permeate the totality of the nursing profession and its future, and are presented clearly and candidly by Tierney (1993).

While readily acknowledging the need for and the advantages of multi-disciplinary research, she makes a plea for preserving the identity of nursing research.

The current forces in the health care systems the world over must be taken seriously. Through the emphasis on cost containment, nursing research can be either enlivened or annihilated. It is the professional responsibility of nurses to encourage the former and prevent the latter. The Centre for Policy in Nursing Research can be expected to help, one of its key policies being to 'identify and articulate key policies in nursing research' (CPNR, 1997).

New opportunities for the development of nursing research abound and they must be grasped urgently. If academic researchers can become more sensitive to professional needs, and if professionals can become more sensitive to the need for scientific enquiry, the future for professional nursing – for the care of patients, for the education of nurses and for the management of nursing services – is exciting and justifies optimism.

References

Bassett, C. (1992) The integration of research in the clinical setting: Obstacles and solutions. A review of the literature. *Nursing Practice* **6** (1): 4–8.

Chief Scientist Office (1993) *Health Service in Scotland*. Scottish Office, Home and Health Department.

Clamp, C.G.L. (1994) *Resources for Nursing Research*, 2nd edn. An annotated bibliography. London: Library Association Publishing.

Closs, G.J. (1994) What's so awful about science? *Nurse Researcher* **2** (2): 69–83.

Closs, G.J. (1997) Science now more than ever. *Clinical Effectiveness* **1** (2): 61–3.

Closs, G.J. & Cheater, F.H. (1994) Utilisation of nursing research: culture, interest and support. *Journal of Advanced Nursing* **19** (4): 762–73.

Committee on Nursing (1972). *Report of the Committee on Nursing*. London: HMSO.

Cormack, D. (1979) Knowledge for what? Janforum. *Journal of Advanced Nursing* **4**: 93–4.

CPNR (1997) *Annual Report 1996/97*. London: Centre for Policy in Nursing Research.

Department of Health (1991) *Research for Health*. London: HMSO.

Department of Health (1993a) *The Patient's Charter*. London: HMSO.

Department of Health (1993b) *Report of the Taskforce on the Strategy for Research in Nursing, Midwifery and Health Visiting*. London: HMSO.

Department of Health (1997) *The New NHS, Modern-Dependable*. Cmnd 3807. London: HMSO.

Department of Health (1998) *Our Healthier Nation – A Contract for Health*. Cmnd 3852. London: HMSO.

English, S. (1994) Nursing as a research-based profession: 22 years after Briggs. *British Journal of Nursing*, **3** (8): 402–40.

ICN (1985) *Guidelines for Nursing Research Development*. Geneva: International Council of Nurses.

Kendall S. (1997) What do we mean by Evidence? Implications for primary health care nursing. *Journal of Interprofessional Care* **11**, (1): 23–33.

King, M., Stinson, S.M. & Mills, K. (eds) (1993) *Proceedings of the First International Conference on Community Health Nursing Research*. Edmonton, Canada: Edmonton Health Board.

Macleod Clark, J. & Hockey, L. (1989) *Further Research for Nursing*. London: Scutari Press.

Montgomery Robinson, K.M., Hilton, A. & Clark, E. (1991) What is research? *Research Awareness Module 3*. Distance Learning Centre, South Bank Polytechnic.

Mulhall A. (1995) Nursing research: what difference does it make? *Journal of Advanced Nursing* **10**: 576–83.

NBS (1994) *Advancing Standards*. Edinburgh: National Board for Nursing, Midwifery and Health Visiting for Scotland.

Newell, R. (1997) Towards clinical effectiveness in nursing. *Clinical Effectiveness in Nursing* **1**: 11–12.

The Scottish Office Department of Health (1998) *Research Strategy for the National Health Service in Scotland*. London: The Stationery Office.

Tierney, A. (1993) Challenges for nursing research in an era dominated by Health Services reform and cost containment. *Clinical Nursing Research* **2**: (4): 382–95.

UKCC (1984) *Code of Professional Conduct for the Nurse, Midwife and Health Visitor*. London: United Kingdom Central Council for Nursing, Midwifery and Health Visiting.

UKCC (1986) *Project 2000: A New Preparation for Practice*. London: United Kingdom Central Council for Nursing, Midwifery and Health Visiting.

UKCC (1994) *The Future of Professional Practice: The Council's Standards for Education and Practice following Registration*. London: United Kingdom Central Council for Nursing, Midwifery and Health Visiting.

Watt, G.C.M. (1993) Making research make a difference. *Health Bulletin* **51** (3). London: Scottish Office, HMSO.

CHAPTER 2

Common terms and concepts in research

Sam Porter and Diana E. Carter

This chapter introduces and provides explanations of some of the terms and concepts frequently used by researchers and which the reader is likely to encounter when reading published research reports.

Research

Research is a systematic investigation of situations, events, objects or people and their characteristics or behaviours which may be conducted to validate old knowledge or generate new knowledge. Researchers use the term *variables* to refer to the attributes, properties and/or characteristics of the individuals, events or objects that are examined in a study. An *operational definition* of each variable to be examined is developed so that the variable can be explored, described or measured. Much research in nursing, midwifery and health visiting is conducted to find answers to clinical questions, to solve practice-related problems, to facilitate decision-making, or to predict or control outcomes of certain nursing interventions. This type of *nursing research* is referred to as *applied research* in contrast to *basic research*, the findings of which are frequently not directly useful in practice but which add to the profession's body of knowledge and may serve as a springboard to future applied research. *Evidence-based nursing midwifery* involves clinicians basing their practice on the best evidence available (Cullum, 1998) rather than, as has often been the case, relying on intuition, trial and error, and personal experience. Quality research is the source of this evidence.

Replication studies

Some research studies *replicate* or repeat the work of previous researchers, although it should be appreciated that because investigators, settings and subjects change over time it is not possible to repeat the original study exactly. In some instances the researcher may have deliberately made modifications of the original study in an attempt to improve its quality. Replication may be performed for a number of reasons:

(1) to determine whether the findings apply in different settings;
(2) to challenge the findings or interpretations of previous studies;
(3) to determine whether the findings from the replication study are consistent with the original findings.

If the findings from a replication study are consistent with those of earlier studies there is a greater probability that these findings are an accurate reflection of reality and thus useful in practice. A useful example of replication can be seen in Cornock's (1998) study of UK nurses' and patients' perceptions of the stress experienced by patients in the intensive care environment, which was a replication of a study that had been carried out in America. The overall outcomes of Cornock's (1998) study were found to be similar to those of the earlier study.

Research aim, objectives, questions

A research aim is a general statement of the purpose of the study; it is then broken down into specific objectives to be achieved or research questions to be answered by the study. For example, Mackin & Sinclair (1998) stated that the aim of their study was to explore midwives' perceptions of stress while working in the labour ward. They then developed six, more specific objectives or statements expressed in the present tense, of their intentions which included: measuring midwives' perceived stress levels and their perceptions of the effects of stress; identification of professional and personal sources of stress; and identification of stress-relieving methods and sources of support for midwives in labour wards. Some researchers specify questions which the research is designed to answer. Like research objectives, questions are worded in the present tense and usually focus on the variables being investigated. The relationships that might exist among variables may also be included in research questions.

(Types of research)

Retrospective and prospective research

A research study may be either *retrospective* or *prospective*. Retrospective studies investigate events that have already happened in an attempt to describe and understand those events, whereas prospective studies investigate what might happen in the future. The study of middle-aged men's smoking habits by Koivula & Paunonen (1998) is a particularly interesting one in this respect in that it consists of both retrospective and prospective elements – retrospective in the sense that data provided some understanding of the factors that might be associated with men's decisions to start smoking, and their experiences of giving up the habit, and prospective in that it sought to describe the likelihood of current smokers attempting to stop smoking in the future.

Historical research

Historical research focuses on past events, examining the relationship between historical variables. Given that historical variables are not amenable to the sort of control that contemporary variables might be, the historical researcher focuses on contextualizing variables in relation to others so as to understand how their interaction affected events and chronological processes.

Quantitative and qualitative research

A research study may be classified according to whether it is a quantitative or a qualitative study, although in practice many studies involve both approaches. *Quantitative research* is a formal, objective, systematic process for obtaining quantifiable information about the world, presented in numerical form and analysed through the use of statistics. It is used to describe and test relationships and to examine cause-and-effect relationships (see Chapter 14). *Qualitative research* uses human speech or writing as data, rather than numbers. More generally, qualitative research is used as an umbrella term for those strategies that seek to explain human behaviour in terms of the reasons people have for behaving in the way they do. Rather than aiming to uncover relations of cause-and-effect, qualitative research seeks to uncover the understandings and motives that lead to certain actions. Qualitative research methods include participant observation, in-depth interviews, oral histories and conversational analysis.

The approach adopted by a researcher will depend on the nature of the issue being investigated and on the type of data required. For example, the decision by Wilkes & Wallis (1998) to use a qualitative approach to describing professional nursing care was based on previous researchers' reported difficulties in describing this phenomenon through quantitative approaches.

Grounded theory

Grounded theory is an inductive method of analysis used by qualitative researchers. (*Induction* is the process whereby a general rule is inferred from a series of empirical findings, whereas *deduction* is the process of developing specific predictions from general principles. *Empirical* is a term which refers to that which is discovered through systematic observation or experimentation, rather than by theoretical or speculative methods.) With grounded theory, data are approached without a preconceived framework or theoretical position. Instead, theory is built up gradually from analysis of the data gathered, usually from *ethnographic* or documentary research. Rather than research being carried out in a linear fashion, grounded theory involves the concurrent gathering, organization and analysis of data. Organization and analysis involves the constant comparison of every element of the data with other elements until a model emerges that is capable of explaining variation in the data.

Ethnography

This refers to the direct study of people in their natural, everyday settings. It is a term that is often used synonymously with participant observation, but in some respects it is a wider term, which includes the research strategy of ethnographic or *in-depth interviewing*, where people are allowed to tell their own stories about the understandings and motivations that lead them to act in the ways that they do.

In-depth interviews

This form of interview is used in qualitative research, the aim being to give respondents the opportunity to describe their experiences in their own words. In order to ensure that the data reflect the respondents' concerns, prior organization of the *interview schedule* is minimized. The interview schedule is a research instrument used to structure the interview and specify the order and wording of the questions to be asked of respondents. Some in-depth interviews have a loose schedule and are referred to as *semi-structured interviews*, while others may eschew any sort of predetermined schedule bar identification of general themes to be discussed, in which case they are referred to as *unstructured interviews*.

Descriptive research

As the term implies, *descriptive research* involves the collection of data that will provide an account or description of individuals, groups or situations that are the focus of interest to the researcher, and, as explained in Chapter 18, may be either quantitative or qualitative. Using questionnaires, interviews, observation schedules and check-lists to gather information, this type of research describes what exists and may help to uncover new facts and meaning, thus providing a knowledge base which can act as a springboard for correlational and experimental studies.

Correlation research

Correlational research studies go beyond simply describing what exists and systematically investigate relations between two or more variables of interest. Such studies only describe and attempt to explain the nature of relationships that exist and do not examine causality. The study of the relationship between nurses' and patients' pain scores at different times post-operatively, and the amount of opioid analgesia received by patients following coronary artery bypass grafting (CABG), which was undertaken by Ferguson *et al.* (1997), is an example of a descriptive correlational study. Using a numerical rating system patients and nurses independently scored the patients' pain intensity and pain distress. Analysis of the data involved statistical correlation that described the relationship between the variables and led the researchers to conclude that patients in the intensive care unit following CABG can experience considerable pain which is not always relieved. Having established this relationship, the researchers could then undertake an experimental study to determine the cause and effect.

Experimental research

Experimental research involves observation for a scientific purpose, usually to test cause-and-effect relationships between variables under conditions which, as far as possible, are controlled by the researcher. The classic research design of an experiment involves selection of subjects who are randomly allocated to either the *experimental group* or the *control group*. Only the experimental group are exposed during the course of the study to the variable thought to be the cause of the effect. Some experimental studies lack one or both of these essential properties of randomization and a control group and are more correctly referred to as *quasi-experiments*. Callaghan & Trapp (1998) acknowledged that their study was a quasi-experiment, pointing out that the control group was non-randomized and referring to this group as a comparison group.

Double-blind selection

This is a method of selecting whether or not a research subject is to be allocated to the control group or the experimental group, whereby neither the researcher nor the research subject is aware of the group to which the subject has been allocated. The identity of the members of each group is only uncovered after the empirical stage of the research has been completed, thus minimizing the possibility of subject or researcher *bias* which could distort the findings. Double-blind selection is often used in *randomized controlled trials* which are designed to test the efficacy of a form of treatment, often pharmaceutical, whereby those research subjects who are assessed to have the potential to benefit from the treatment are randomly allocated to either the control group who receive a *placebo* rather than the active treatment, or the experimental group who receive the treatment.

Independent and dependent variables

The variable that is hypothesized to be the causal factor in the relationship that is being examined is referred to as the *independent variable*, and is manipulated during the experiment in order to see if it has any measurable effect on the *dependent variable*. For example, in a comparative study of two depot injection techniques (the 'air bubble' and the 'Z-track') by MacGabhann (1998) the injection technique was the independent variable while complications of the injection technique, which included the incidence and degree of medication seepage, skin lesions, degree of pain and irritation experienced at the injection site, were dependent variables. *Extraneous variables* are variables that confound the relationship between the independent and dependent variables and they need to be controlled either through the research design or by statistical procedures. In the above study it is possible that the results were influenced by extraneous or *confounding* variables such as patients' age, weight and general condition.

Hypotheses

A *hypothesis* is a proposition that identifies a relationship between two variables and sometimes advances an explanation for that relationship. Hypotheses are usually predictive in that they have the form 'if X occurs then Y will occur', X relating to the manipulation of the independent variable and Y relating to the response of the dependent variable. For example, Walker (1998) hypothesized 'that patients receiving intramuscular analgesia will report higher pain scores than patients receiving patient-controlled analgesia or epidural analgesia'. In this instance the independent variable was the method of analgesia administration while the dependent variable was the patients' reported pain scores.

Action research

Action research is not simply concerned with understanding a problem, but also with attempting to solve it. It involves the researcher working with research participants to analyse the situation they wish to change, and planning how to change it. For action research to be successful, its findings have to be useful to the research participants. The use of the term *participant* is significant here, in that the term *research subject* is rejected because it implies a passive role for those being researched, whereas all those involved in action research are seen as taking an active role.

Literature review

This is a critical review of previous literature relating to a research topic, the aim of which is to prepare the ground for new research. It provides the researcher and the reader with knowledge of the field being researched and contextualizes the research problem being considered. The literature review may identify gaps in the previous literature that the new research can address, or may suggest research to be replicated. Inductive methods of research, most notably *grounded theory*, tend to place less significance on the role of the literature review.

Frame of reference

A frame of reference provides an abstract and logical structure to a study which enables the researcher to link the study findings to nursing's existing body of knowledge, thereby providing a context for interpretation of the findings and making possible the development of new theory or improvement of existing theory. It is the structure within which a study is developed and serves to link the components of the study together. A *conceptual framework* is developed through identification, definition and linkage of the concepts of interest which are selected for study from the researcher's experience or from theories or earlier studies and is used by researchers investigating new areas of nursing or areas in which existing theory is inadequate. Thus, exploratory and descriptive research involves the development of conceptual frameworks as a frame of reference. Barrett & Myrick (1998) developed a conceptual framework to guide their exploratory study of preceptor/preceptee job satisfaction, having concluded from their review of the literature that there was a lack of agreement on the definition and determinants of job satisfaction. A *theoretical framework* is a frame of reference that is derived from an existing theory which provides a general, abstract explanation of the interrelationships of the concepts to be investigated in the testing of a theory. Koivula & Paunonen (1998) developed a theoretical framework for their study of middle-aged men's experiences of and attitudes towards smoking.

Population and sampling

The term *population* refers to the entire class of cases to which the researcher wishes to generalize her research. For example, the population for a national study investigating registered nurses' experiences of caring for patients in the terminal stage of illness might comprise all currently practising registered nurses. At a different level, the researcher might be interested only in the experiences of nurses within one health board area, in which case the population would be all practising registered nurses within that area. Even at this level, unless the target population is relatively small, the researcher would be unlikely to be able to include all nurses who fulfil the criteria for selection and has instead to select a *sample*.

Sampling

A sample is the proportion of the defined population who are selected to participate in the study and is intended to reflect all the characteristics of that population. These elements of the population from whom the researcher seeks to collect data are sometimes referred to as the *selected sample*. It is frequently the case that not all those who are selected actually participate in the study. For example, in the case of a study which involves data collection by means of a mailed questionnaire, some of the selected sample may refuse to participate, some may not receive the questionnaire which the researcher mailed to them, while others will receive the mailing but forget to complete and return the form. The sample who actually participate and produce data are referred to as the *data-producing sample*. In reporting the findings of a study, researchers often refer to the individuals who comprise this sample as 'participants', 'subjects' or 'respondents'. The purpose of selecting a sample is that it can be researched to a greater depth than could the population as a whole.

Sample selection

How a sample is selected in an important aspect of any study. Ideally, the sample should be representative of the population from which it has been selected so that the results of the research can be inferred to apply to all cases in the population. A *random sample*, provided it is large enough, will produce a sample that is most representative of a population because each member of the population has an equal chance of being selected. Other methods of sampling include *stratified random sampling*, whereby the population is divided into strata using variables such as gender, age, social class, and diagnosis, and samples of each strata are then randomly selected. Sampling methods in which some members of the population do not have an equal chance of being selected are also used by researchers, and include *accidental sampling, quota sampling*, and *purposive sampling. Snowball sampling*, which is a method of attaining a sample whereby subjects are selected on the basis of recommendations or introductions made by earlier research subjects, is often used when access to the population under research is difficult, for example, illegal drug users. Sampling is dealt with in more detail in Chapter 22.

Pilot study

Many researchers conduct a pilot study as a preliminary to the actual study. A pilot study is a smaller version of the proposed study which provides a trial run before embarking on the actual study. A pilot study can serve a number of purposes:

1. It facilitates the testing of the adequacy of the research design and logistics of the main study and may help the researcher to identify problems with the study design which can be rectified before embarking on the actual study.

2. It gives the researcher experience of administering the data-collecting instrument to the subjects.
3. It helps to determine whether the instrument is collecting the type of data required and whether the subjects are able to use those data.
4. It provides an opportunity for analysing the research data.

Walker (1998) conducted a pilot study prior to her investigation of orthopaedic patients' reporting of pain management. This revealed that some of the patients did not understand the phraseology of the questions in the questionnaire that was to be used to allow reporting and appraisal of their pain management. Walker was then able to amend the questionnaire prior to the main study. In some instances a pilot study may be considered unnecessary, as in the case of a study where the method and techniques are familiar to the researcher and the instrument is a standard one which has been used previously with the population of the research.

Measurement

Research involves the collection of data that are used to assess or measure the subjects of the study in relation to the variables of interest. A number of scales are used for this purpose.

Nominal scale

This is perhaps more accurately described as a *categorization* than a scale, in that data are organized according to certain categories or characteristics which the subjects may or may not possess and which are not amenable to rank ordering. This means that the differences between them are not measurable. An example of a nominal level of measurement would be categorization of subjects according to marital status, in that the categories single, married, divorced and widowed are not amenable to ranking of magnitude – you cannot say that being divorced is twice as great as being married.

Ordinal scale

An ordinal scale is more informative than a nominal scale. It is a measuring scale used to categorize data in rank order according to a certain characteristic, although it cannot measure precisely the difference between them in relation to that characteristic. For example, a scale measuring the ability of clients to care for themselves would be able to differentiate greater or lesser capacities to self-care, but would not be able to state exactly how much clients differ.

Interval scale

This measuring scale can both process data in rank order according to a certain characteristic and measure the difference between them in relation to that characteristic. Measurement of difference is possible because points on the scale are ordered in an equal and measurable gradation. However, the difference measured in interval scales is not proportionate because these scales involve the arbitrary selection of a zero point. This means, for instance, that a point twice as high as another on the scale does not signify twice the magnitude of the characteristic. For example, in the measurement of temperature, because zero Celsius is arbitrarily chosen, with temperatures existing below as well as above zero, 40 degrees Celsius is not twice as hot as 20 degrees.

Ratio scale

A ratio scale can both process data in rank order according to a certain characteristic, and measure the difference between them in relation to that characteristic in a proportionate manner. Measurement of difference is possible because the points on the scale are ordered in an equal and measurable gradation. Proportionate measurement of difference is possible because the scale has a non-arbitrary zero point. This means that a point that is twice as high as another on the scale reflects twice the magnitude of that characteristic. For example, an age scale has a zero point of birth, so that a 40 year old can be said to be twice as old as someone who is 20 years old.

Reliability and validity

Reliability is a term used in reference to the accuracy of the data in terms of their stability or repeatability. Thus, an instrument that is administered in the same circumstances on two separate occasions should provide identical data.

Validity is another term that will be encountered when reading research reports. It refers to the extent to which an instrument actually does what it purports to do and is dependent upon, but independent of, reliability: dependent in the sense that reliability is a necessary precondition for validity, yet independent in the sense that even perfect reliability tells you only that perfect validity is possible. (It actually tells nothing of the extent to which validity has been achieved!) Reliability and validity are discussed in more detail in Chapter 3.

Objectivity

Ideally, all instruments are completely objective and this means that the data that are obtained are a function of what is being measured. However, a number of factors can impede the realization of this ideal: (1) the interpersonal relationships in the research situation as face-to-face interviewing is particularly sensitive to the loss of objectivity; (2) the extent to which the researcher plays an active role in determining the nature of the data as, for example, in observational studies; (3) the nature of the instructions printed on paper-and-pencil instruments as instructions should provide the necessary information on how to complete the instrument but should not in any way suggest the content of responses. The findings of observational studies may be biased by *observer effect* (sometimes referred to as the *Hawthorne effect*) whereby those who are being observed alter their usual behaviour in order to create a more favourable impression (Holyoake, 1998), and steps should to be taken to minimize this.

Objectivity is a judgement that the researcher must make; it is also a judgement that the reader makes in evaluating the research situation, the directions and the nature of the instrument.

Results

The results of a study are based on the analysis of the data collected (see Part II (D): Chapters 30–33). The form of presentation of the results will depend on the nature of the study and the type of data collected. Qualitative researchers generally present their findings in textual format thereby preserving the richness of their qualitative data, while data from quantitative studies are frequently presented in tables, graphs, pie charts, and other visually stimulating ways which serve to enhance the clarity of presentation (Chapter 34). Statistical methods are often applied to quantitative data so that the data can be summarized and easily presented; this also helps the researcher to arrive at legitimate conclusions and reduce the element of subjective bias which anyone analysing the research findings will inevitably bring to them.

Researchers should state the degree of confidence that can be placed in the results. This is usually stated in terms of *probability*; for example, 'the probability is less than 1 in 20 that this result could have occurred by chance'. The degree of confidence in this instance is that if the research were to be repeated 20 times under exactly the same conditions, the same result would be expected on at least 19 occasions (or, if repeated 100 times, in at least 95). Clearly, the higher the level of confidence which the statistical analysis will allow to be stated, the more certain one can be that the results could not have occurred by chance.

Generalization

Generalization, which is an aim of research, involves extending the implications of the findings in the study sample to the larger population from which that sample was drawn. The extent to which the researcher can generalize on the basis of one piece of research will depend on a number of factors and on the extent to which they have been taken into account. Asking the following questions of a research report will help you to judge whether generalization of the findings is possible:

1. Was the sample randomly selected and representative of all individuals to whom the findings might apply? What size was the sample?
2. Were all the variables that might have influenced the results accounted for? For example, in an experimental study were all the subjects exposed to the same research conditions?
3. Were the data collected under the same conditions for all subjects?
4. Were the data-collecting instruments valid and reliable? Does the report provide enough information about validity and reliability to enable you to judge?
5. Are the results of the research presented in full, were appropriate statistical methods used and were the results stated with a high level of confidence?
6. Does the research report give enough information for others to be able to repeat the research if they wish to?

This chapter has defined and briefly explained a number of terms and concepts used by researchers, and many of these terms and concepts will be re-visited in later chapters.

References

Barrett, C. & Myrick, F. (1998) Job satisfaction in preceptorship and its effect on the clinical performance of the preceptee. *Journal of Advanced Nursing* **27** (2): 364–71.

Callaghan, S. & Trapp, M. (1998) Evaluating two dressings for the prevention of nasal bridge pressure sores. *Professional Nurse* **13** (6): 361–4.

Cornock, M. (1998) Stress and the intensive care patient: perceptions of patients and nurses. *Journal of Advanced Nursing* **27** (3): 518–27.

Cullum, N. (1998) Getting to grips with research evidence. *Nursing Times* **94** (21): 60–1.

Ferguson, J., Gilroy, D. & Puntillo, K. (1997) Dimensions of pain and analgesia administration associated with coronary artery bypass grafting in an Australian intensive care unit. *Journal of Advanced Nursing* **26** (6): 1065–72.

Holyoake, D. (1998) Observing nurse–patient interaction. *Nursing Standard* **12** (29): 35–8.

Koivula, M. & Paunonen, M. (1998) Smoking habits among Finnish middle-aged men: experiences and attitudes. *Journal of Advanced Nursing* **27** (2): 327–34.

MacGabhann, L. (1998) A comparison of two depot injection techniques. *Nursing Standard* **12** (37): 39–41.

Mackin, P. & Sinclair, M. (1998) Labour ward midwives' perceptions of stress. *Journal of Advanced Nursing* **27** (5): 986–91.

Walker, S. (1998) Orthopaedic patients' reporting of pain management. *Nursing Standard* **12** (46): 43–7.

Wilkes, L.M. & Wallis, M.C. (1998) A model of professional nurse caring: nursing students' experience. *Journal of Advanced Nursing* **27** (3): 582–9.

CHAPTER 3

Validity and reliability

Diana E. Carter and Sam Porter

Validity and reliability defined

Validity and reliability are the criteria upon which the veracity and credibility of research findings are judged and are important in all research although the methods of achieving these qualities will vary depending of the type of research. Any measuring instrument – whether this is a piece of equipment or a data-collecting tool such as a rating scale, questionnaire, observation or interview schedule – must essentially be valid and reliable. *Validity* underpins the entire research process and refers to the degree to which an instrument measures what it is supposed to be measuring, while *reliability* refers to the degree of consistency or accuracy with which the instrument (used under similar conditions) measures the attribute under investigation. For example, to measure a person's body temperature you would use a thermometer (a valid instrument), but if the thermometer is not used correctly, or if the person reading the thermometer makes an error, then the measurement will be unreliable.

The relationship between validity and reliability

In order to be valid a measurement must be reliable or, put another way, reliability is a precondition for validity in that an unreliable measure cannot be valid. However, it is important to appreciate that reliability does not guarantee validity. The analogy of the marksman shooting at a target is often used to illustrate this relationship, as shown in Fig. 3.1. To be valid an instrument must measure the concept of interest. Assuming that the purpose of a measure is to hit the bull's-eye, it can be seen in Fig. 3.1 that in the first instance the shots (using the same instrument) are very widely scattered. There is no reliability and therefore no validity. On the second target, while the shots are clustered around the same point demonstrating that reliability has been achieved, validity has not been achieved as they are not hitting the intended spot. Finally, in the third target, the measure is both reliable and valid.

Different research approaches place different emphasis on the attributes of

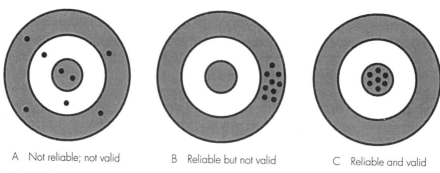

A   Not reliable; not valid   B   Reliable but not valid   C   Reliable and valid

Fig. 3.1   Illustration of validity and reliability.

validity and reliability. Quantitative research approaches, which generally use structured techniques of data collection (e.g. questionnaires), place greater emphasis on validity and reliability than qualitative studies, where researchers generally know from the outset that they are not going to get consistent responses to the questions they ask. However, qualitative researchers may argue that their findings may be more valid than those of quantitative studies as the latter tend (to varying degrees) to decontextualize the subject being researched. The next section in this chapter will address the techniques and methods used in quantitative research to determine validity and reliability.

Validity in quantitative research

Internal and external validity

As a measure of truth or accuracy, validity is important throughout the research process and is also relevant to the overall study design. *Internal validity*, which is addressed more frequently in experimental studies examining causality than in other studies, is the extent to which the effects that are detected in the study are a true reflection of reality rather than the result of extraneous variables.

External validity concerns the philosophical question of whether the findings of the study can be generalized beyond the sample from which they were derived and involves both *population* and *ecological* validity. Population validity relates to whether the results of a particular study can be applied (generalized) to different groups of people. In this context it is important to ensure that the sample is selected in such a way as to ensure that it is representative of the population from which it is drawn. This is sometimes referred to as population validity, further details of which can be found in Chapter 22. Ecological validity, which focuses on whether the results of a study would apply in other places and contexts, is often difficult to establish given that many experimental studies are conducted in an artificial setting which, by virtue of definition, is not the same as real life.

Validity of measuring instruments

It is important to ensure that data-collecting instruments not only yield data relevant to the problem being studied but also measure what they purport to measure, and that any differences among the study sample in terms of the measured attribute reflect true differences among those individuals. If a measure lacks validity it will not mean what you think it means.

The concept being investigated (measured) must be clearly defined, but owing to the abstract nature of many concepts, such as patient satisfaction, comfort, and distress, this is not always easy to achieve. Demonstrating the validity of an instrument would be easier if there was a simple statistical test or formula that could be applied. There are different dimensions to the validity of a measure and it is useful to consider these using Neale & Liebert's (1986) 'three Cs': content validity, criterion validity and construct validity.

Content validity

Content validity is concerned with the extent to which the measure adequately covers the various dimensions of the concept under investigation. At the simplest level there is *face validity*, which involves forming a subjective impression of whether 'on the face of it' the research instrument appears to measure what it is supposed to measure. The rigour of this approach can be enhanced by asking for expert opinion and/or searching the literature for information against which to compare the *content* of the instrument. Dunning & Martin (1998), in their investigation of patients' beliefs about diabetes and diabetic complications, pilot tested their questionnaire with 40 subjects in an attempt to establish face validity and also sought the opinions of a panel of experts in diabetes education and questionnaire design to establish content validity. Ultimately, however, a judgement had to be made in terms of whether or not the content of the questionnaire was appropriate to its intended purpose.

Criterion validity

Concurrent and predictive validity are two types of criterion validity. Concurrent validity uses an already existing and well-accepted measure against which the performance of the new measure can be compared. If, for example, you have developed what you consider to be a quicker (and possibly cheaper) tool for measuring patient satisfaction with care than those currently available, its performance could be assessed against existing available instruments.

As the name suggests, predictive validity assesses the degree to which a measure can predict a future event of interest – for example, pressure sore risk assessment tools. However, an interesting article by Edwards (1994) draws attention to the fact that scrutiny of these tools/scales suggests that problems exist with both the validity and reliability of many of them.

Construct validity

While criterion validity is based on pragmatic rather than theoretical considerations, construct validity tests the link between a measure and the underlying theory. Construct validity relates to the fit between the conceptual definitions and the operational definitions of the variables being studied; that is, operational definitions (the methods of measurement) need to validly reflect the theoretical constructs. While this is generally considered to be the most important form of validity as it provides a test of a measure and of the theory upon which it is based, it is also the most difficult to establish.

Reliability in quantitative research

Reliability is a precondition for validity in that an unreliable measure cannot be valid. It is concerned with the extent to which a measure produces consistent results. While absolute reliability is theoretically possible, some degree of inconsistency is present in all measurement procedures – for example, it is unlikely that over many measurements temperature would be recorded as exactly the same even if the actual temperature remained constant. Errors of this type are known as *random errors* and have an effect on reliability. *Constant errors* may also occur if, for example, the thermometer being used always recorded a temperature that was two degree higher than the true temperature. Because constant errors are consistent it is generally accepted that they affect validity more than reliability.

Errors and inconsistency

The reliability of data is always threatened by the possibility of errors and inconsistencies. Errors which are randomly distributed in a large group of study subjects will not affect the validity of measurements as they will tend to offset each other, whereas errors that are consistently piled in one direction will bias the study. However, if a measurement is required for the diagnosis of an individual's nursing problems/needs, this unreliability cannot be tolerated as it will have a negative effect on the nursing care that the patient receives.

Sources of error

The main stage at which random errors affect reliability is during data collection, and many factors can be identified, as outlined in Table 3.1. Inconsistencies of

Table 3.1　Sources of random errors

Sources of error (unreliability)	Examples
Environmental factors	Noise Light Location
Subject-related	Lack of understanding Subject 'reactivity' to the observer's presence Transitory personal factors such as mood, anxiety, tiredness
Instrument-related	Defects in physical measuring instruments Wording defects in pen-and-paper instruments causing lack of clarity, resulting in respondents providing different responses due to differing interpretations of questions asked Instrument format: open-ended/closed questions on the same topic may be answered differently Response sampling errors as a result of the sampling items used to measure an attribute (e.g. which questions are included in knowledge test)
Researcher-related	Psychological biases affecting the reading of measurements Variations in method of administration of data-collecting instrument from one subject to the next

this type – known as unreliability – also affect validity. However, even if these sources of error were controlled there is no guarantee that the measurement would be valid. Validity must be assessed independently on its own merits.

Assessing reliability

Whereas determining validity can prove difficult, reliability can be assessed with attention generally paid to *stability, consistency* and *equivalence*, which are aspects of the concept of reliability. A reliability coefficient is a way in which different levels of reliability can be numerically indicated – the higher the level the greater the confidence in the reliability of the instrument.

Testing for stability: the test–retest method

The stability of a measure relates to the extent to which repeated administration of the instrument produces the same results. For example, if a questionnaire designed to measure individuals' knowledge of a particular subject was administered on two occasions, then, provided there had been no opportunity for those individuals to increase their knowledge in the interval between tests, reliability would be demonstrated by achieving the same results on each occasion. Assuming that the variables under study will remain constant over time, the test/measure is repeated and the different results compared by computing a *reliability coefficient*, which is a numerical index (between 0.00 and 1.00) of the test's reliability. The higher the reliability coefficient, the higher the stability, thus a score of 0.80 indicates a more reliable instrument than a score of 0.50. It is generally accepted that a reliability coefficient above 0.70 is satisfactory, although it must be emphasized that if clinical decisions are to be based on the results of the measure then a higher reliability may be required. McLaughlin (1997) calculated a reliability coefficient of 0.78 for the questionnaire used in her study of student nurses' attitudes towards mentally ill people and considered that this reflected adequate reliability of the instrument.

Testing for internal consistency: the split-half/odd–even method

Internal consistency is sometimes referred to as *homogeneity* and is concerned with the extent to which the items within an instrument actually measure the variable that is being investigated. The split-half method involves calculating the individual's score on half the items and comparing this with his score on the other half. It assumes that items are distributed randomly and that the scores on the two halves should be very similar. The extent to which they differ is an indication of the unreliability of the measure. An inherent difficulty is that different 'splits' can result in different reliability estimates. For this reason the split-half approach is increasingly being replaced by tests that compensate for this, the most widely used being *Cronbach's alpha* which produces a numerical index between 0.00 and 1.00 and is interpreted in the same way as other reliability coefficients. Barrett & Myrick (1998) used Cronbach's alpha to compute a measure of reliability for each of the subscales used in their study and concluded that the alpha coefficients, which ranged from a low of 0.844 to a high of 0.978, indicated a high reliability of the subscales. Similarly, Cronbach's alpha was used by Foxall *et al.* (1998) to estimate the reliability of the proficiency scale which they developed to examine ethnic differences in breast self-examination practices between African American nurses and Caucasian nurses. Their scale revealed a reliability coefficient of 0.86 for the African American nurses and 0.85 for Caucasian nurses.

Testing for equivalence: parallel tests and interrater reliability

Equivalence involves comparing the extent to which two versions of the same paper-and-pencil instrument, or two observers measuring the same event, produce the same result. If, for example, you have developed a questionnaire its reliability can be estimated by measuring the degree of equivalence between the results of administering this instrument and the results achieved by administering a parallel instrument to the subjects about the same time. Using alternate or parallel forms of the same test provides a check on the consistency or equivalence of different measuring instruments. The results of a new test can be compared with those of a test previously shown to be reliable and valid. Determining interrater (or interobserver) reliability involves the simultaneous recording of the same event by two independent trained observers and computing an index of equivalence or agreement using correlational techniques. Callaghan & Trapp (1998) used a wound-assessment tool in their study, which evaluated two dressings for the prevention of nasal bridge pressure caused by the facial mask in patients receiving intermittent positive pressure ventilation. To assess the tool's reliability three senior nurses independently assessed a number of patients' nasal bridges for inflammation of the epidermis on entry to the study and on Day 1 of the study with 100% agreement. Thus, interrater reliability was established for the three nurses using the wound-assessment tool in the study.

It is important to appreciate that reliability of an instrument is not a property of the instrument *per se*, but rather of the instrument when administered to a certain sample under certain conditions. For example, an instrument which has been shown to be reliable for use with nurses in the UK may not be reliable for use with nurses in the USA given the differences in how nursing is practised in these two countries. Interestingly, a small, local reliability study of the wound-assessment tool used by Callaghan & Trapp (1998) (which was completed after the researchers commenced their study) failed on that occasion to demonstrate interrater reliability.

Validity and reliability in qualitative research

As with most things in qualitative research, issues surrounding the criteria of validity and reliability are more ambiguous and contested than they are in relation to quantitative research. Perhaps the best way to demonstrate this is to show some of the questions that might arise in the mind of a reader of qualitative research.

Questioning validity

Let us start with the issue of external validity – whether or not the findings of a piece of research can be generalized beyond the sample from which it was derived. One of the characteristics of qualitative research methods, such as in-depth interviews, is that they take a lot of time and effort to conduct, transcribe and analyse. As a result, with the same resources, the qualitative researcher is usually able to gain data on far fewer subjects that can a quantitative researcher. This very practical limitation has significant effects on the validity claims that qualitative research can make. Imagine that a qualitative researcher conducts 40 hour-long interviews with people with asthma to find out how the disease affects their everyday lives. These interviews would generate a huge amount of data, yet how externally valid could we adjudge these data to be? Of the millions of people who suffer from asthma, only 40 have been selected. How could we know that the experiences they recounted were shared by a significant proportion of the population of asthma sufferers? Does this mean that qualitative data can only tell us about the lives of the people actually studied? In short, we see here that the issue of the generalizability of qualitative data is a thorny one.

It might be thought that problems of external validity in qualitative compared to quantitative research are made up for by its superior capacity to be internally valid. After all, while few subjects may be researched, the information gained from each subject is far deeper and richer than the information about a subject that tends to be gleaned by quantitative methods. Unfortunately, in some respects, problems here are even more profound.

As has already been noted, internal validity relates to the degree to which the data gathered in a study are a true reflection of reality. One of the distinctive aspects of qualitative research is that qualitative data consist not of 'objective' facts, but of people's interpretations. This engenders a number of problems in relation to validity, among which is that reality (whatever that may be) is often at least twice removed from the reader of the research. First you have the accounts of the research subjects. In all likelihood, different subjects will interpret the same events and processes in different and sometimes contradictory ways. In such cases, how are we to decide which interpretations best reflect reality? Indeed, does such a question even make sense, given that we are looking at perceptions rather than at that which is perceived?

Secondly, data are processed through the interpretations of the researcher. How do we know that the researcher is not using the data to grind a particular axe? For example, if the researcher is unsympathetic to the group of people she is researching, how can we tell whether or not she has selected the most damning data to present and excised more favourable information? Even if the researcher is scrupulously neutral in her treatment of researcher subjects, how can we know the degree to which the data, which in qualitative research are often notoriously messy and contradictory, have been altered to enable the researcher to give a coherent account of her findings? These are only a few of the questions that might be asked in relation to the internal validity of qualitative research; however, they demonstrate the degree of difficulty that this criterion presents to researchers and readers. In the absence of statistical procedures for data processing, such as exist in quantitative research, how can readers be persuaded that what they read is an accurate reflection of the reality that is purportedly described?

Questioning reliability

The criterion of reliability is beset by similar problems to those of validity in qualitative research. It will be remembered that reliability relates to the constancy of findings that a research instrument is capable of engendering when used u..... similar conditions. One of the major issues here for qualitative researchers is the absence of similar conditions. Take, for example, unstructured interviews: these are dynamic encounters between an active interpreting subject and an active interpreting researcher. In such circumstances, no interview, even with the same two people participating, will ever be the same. As Holstein & Gubrium (1997) stated: 'One cannot simply expect answers on one occasion to replicate those on another because they emerge from different circumstances of production.'

Qualitative approaches to validity and reliability

Unfortunately, there is no consensus among qualitative methodologists on how to tackle the problem of validity and reliability in qualitative research. As Hammersley (1992) has noted, there are three basic positions in relation to assessing qualitative research. The first approach argues that qualitative research should be judged on the same basis as quantitative research. At the opposite end of the spectrum it is argued that the character of qualitative research means that it is not possible to apply criteria to judge it. The third approach is median and argues that it is *possible* to develop criteria for judging qualitative research, but because qualitative research represents an alternative paradigm of knowledge acquisition to quantitative research, the criteria used cannot simply mimic those used to test quantitative studies.

In some respects the title of this chapter entails an implicit acceptance of the first approach. The criteria of validity and reliability were developed within the quantitative paradigm. Using the same terms in relation to qualitative research involves the assumption that the same criteria can be used to judge that type of research. The problem with this approach is that there is a tendency to shoe-horn concepts and language developed in a radically different context into the language and conceptual frameworks that underpin qualitative research (Leinenger, 1994). Primarily, the search for unequivocal empirical knowledge, and the use of criteria to judge whether this has been attained, sits ill with qualitative research's focus on the meanings people have, in that those meanings will differ from person to person. In their focus on human subjectivity, qualitative researchers must accept that there is no one 'truth' about the phenomena they are examining, merely the numerous interpretations of that phenomena made by the subjects of their research.

This denial of the possibility of unequivocal knowledge in qualitative research has led some commentators to argue that there are no criteria that can be adopted to assess the degree to which research results reflect reality:

'To accept that social reality is mind-constructed and that there are multiple realities is to deny that there are any "givens" upon which to found knowledge. If one accepts these assumptions, different claims about reality result not from incorrect procedures but may simply be the case of one investigator's interpretation of reality versus another's.' (Smith, 1984: 383)

Space precludes a discussion of the various philosophical debates surrounding this radical critique of the possibility of knowledge. Suffice it to say that such a position denies us any basis upon which to decide between safe and unsafe research, and, if accepted, would mean that qualitative research could have no role in informing nursing knowledge.

Other commentators have regarded this fundamental rejection of criteria as an instance of throwing the baby out with the bath water. While qualitative researchers may not be able to use the same criteria as their quantitative colleagues, this does not mean that qualitative research reports are beyond any sort of rational assessment of their validity. Such a position, while attempting to develop criteria by which to judge qualitative research, eschews use of the quantitative blueprint of validity and reliability. This is often reflected in the use of alternative terms, such as credibility, to describe the criteria to be applied to qualitative research.

Credibility

One of the best-known approaches to judging the credibility of qualitative research was developed by Schutz (1962), the social phenomenologist. Schutz described his most important criterion as the postulate of adequacy, which states, in Phillipson's (1972) paraphrasing, that:

'...each term or concept in the model of action must be constructed so that an act actually performed in the world in the way indicated by the construct would be understandable *for the actor himself* and for his fellow men in terms of commonsense schemes of interpretation. This ensures consistency of social scientific constructs with those of everyday commonsense experience.' (Emphasis in original)

In other words, the credibility of qualitative claims about the group of people under consideration depends upon the group finding the descriptions and explanations of their lives recognizable and understandable. The logic of this criterion is that if the aim of qualitative research is to illuminate and explain other people's understandings of the world, then the information presented in a qualitative research report must be compatible with those understandings. That this is the case can only be ascertained by going back to the sources of those understandings.

While such a criterion may seem eminently sensible, it is not without its problems, which come into starkest focus when we consider the issue of critical research. For example, a piece of research into an institution catering for people with learning disabilities discovered that the attitude of staff members to clients was less than caring. Would this research be adjudged invalid because staff, when presented with the findings, denied that they recognized the attitudes and understandings attributed to them? When we are dealing with the possibilities of power and oppression, those who may openly display that power and oppression will have a vested interest in denying that they do. In health care situations, which are supposedly animated by a caring ethos, the motivation to deny recognition of uncaring attitudes and actions becomes all the more acute.

Since Schutz (1962) there have been numerous attempts to construct criteria for the credibility of qualitative research. Here we have space to consider one of these, as set out by Brewer (1994). Brewer argues that, in the absence of statistical tests to check the qualitative researcher's findings, the confidence of the reader that those findings adequately reflect the nature of the social world under consideration depends upon her being persuaded of the researcher's integrity and good practice. Brewer lists six injunctions for good practice:

1. Establishing the relevance and representativeness of the setting under study.
2. Identifying the features of the research area addressed and those they left out, and discussing the possible implications of these choices.
3. Identifying the theoretical framework of the research, along with the broader values and commitments to which the researcher adheres.
4. Establishing the researcher's integrity by outlining:
   (i)   the amount and quality of empirical material gained;
   (ii) the researcher's background in relation to the setting of the research;
   (iii) the researcher's experiences during the research, especially any constraints encountered;
   (iv) the strengths and weaknesses of the research design and strategy.
5. Establishing the authority of the data by:
   (i)   discussing problems that arose in the research;
   (ii) outlining the grounds on which data were categorized, and identifying whether the categories used were those of the respondents or the researcher;
   (iii) discussing alternative explanations or ways of organizing the data;
   (iv) producing sufficient extracts from the data to allow the reader to decide whether the researcher's interpretation of the data is a reasonable one;
   (v)   discussing power relations between the researcher and her research subjects – for example, how ethnic, class or gender differences might have affected the research dynamic.
6. Demonstrating the complexity of the data by:
   (i)   discussing negative cases that fall outside the categories developed;
   (ii) showing the multiple and often contradictory descriptions supplied by the respondents themselves;
   (iii) stressing the context of respondents' accounts and discussing how that context might influence accounts.

The point of Brewer's (1994) sensible suggestions for establishing the credibility of qualitative research is not to provide cast iron guarantees, but to ensure that the reader of research can make an informed interpretation. Rather than seeing this state of affairs as a weakness, it can equally be seen as beneficial to the pursuit of knowledge in that it encourages reflexivity and critical thinking, instead of passive reception of research claims.

Conclusions

This chapter has discussed the concepts of validity and reliability and has highlighted some of the methods which researchers may employ in their attempts to ensure that their data possess these attributes. Published research frequently fails to mention the attempts that were made by the researcher to establish validity and reliability; and without such detail the reader cannot assume that the data meet the intended criteria. It is worth remembering that research data and findings will only be as valid and as reliable as the validity and reliability of the instruments used to gather those data, or generate those findings, and that while conclusive guarantees of validity and reliability may not be possible, researchers must be as rigorous as possible in their attempts to meet these requirements and should be explicit about their attempts to do so.

References

Barrett, C. & Myrick, F. (1998) Job satisfaction in preceptorship and its effect on the clinical performance of the preceptee. *Journal of Advanced Nursing* **27** (2): 364–71.

Brewer, J.D. (1994) The ethnographic critique of ethnography: sectarianism in the RUC. *Sociology* **28** (1): 231–44.

Callaghan, S. & Trapp, M. (1998) Evaluating two dressings for the prevention of nasal bridge pressure sore. *Professional Nurse* **13** (6): 361–4.

Dunning, P. & Martin, M. (1998) Beliefs about diabetes and diabetic complications. *Professional Nurse* **13** (7): 429–34.

Edwards, M. (1994) The rationale for the use of risk calculators in pressure sore prevention, and the evidence of the reliability and validity of published scales. *Journal of Advanced Nursing* **20** (2): 288–96.

Foxall, M.J., Barron, C.R. & Houfek, J. (1998) Ethnic differences in breast self-examination practice and health beliefs. *Journal of Advanced Nursing* **27** (2): 419–28.

Hammersley, M. (1992) *What's Wrong with Ethnography?* London: Routledge.

Holstein, J.A. & Gubrium, J.F. (1997) Active interviewing. In D. Silverman (ed.) *Qualitative Research: Theory, Method and Practice*. London: Sage.

Leinenger, M. (1994) Evaluation criteria and critique in qualitative research. In J. Morse (ed.) *Critical Issues in Qualitative Research Methods*. Thousand Oaks: Sage.

McLaughlin, C. (1997) The effects of classroom theory and contact with patients on the attitudes of student nurses towards mentally ill people. *Journal of Advanced Nursing* **26** (6): 1221–8.

Neale, J.M. & Liebert, R.M. (1986) *Science and Behaviour: An Introduction to Methods of Research*, 3rd edition. New Jersey: Prentice Hall.

Phillipson, M. (1972) Phenomenological philosophy and sociology. In P. Filmer, M. Phillipson, D. Silverman & D. Walsh (eds) *New Directions in Sociological Theory*. London: Collier-Macmillan.

Schutz, A. (1962) *Collected Papers*, Vol. I. Den Haag: Nijhoff.

Smith, J. (1984) The problem of criteria for judging interpretive inquiry. *Educational Evaluation and Policy Analysis* 6 (4): 379–91.

CHAPTER 4

Agencies supportive to research

Senga Bond

This chapter is devoted to sources of support for those who wish to begin to carry out research. Of course, research efforts extend from large-scale multi-disciplinary, multi-centre projects involving major financial and manpower resources, to those which can be done by an individual requiring little more than a notebook, a pencil and lots of time. It is well nigh impossible for anyone to carry out good research without support. Different forms of assistance are appropriate for all types of research and all research workers, whatever the stage of their research career. However, for those at the earlier stages, it is of the utmost importance to obtain good advice as well as the means to support the research.

Let us assume you have the motivation, interest, and a bright idea and want to embark on research but lack the knowledge of where to begin. The fact that you are reading this book would suggest that you are on the right track! Books like this are a useful source of ideas but because they are not interactive in the same way as people, they are at best only a partial answer. Doing research is an intellectual craft activity and no one learns their craft from books. If we posed the question, 'Why do I want help?' it might be answered in a number of ways, including:

- education for research
- supervision
- advice about a specific project
- kindred spirits to provide emotional sustenance
- financial support
- information resources.

Education for research

Some aspects of research are generally included as a small component of most diploma and degree level nursing courses, and there are many short 'research appreciation' courses as well as longer forms of research preparation at diploma, masters and doctorate levels. While you may have had some introduction to research ideas and to research studies, it may be worth considering extended research training. Courses in research methods are available in many higher educational institutions as well as distance learning through the Open University, for example. It is generally easier to obtain time off work for a part-time day/evening course, but it is often more beneficial to be able to concentrate on full-time study if it can be arranged. The calendars of universities and colleges should provide details of whether suitable courses are available, and their entry requirements. It may be that research does not feature in the course title – for example, MSc Health Sciences – and so course content needs to be examined carefully. Appropriate courses may be found in nursing departments, in social sciences, public health or in health services research departments. Some provide an option which permits progress from diploma to higher degree.

A traditional way to obtain research education is to register for a higher degree after having secured a good quality first degree. Depending on the level of research education in the first degree, it may be advantageous to combine a Master or Doctor of Philosophy (MPhil/PhD) with some formal research teaching within a masters or similar level of taught course. For those who are serious about pursuing a career which includes research, completion of a doctorate is now almost mandatory and is better obtained at the earliest opportunity.

Information about local courses and study opportunities should be available from the Research and Development (R&D) manager in your local NHS Trusts. This person may know people who have attended courses and are able to offer some insight into what the courses offer. Many universities advertise research study opportunities in the professional press (for example, *Health Services Journal*) or the national press (for example, *Guardian Education* or the *Times Higher Education Supplement*).

Rather than embark on formal research training you may be guided in the direction of a 'research appreciation' course. These courses offer little preparation for those with a serious intention to do research and are oriented more for 'consumers' and 'participants' in research, to raise awareness and interest at a very superficial level. One advantage of doing a formal research methods course is to assist those who have found research interesting in an undergraduate pro-gramme to decide whether they have the motivation and ability to proceed to carry out research. While taking a higher degree may delay the start of an interesting project, it is essential in laying down a good foundation from which to proceed. It is for this reason that students embarking on a higher degree by research are advised to participate in a general methods course first, or as part of their higher degree, so that as well as learning through a project using a particular method, they can extend their knowledge to other methods and techniques used in research.

Advanced research training at post-doctoral level is also advised for those whose career intentions include research. This means that it takes at least ten years of academic training to reach the first rung of the research ladder to gen-erate research income from peer-reviewed sources.

Supervision

Those who embark on a formal research course will be allocated a supervisor. It is very important that supervision relates to the methodological aspects of the study, to the practical aspects of planning and conducting the research, as well as to its subject matter. If there is a need for supervision in the substantive topic from a nutritionist or a psychologist or nurse expert in the subject of the study, then two supervisors are needed. Supervisors are there to discuss, challenge, guide and offer advice, not to do the project. They need to be asked for help and are encouraged to assist when students have done some preparation and thought through the problems of conducting the research at theoretical, methodological and practical levels. Most supervisors, especially if they are good and hence in demand, will have heavy requests for their time. However, if they are faced with a keen student who is well prepared, then demands are more likely to be met. Most higher educational institutions now prepare guidance for students and supervisors in managing projects and the supervision process. They are expected to set clear work targets and meet them. Choosing your supervisor wisely can make all the difference in benefiting from research training, and supervisors should have substantial research experience before assuming the task of supervision. It is wise to check their credentials and the experiences of previous students.

Advice about a specific project

Of course the need for advice could be at any stage of the research process, but in general terms the earlier advice is sought the better. Recognizing the need for advice could be in working on a project that inspires you, but you are not sure what to do next. As a formal supportive agency, this is the kind of work for which an R&D adviser or other person with a research advisory remit in the health service would be the first port of call. This person should have a sufficiently broad overview of research to enable you to refine your ideas and begin to formulate possible directions for the project. It is important to bear in mind that it is not possible for any one individual to have detailed knowledge of every research problem with which she is faced, but nurses in research advisory roles should be able to assist you sufficiently to enable you to prepare to consult with someone with more specialist knowledge if this is warranted.

Regional NHS Executive R&D Directorates have often funded University Departments or staff within the NHS to offer a research advisory service. Your local NHS library or Trust R&D manager should have a directory of names and locations and these are also available on the Web pages of every Regional R&D office (see end of chapter for sites). With R&D investment in the NHS in recent years it is likely that there will be someone locally whose job it is to provide research advice to NHS staff. In Scotland research networks have been created to cover the whole of the country and to offer advice to those wishing to conduct health-related research. Sometimes specific research advisory mechanisms have been developed for nurses to assist them to get a toe-hold into research.

These local resources may not be specifically for nurses nor are they provided by nurses themselves, but can come from a diverse range of scientific backgrounds. Whatever their background, the personal recommendation of someone who is helpful is by far the best way of securing useful contacts. The message is: begin where you are and use whatever talent is available locally before proceeding further. It is always appreciated if you arrive with well-considered questions and have prepared your material for the meeting.

Kindred spirits to provide emotional sustenance

Another type of support, which is rather different from specific advice or supervision for your project, is to find like-minded individuals who are carrying out research and facing similar problems. It is probably a universal finding that research workers at some point in developing or carrying out a project feel isolated, dejected, and ready to give up. At such times it is useful to share your experience with someone who may have gone through, or be in the process of facing, the same distress. This is when membership of an informal or formal research group may be useful. There may be local research interest groups near you and these serve several functions. As one of their strengths, they bring together people who have a general interest in learning about and supporting research. On the whole you are likely to find others with research interests very willing to help and listen, and offer support of different kinds. In this regard the Research Networks in Scotland serve a useful function in bringing together people from a range of backgrounds and interests.

Other benefits to be gained from membership of a local research group are, for example, hearing of current developments in research (nationally as well as locally), learning how others have gone about research, and discovering how they have attempted to overcome their particular difficulties. By providing an informal setting to discuss research issues generally, research meetings can be very positive occasions for those planning to begin, or already engaged in, research. Less formal get-togethers of nurses involved in research are also useful. Sometimes an informal lunchtime gathering is sufficient to air a difficulty and regain vital energies which may be dwindling.

At a national level the conferences arranged by nursing organizations, including the annual conference of the RCN Research Society or specific clinical groups, provide occasions for hearing research workers talk about their work. This is most effectively done at residential conferences where there are opportunities for networking as well as hearing about recent developments, and special interest groups can meet to discuss particular issues.

The other kind of non-nursing groups and associations that may be worth considering are those with a more specific focus of interest; examples would be the Society for Tissue Viability, the British Society of Gerontology, the Society for Research in Rehabilitation, and the Society for Social Medicine. While some of these are not specifically research groups, a major interest is the discussion of current research and methods in their respective fields. These groups would be of major importance in keeping abreast of developments that are broader than nursing and maintaining current awareness of findings and methods. Membership of such a group would bring you into contact with others who share an interest in a narrower substantive field. Gradually professional nursing groups, like the RCN societies, are developing research-oriented themes in their conferences and professional meetings, and are therefore a focal point for researchers and clinical practitioners alike.

Financial support

Financial assistance may be sought for research education or for funding a specific project. The opportunities available for research education described above may also carry certain remuneration. The funds apportioned to research education within the health service is highly variable. While all NHS Executive R&D Directors are committed to supporting the research infrastructure, how they do so varies, and obtaining funding is generally in open competition, with nurses competing with other disciplines for different levels of funding to pay for anything ranging from a short course on a specific research method through to three-year PhD research support and salary. NHS Trusts also differ in the amount of funding made available for research training, with some regarding funding of research training as appropriate, while others do not. With training budgets devolved into clinical directorates it is reputed to be increasingly difficult to fund research training.

In financial terms, much more money is available for funding individual projects than for research training. In nursing the problem is not that there is not the funding but that there is a shortfall in the number of nurses with the experience needed to attract it. Grant-awarding bodies are unlikely to fund research proposed by an inexperienced would-be researcher with no evidence of her capability of managing a research project. It is naive to expect funding without a track record, so how does one's request ever get considered?

There are no short answers. Traditionally, individuals build up research credibility by working with experienced researchers and learning the craft from them. By so doing one gradually develops a reputation sufficient to enable grants to be awarded on the basis of sound proposals. Research budgets are available to nurses in all of the health-related charities as well as central government research funds, the NHS Executive Regional R&D budgets and the Medical and Economic and Social Research Councils. Funds are not earmarked for nurses but are open to competition on the basis of the quality of the proposal. In some respects nurses are disadvantaged by the membership of many funding bodies being medically rather than health oriented and having a preference for particular approaches to research.

Many research-funding sources operate in 'response mode' – that is, they will respond to proposals originating from the applicants. However, increasingly, priority areas are being identified and proposals invited in line with specified topics. This is not a bar to nurses applying for funding as long as their proposals are in line with what is requested. It is important, therefore, to know the priorities of different funding agencies and to ensure that proposals are appropriately targeted.

To assist novices some NHS R&D offices make small amounts of money available, for example £5000–£10 000, which do not have to go through the usual peer review process for those new to research. Intermediate level grants then are pitched at £25 000–£50 000 over one to two years, while larger grants are also available. To obtain a small grant the project being prepared has to be seen as pilot work leading to a more substantial research project. It may be available to assist in funding higher degree work, but will not be awarded unless what is being prepared is of high quality and feasible with the resources being asked for.

A directory of grant-giving bodies specifically for nursing is provided in the *Directory of Nursing Charities* (Queen's Nursing Institute, 1993). Many of these provide small amounts of money for educational purposes but some also indicate a willingness to finance research projects. Other sources of availability of grants for research are listed at the end of the chapter.

Finance for research may also be attracted from industry and commerce, particularly the pharmaceutical companies and those devoted to other health products. Some companies, like 3M, Smith & Nephew and Maws, annually award scholarships but *ad hoc* projects may also be funded. Commercial concerns could probably be more widely used than they are, but ethical considerations sometimes intervene.

Chapter 10 in this volume deals with writing a proposal, which is only one facet of attracting research money. The proposal, irrespective of its scientific merits, must prove sufficiently appealing to attract sponsorship and there is an art in preparing such a submission. Novices typically would be advised not to do this but just to gain some experience of working as a research assistant before bidding for independent research funds.

Information resources

While information resources have been placed last, they are by no means least in importance. Anyone wishing to carry out research will need to know what has already been published on the topic. For this reason libraries and other information services are integral to research development. Chapter 8 describes major sources of research information which are increasingly accessible through on-line computer facilities.

While using these abstracting and indexing sources is important for individuals to keep abreast of current literature, group efforts to share knowledge and reading can be stimulating and beneficial. In some clinical and academic departments, journal clubs meet on a regular basis to discuss recent important publications and to inform participants of useful papers and books which have been identified. By allocating particular journals to members and sharing the reading, an enormous amount of scanning can be shared and useful items located which might otherwise have been missed. Journal clubs have the added advantage of encouraging discussion, learning how others regard methods and findings, and generally sharpening research awareness. An active journal club demonstrates to others the importance placed on knowing what is happening nationally and internationally. They are, therefore, as important for 'users' as for 'doers' of research.

Conclusions

No matter who it is, or the degree of development in their research career, some forms of support are necessary to carry out research. This chapter has done little more than indicate some of the sources of such support in getting started. It would be easy to consider support purely in financial terms – for example, for research education or to fund a project to buy staff time or materials. This is only part of the story. Just as important are sources of support which are sustaining in both intellectual and emotional terms. One has only to read the acknowledgements section of any thesis to find reference to the assistance given by supervisors and colleagues, not to mention long-suffering family and patients. Often it is the generosity of others in terms of their time, intellectual application, and listening ability, as well as their skills in motivating and encouraging others to write proposals and reports, which enable research to succeed.

The research community itself is perhaps the most important supportive agency. Researchers, by their willingness to give the same encouragement and assistance to others which they themselves have received, are an important source of mutual support. Used wisely they are of incalculable benefit.

Useful addresses

The RCN's research co-ordinating centre Web page at http://www.man.ac.uk/rcn/ is probably the single most useful source of, and access to, relevant information. This site offers links not only to information about research activities in the RCN but to R&D in all of the English Health Regions, Northern Ireland, Wales and Scotland, providing details of their local research networks, funding opportunities, training and support units.

There are also links to the register of completed and ongoing research projects funded by the NHS (http://www.doh.gov.uk/nrr.htm), to the main NHS research programmes and to the Web pages of some research organizations. Accessing this site offers a very quick route into a great deal of useful information.

The Foundation of Nursing Studies at 32 Buckingham Palace Road, London, SW1 0RE (tel. 0171 233 5759; e-mail admin@fons.org) is a useful organization for those who are interested more in the application of research in practice. They offer courses and funding for research implementation projects.

Useful sources of research grants

Association of Medical Research Charities (1998) *Handbook of the Association of Medical Research Charities*. London: British Heart Foundation.
Charities Aid Foundation (1998) *Directory of Grant Making Trusts* (16th edn). London.
Queen's Nursing Institute (1993) *Directory of Nursing Charities*. London.
Waterlow Information Services (1998) *Charity Choice*. London.

Useful web sites

http://www.leeds.ac.uk/rdinfo
http://www.man.ac.uk/rcn/rcnfunding.htm

CHAPTER 5

Ethical issues in research

Hazel E. McHaffie

Consider, if you will, two scenarios.

1. Joseph Lyons is struggling. He is an inpatient on a medical ward following a stroke. For some time he has had difficulty with bladder control largely because of his slowness in movement. The nurse seeing him struggling will instinctively come to his aid, attend to his needs, and prevent unhappiness. The researcher observing Mr Lyons may well simply watch, wait to see how long it will take someone to respond to his needs, note his distress, record the nurses' reaction to another wet bed, and analyse the possible causes and effects of the various components of this experience. For the researcher, who is also a nurse, a dilemma will present. What are the boundaries of her responsibility?

2. Robin Allen is a nurse working as a clinical specialist in a busy intensive care unit. He agrees to participate in a study looking at the impact of personal experience of loss and bereavement on professional attitudes and behaviours. During the course of his interview he discloses that he has lost three partners who died from AIDS-related illnesses. He further admits that none of his colleagues knows that he himself is HIV positive. What should the researcher do with this information?

In nursing, midwifery and health visiting, research depends for its success on careful observation, contemplation, recording and analysis, but this may involve hearing and seeing things about which others do not know. The contract a researcher has with a participant allows confidences to be given which would compel a clinician to act. Respondents are not unaware of the opportunities: sharing troubling thoughts and experiences can be therapeutic. Thus, for example, if a safe and confiding atmosphere is provided, a mother may well tell a researcher that she has harmed her baby; a teenager may report that she is being abused. To divulge that information to a health visitor or a social worker has obvious ramifications and possible penalties, but for the researcher in receipt of these confidences there are difficult decisions to be made about how to respond and burdens of a different nature (McHaffie, 1996).

A range of ethical problems present themselves not only to those actively engaged in research but to clinicians whose patients are involved in projects, to educators and to managers. By definition, where a dilemma presents there are no easy answers. It may be necessary to weigh up present safety, long-term benefit, or the conflicting interests of different parties against the integrity of the research. Simply because there are few concrete points of reference the decisions can be difficult and worrying.

Ethics is a brand of philosophy which deals with thinking about morality. In assessing the morality of a person's conduct we make a judgement about whether something is right or wrong. Each of us has our own values, beliefs and standards and this very diversity complicates matters. Codes and official guidelines only take us so far. We are each individually accountable for our practice and must be able to justify the decisions we make.

Responsibilities of all nurses, midwives and health visitors

Enormous strides have been made in the scientific, technological and social developments of health care in recent years. Emerging ethical dilemmas have exercised the minds of many. Fundamentally the biomedical ethical principles underpinning practice remain unchanged: respect for autonomy, and the principles of doing no harm, doing good and acting justly (Beauchamp & Childress, 1989). Professional advice has become more expansive but is consistent with these basic tenets (British Medical Association, 1993; Royal College of Nursing, 1993; UKCC, 1996).

The United Kingdom Central Council for Nursing, Midwifery and Health Visiting, in its *Code of Conduct* (UKCC, 1992), requires all its practitioners to 'safeguard and promote the interests of individual patients and clients'. In its 16 items it clearly places responsibility with the individual: it is no defence that someone else gave the instruction, or that one was an innocent bystander. Acts and omissions alike incur censure. The professional bodies reinforce this responsibility, applying it to research as well as to clinical practice (Royal College of Nursing, 1993; Royal College of Midwives, 1989; International Confederation of Midwives, 1993). Indeed, the Royal College of Nursing document, *Ethics Related to Research in Nursing*, spells out the issues clearly and comprehensively.

Individual professional accountability

Practising nurses and midwives can be caught up in the ethical issues around research without ever being actively involved in the process itself. Simply because their patients/clients become participants, they inherit a special responsibility. Research can be detrimental and the clinician has a specific obligation to ensure that nothing jeopardizes the well-being of those in her care.

Good practice should be based wherever possible on sound evidence. It is not ethically acceptable to follow tradition or received wisdom without question. In order to practise safely and well, every practitioner needs to be aware of the research in her field of practice and able to use it effectively. However, not all research is valuable and usable. Being personally accountable involves discrimination, which means being able to read, critically evaluate and effectively utilize reports of studies.

A fundamental requirement in any endeavour is to possess the knowledge and skills that are compatible with the demands of the task. It is important to recognize the limits of one's competence and not to take on tasks unless they can be carried out in a safe and skilled manner. Research is a skilled occupation, just as clinical practice and education are. It should not be thought that it can just be 'picked up' without the advice and help of experts.

Where clinicians are asked to be actively involved, even at a minimal level, in the research process they must be acquainted with what the procedures involve. Thus, if they are asked to witness the signing of a document giving informed consent, they should satisfy themselves that the patient has fully understood the risks involved and understands that he has the right to withdraw at any point without influencing in any way his therapeutic management.

Nurses and midwives are not infrequently employed as data collectors. Given the clinical load they already carry, it is vital that this additional role is not detrimental to the well-being of their patients. They are obliged to state if this is the case. As at all other levels of involvement, if they undertake data collection, they are bound by the same ethical principles incumbent on all researchers. Integrity and accuracy are mandatory. Clearly the success of the research is dependent on the willingness, accuracy and conscientiousness of such data collectors.

Particular tensions may present with this dual role. Confidential information may be acquired as part of being a clinician or in the course of data collection. Such information must not be divulged outside the sphere in which it was collected except with the express permission of the respondent himself. As we have already seen, conflicts of interests can place the researcher in an unenviable position.

Responsibilities of the researcher

Personal integrity

Researchers are bound by their professional codes as well as the guidance provided for the conduct of research in general. Intellectual honesty and integrity are required at each level of the enquiry.

There is an initial obligation to ensure that the work they are proposing is appropriate. It is not appropriate, for example, to conduct a study which does nothing to contribute to further knowledge; to do it for the wrong reasons; or to carry out tasks for which one is inadequately prepared. This may sound perfectly straightforward. In reality conflicts may arise even here. Sometimes the requirements of an academic institution may not concur with those of clinical practice. On occasion the research budget does not permit expert methodological, computing or statistical advice and a researcher falls back on books and secondhand advice. These are compromises and force uneasy decisions.

Recognizing one's personal limitations is essential at every level: few researchers are experts in all methods and in all aspects of the research process. In addition, every individual brings some personal history to an enquiry. Where this might prejudice the work in any way, it should be declared. Even very eminent researchers have taken a subject on board because of their personal agendas: this is not of necessity a bad thing, but it is a potential bias. Both researcher and reader must calculate its effect. Such honesty is part of the requirement for personal integrity and accuracy. By the same token, the effect the researcher may have had on her subjects should be openly acknowledged. If such matters are not made explicit, doubt may be cast on the integrity of other parts of the enquiry.

Conducting research and then allowing the results to gather dust on a shelf is unethical. If the study was needed in the first place, its results should be published and disseminated appropriately. Many subjects as well as data collectors have, over the years, lamented the lack of availability of findings (Hicks, 1994). It is unethical to 'use' people in this way. Where they have contributed time, energy and emotions, they are entitled to some feedback. Funding bodies who resource the enquiries are also due some tangible return for their investment.

The research world operates on a basis of trust, but a worrying level of fraud has been uncovered in recent years (eg. Millar, 1997; Murray, 1998). Indeed, in 1997 a Committee on Publication Ethics was set up specifically to investigate the scale of the problem. Actual examples of fraudulent researchers may be relatively few but they attract severe censure (e.g. Dyer, 1997a, 1997b; McHaffie, in press). Academics are under pressure to publish, to progress their careers; professionals can believe passionately that a certain form of treatment is efficacious and want the medical world to be convinced. For a minority the temptation to manufacture evidence can be hard to resist.

More common than actual falsification of results is the practice of 'doctoring' the reporting to omit those aspects of the project that were less than successful. Not only is this intellectually dishonest, but it carries the grave risk that others will subsequently repeat the errors in judgement. No research project carried out in the natural world can be perfect. It is far better to acknowledge the limitations, delays, unexpected hitches and inappropriate use of tools or ambiguous questions, than to pretend the exercise was perfectly planned and executed, and risk losing credibility and integrity. A conflict may, however, present where the results would be unwelcome to the host organization. If, for example, the research uncovers undesirable practices among some of its nurses, reporting them may offend the hosts. It is important in these circumstances to balance the value of the information, the context and nature of the reporting and the overall message against the damage that may result from the disclosure.

Another aspect of intellectual honesty relates to the extent of the reporting. It is important to present findings which do not support one's hypothesis or hunch as well as those which do. Researchers are scientifically accountable to their peers: the advancement of theory and methods for the profession depends upon their integrity (Clark, 1991; Sandelowski, 1993). Widespread peer review, competent scrutiny and constructive criticism from within the research community, as well as from without, can do much to promote good quality at all stages of any enquiry. Building in such advice is advisable.

Responsibility to participants

Informed consent

In any research which involves human subjects in the United Kingdom, there must be safeguards for their protection. The hazards of radioactive substances or of aggressive drug treatments are obvious. Less well recognized are the emotional, psychological and social harms which might accrue. It can be damaging to be asked insensitive questions. Confidence can be undermined if a subject is left feeling ignorant about a topic. Where a participant is assigned to a control group he can feel disadvantaged if the experimental intervention appears more beneficial.

It is imperative that prospective subjects are warned of the potential risks of involvement before they agree to participate. Of course it is perfectly possible technically to spell out these drawbacks but not to truly inform. If the researcher is to behave ethically, she should give the individual every opportunity to question, to receive accurate information and to reflect on the matter or consult others before committing himself in any way. Wherever possible it is wise to supply written material to accompany verbal information. It should also be made perfectly clear that a patient has an absolute right to decline to participate or to withdraw at any time. No risk of less effective or kindly care should ever be a result of such a refusal – a fact which should be spelled out plainly. Ill people are very vulnerable and feel disempowered. It is imperative that this vulnerability is not exploited in any way.

How and when such consent is obtained matters. To approach a woman in strong labour, or a sedated patient minutes before he goes to theatre for major surgery, is unacceptable. Simple reflection will demonstrate the truth of this statement. Less clear is the issue of how much to tell. For some studies it is not possible to divulge all the information known about the subject. In other cases it would be detrimental to the study for the subjects to know everything about the aims of the project. Take, for example, an investigation of non-accidental injury in children in an Accident and Emergency Department; or a study of the effects of intramuscular vitamin K for newborns; or the behaviours of married men who have sex with men. In all these areas of interest, the quality of data produced might well be jeopardized if too much information is divulged to potential respondents. If the parents think the researcher suspects them of deliberately harming their child, they are not likely to want to talk about the 'accident'. Mothers will be reluctant to expose their babies to possible danger, no matter how remote. Married men might view with dismay the prospect of someone studying homosexuality appearing on their marital doorstep. Where does society's right to accurate information or the funding agency's right to good quality data, or the individual's right to be informed begin and end? Careful judgements must be made.

A fundamental respect for other people should be the guiding principle. Their right to be autonomous should be upheld. In the field of HIV and AIDS the need for a partnership between researchers and subjects has been clearly demonstrated. People with the virus have gone to extreme lengths to ensure that participation in clinical trials does not unfairly discriminate between patients or potentially damage the health of any individual person (Institute of Medical Ethics, 1992). Not all patients, however, have been as articulate or well informed. But again their very vulnerability should make the researcher more vigilant in protecting their interests.

It is sometimes assumed that information collected during the course of providing nursing or midwifery care is available for research purposes. This should not be assumed. If clinical data are to be used for research, permission needs to be sought from the patients and in some cases the person who is in clinical charge of the patient and the authorities by whom the records are held (Dimond, 1990).

The identity of the researcher

Researchers can undertake projects for many and various reasons, but some of these reasons may be questionable. An individual with strong negative homophobic prejudices is probably not an appropriate person to research attitudes to patients who are HIV positive. Someone employed by a drug company may not be able to declare all his findings if they demonstrate that a particular product had unwelcome side-effects. A lay person may not fully comprehend the nuances and culture of a specialized paediatric intensive care unit: interpretation of what she sees may be inaccurate. The identity of the researcher can influence the quality of the design, conduct and recommendations of the study.

It can sometimes seem important to conceal the identity of the researcher. Examples of such disguise can be found in the literature and include researchers pretending to be criminals, police, homosexuals and nursing auxiliaries. Extremely rich data can be obtained in some circumstances where respondents see the incomer as 'one of them'. Indeed such data might be unobtainable in any other way, but serious attention must be given to the rights of those people who disclose information unwittingly for research purposes (Johnson, 1992). Many people have strong moral objections to such deception.

In health care enquiries, the research may well overlap with clinical management. Where the researcher is not involved in delivering the treatment, it is important that the clinicians are aware of their patients' participation. Naturally if an intervention is necessary which includes a new or altered form of treatment, close liaison will be imperative, but the courtesy of informing clinical colleagues should apply even when their permission is not necessary.

Confidentiality and anonymity

During the course of data collection, researchers may be told much that is confidential. They are required to give assurances of confidentiality and anonymity in almost all cases. Indeed the rich quality of data obtained in many studies has only been possible because of such assurances. These confidences must be respected. Where it appears imperative to disclose any such information the explicit permission of the respondent is required. On the surface, this seems beyond question. In practice, conflicts may arise. Information may be disclosed which puts emotional well-being at risk as well as lives. It is very burdensome to be told that a respondent is contemplating suicide; feels she may do violence to her infant; is living off money acquired by immoral or illegal means; or is putting others' safety in danger. Conflicting interests and risks must be balanced and the researcher may make judgements which sometimes weigh heavily. It can be helpful to appoint impartial and experienced advisers to support and guide the front line researcher in any project with potential risks of this nature.

Where there is any possibility that information will be obtained relating to safety, well-being or clinical problems, it is important to establish accepted lines of communication before the event. Who will the researcher tell? Who else will be informed or contacted? How much will be disclosed? Roles and responsibilities will then be clear and appropriate action can be instigated promptly.

Preserving the anonymity of respondents or participating institutions or organizations is another requirement. Individuals may very well not wish to admit that they supported the administration of drugs to end a life peacefully and in a dignified way if such information could be traced back to them. Junior health care professionals may be reluctant to disclose their views on the management of the wards on which they work if they fear identification. Respondents have a right to such protection.

Ethics Committee approval

As part of the protection of people's rights and interests, Local Research Ethics Committees exist for the scrutiny of proposed projects. Each Health Authority (Health Board in Scotland) has a requirement to set up appropriately constituted committees (Department of Health, 1991; Scottish Office Home and Health Department, 1992; Royal College of Physicians, 1996). Some academic institutions also operate their own systems of vigilance. The *modus operandi* of each committee varies, and intending researchers should obtain the necessary information and documentation from the relevant body. Contact information can usually be obtained through the headquarters of the relevant Health Authority/Board. With the advent of Trusts there is a potential for additional problems in accessing subjects and in collaborating between organizations. Commercial and professional sensitivities have added a competitive dimension to the provision of health care and for a variety of reasons managers may be less open with information about their services in the future.

Nevertheless, irrespective of whether the researcher is or is not an employee in the National Health Service, projects involving patients must be scrutinized by ethics committees. Where research subjects are the health care professionals themselves, different areas have differing policies about whether such approval is necessary. Advice from the Health Authority/Board or the Local Research Ethics Committee should be sought.

Ethics committees are made up of representatives from the health professions, individuals with various interests such as law or theology and members of the lay community. Each committee has boundaries relating to the geographical or subject area it will review. Problems do arise, and with the increasing complexity and range of research projects, there is some concern that these ethics committees may withhold approval less to protect potential respondents than to demonstrate their power or because they are unfamiliar with the nature of the enquiry (Pollock & Tilley, 1988; Neuberger, 1991).

Responsibilities of the educator

Research is no longer a tiny component tagged on to the end of courses for nurses, midwives and health visitors to fill in a Friday afternoon slot. It is something which underpins all of health care to a greater or lesser extent, depending on the evidence available. Part of the preparation of its practitioners is to equip them to care well. The quality of the care offered depends on an understanding of what research has shown to be good practice.

If individual clinicians are to be professionally accountable they require the skills accurately and critically to assess the evidence, and educators have a specific responsibility to give them such equipment. However, using research to inform one's practice can be difficult. Resistance, resentment and jealousy can all present barriers to change. It is unacceptable to provide nurses with the knowledge of what needs to be done without the skills to do it. They require skills of negotiation and assertiveness to practise in a world which has a long way still to go in its striving to be research aware and research based.

The increasing inclusion of research components in clinical, management and educational courses at both basic and post-basic levels is to be applauded. However, the requirement that students undertake a small project as part of their course raises problems. Such endeavours are necessarily time limited; they usually have fairly tight geographical limits which carries the threat of overloading respondents in their area; and resources are inevitably constrained. The inexperience of the students may seriously compromise subsequent entry to the field for senior career researchers. Since many of the fundamental principles and skills may be taught in the classroom, it is debatable whether the practice of requiring practical experience in data collection is appropriate.

Responsibilities of the manager

Entering an institution or community to carry out research is a privilege not a right. There are costs and risks to the organization acting as host to such an endeavour. Managers must assess the psychological as well as the financial costs, both direct and indirect. Researchers can impede work, distract staff, create unrest and expose undesirable, unethical and questionable practices.

Those with the authority to sanction or commission research carry a heavy obligation. In negotiating with researchers, clinicians, educators and sponsors they will require great tact and diplomacy. As they have a duty to encourage the conduct of good research in their area of responsibility, it is imperative, therefore, that they understand what is worth while and achievable, and what is feasible given service demands. With the strong pressures on resources and time, it is easy for managers to expect too much too quickly. In the furtherance of sound knowledge, studies must be well conducted with rigorous checks on reliability and validity. It is just as harmful to support all research attempts indiscriminately as to resist research. Some studies simply should not be encouraged. Good communication and liaison with expert researchers will facilitate sound and effective judgements.

Where managers commission research, they have an obligation to respect the right of any individual to refuse to undertake a project if she considers it to be outside her range of competence. There may well be ways of negotiating the involvement of others with the necessary skills. Reservations relating to the feasibility of carrying out the study within existing constraints must also be heard.

There are special duties attending those who simultaneously manage health services and commission research. Data collected for the research must not be used for purposes outside the research endeavour in, for example, disciplinary proceedings. Such material is confidential with specific boundaries. Neither should there be any attempt to probe for identifying information which the researcher has deliberately concealed. Where results call for changes these will need to be assessed in the light of wider knowledge and implemented carefully. Managers have a weighty responsibility to ensure that such changes are recommended by expert reviewers in addition to the researchers who might have a vested interest in their own project.

Special protection should be ensured for the vulnerable, and this applies at the level of conducting the enquiry as well as reporting the results. The interests of patients, the staff and the service must not be compromised by the demands of the research undertaken.

The effect of research on the community

Participants in research are part of a wider community. Their involvement in enquiries can cause problems, and managers need to be alive to the possibility of complications.

Where the health care professionals themselves are involved as participants there may be implications if they are withdrawn from the service temporarily or are required to take on additional work or given specific opportunities not available to all. Frustrations and resentments may result.

Feelings of envy or resistance can quickly accumulate if specific groups are frequently targeted for research. The enormous sums of money projected into research relating to HIV and AIDS represent a case in point. Provision of resources in various forms is seen to be discriminating in favour of a select group and at the expense of other specialities who feel they are at least equally deserving. For the communities so over-researched there can be negative as well as positive results. A sense of elitism can be counteracted by a tendency to self-criticism, introspection and doubt, as well as fatigue and lack of enthusiasm.

Conclusions

Ethical dilemmas result from conflicting values. They can relate to whether or not to do the research, the subject to be studied and the actual conduct of the enquiry. Difficulties can present at both a personal and a professional level.

Judgements about what is right conduct lie on a continuum ranging from the clearly unethical to the clearly ethical. Individual tolerances vary, and people's values and attitudes change over time. The issues are not often all black or all white.

Not only those conducting the research, but also nurses, midwives and health visitors involved at the level of protecting the people in their care, require to be sensitive to these issues. They must be prepared to defend what is ethical, renounce the indefensible and support each other in the move towards sound knowledge-based practice.

References

Beauchamp, T.L. & Childress, J.F. (1989) *Principles of Biomedical Ethics*, 3rd edn. Oxford: Oxford University Press.

British Medical Association (1993) *Medical Ethics Today. Its Practice and Philosophy*. London: British Medical Journal Publishing Group.

Clark, E. (1991) *Evaluating Research*. Module 10 in Research Awareness programme. London: Distance Learning Centre, South Bank Polytechnic.

Department of Health (1991) *Local Research Ethics Committees*. London: HMSO.

Dimond, B. (1990) Legal aspects of research. *Nursing Standard* **4** (39): 44–6.

Dyer, C. (1997a) Consultant struck off over research fraud. *British Medical Journal* **314**: 205.

Dyer, C. (1997b) ME researcher accused of cooking the books. *British Medical Journal* **314**: 271.

Hicks, C. (1994) Bridging the gap between research and practice: An assessment of the value of a study day in developing critical research reading skills in midwives. *Midwifery* **10**: 18–25.

Institute of Medical Ethics (1992) AIDS, ethics, and clinical trials. *British Medical Journal* **305**, 699–701.

International Confederation of Midwives (1993) *International Code of Ethics for Midwives*. London: International Confederation of Midwives.

Johnson, M. (1992) A silent conspiracy? Some ethical issues of participant observation in nursing research. *International Journal of Nursing Studies* **29** (2): 213–23.

McHaffie, H.E. (1996) Researching sensitive issues. In L. Frith (ed.) *Ethics and Midwifery. Issues in Contemporary Practice*. Oxford: Butterworth-Heinemann: 258–73.

McHaffie, H.E. (in press) Ethics and good practice. In S. Proctor & M. Renfrew (eds) *Informing Practice in Midwifery*. London: Ballière Tindall.

Millar, B. (1997) Honesty on trial. *Nursing Times* **93** (35): 10–11.

Murray, I. (1998) Journals want watchdog on research fraud. *The Times*, London. 5 June: 13.

Neuberger, J. (1991) *Ethics and Health Care*. London: King's Fund.

Pollock, L. & Tilley, S. (1988) Submitting for approval. *Senior Nurse* **8** (5): 24–5.

Royal College of Midwives (1989) *Practical Guidance for Midwives Facing Ethical or Moral Dilemmas*. London: Royal College of Midwives.

Royal College of Nursing (1993) *Ethics Related to Research in Nursing*. London: Royal College of Nursing.

Royal College of Physicians (1996) *Guidelines on the Practice of Ethics Committees in Medical Research involving Human Subjects*. London: Royal College of Physicians.

Sandelowski, M. (1993) Rigor or rigor mortis: the problem of rigor in qualitative research revisited. *Advances in Nursing Science* **16** (2): 1–8.

Scottish Office Home and Health Department (1992) *Local Research Ethics Committees*. Edinburgh: HMSO.

UKCC (1992) *Code of Conduct for Nurses, Midwives and Health Visitors*. London: United Kingdom Central Council for Nursing, Midwifery and Health Visiting.

UKCC (1996) *Guidelines for Professional Practice*. London: United Kingdom Central Council for Nursing, Midwifery and Health Visiting.

CHAPTER 6

An overview of the research process

Desmond F.S. Cormack

Irrespective of the discipline in which research is undertaken, the series and sequence of steps are essentially the same. What will differ between disciplines such as nursing/midwifery and psychology, for example, will be the subject of the research rather than its structure or process. The research process discussed in Part II of this book is a description of what is commonly referred to as 'the scientific method'. The strength of the scientific method as an approach to problem-solving is that it optimizes the possibility of arriving at the most 'correct', although rarely perfect, solution. Thus, subjectivity is reduced and objectivity is increased in the examination of a particular issue or the asking of a specific question.

An understanding of the research process is not, of itself, sufficient to enable its application. The topics discussed in the first six chapters of the book, for example, are each important in the development of research skills. Similarly, the subjects described in the final chapter are of importance in relation to undertaking, participating in, and using research. Part II cannot be seen in isolation from other parts of this book; it is merely one distinct phase in a number of interrelated parts of understanding the nature, purpose and structure of research. A knowledge of research principles will not, of itself, make a skilled researcher. The need for appropriate guidance and supervision during all stages of the research experience is of considerable importance.

As with many activities which require a high level of knowledge and skill, the knowledge and skill required to undertake research can be learned. They are learned in a number of ways: being told by others, discussing the subject with others, reading about the subject, and by doing a piece of research. Although all educational methods are of value, the ability to undertake research – like riding a bicycle – is never fully developed until practical experience is obtained.

To some extent, but by no means always, the phases of the research process are sequential, with many studies tending to follow a similar series of steps in a similar order. However, the content and structure of this chapter, indeed the entire book, is not intended to suggest that there exists an identical blueprint for all pieces of research. Rather it presents a series of general principles which will be modified to meet the needs of individual researchers and, more particularly, to reflect the research design used. Indeed, it is correct to regard the research design as being *the* deciding factor in determining the shape and sequence of the application of the research process. Part II of this book presents the sequence of steps in the order in which they are frequently undertaken. However, as will be demonstrated in this chapter, there is considerable overlap, interrelationship and possibly some variation in the sequence of events. Figure 6.1 shows the outline of the research process in terms of each of the phases to be considered and also identifies the chapter(s) dealing with each phase.

The interrelationships of the various phases of research are many and complex. Figure 6.1 is not intended to demonstrate all these possible relationships; rather it is intended to show the existence of some of them. Although Chapters 7–35 may

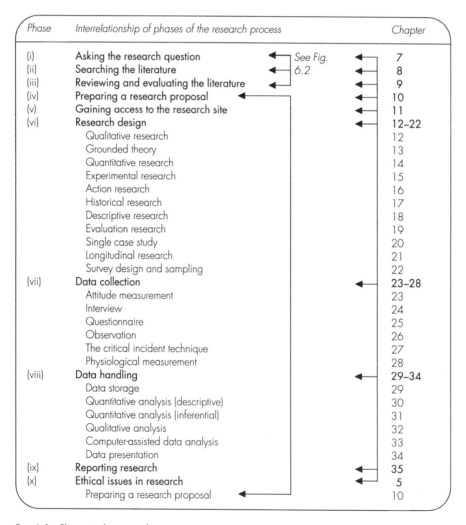

Fig. 6.1 Phases in the research process.

appear to present the process as a series of relatively isolated phases, in practice they overlap.

Asking the research question

Although phase (i) is often regarded as the first formal part of the research process, a number of factors and experiences precede it. It is unlikely, for example, that a potential researcher will suddenly decide that a particular subject should become the focus of a research-based study. It is more probable that, in the course of professional experience and activity, a problem area will slowly emerge as a possibility for a research project. For example, a nurse may have suspected for a long time that the design and height of hospital beds prevents nurses from lifting a patient 'properly', thus placing both patient and nurse at risk. Similarly, an experienced midwife may suspect that all is not well with the methods used to teach students how best to develop and use interpersonal skills. These examples, in themselves, are not formal research questions, they need to be developed, refined and made specific, as described in Chapter 7. Every trained nurse and midwife, therefore, has the experience with which to start to participate in the research process.

It may well be that the ability to think in this enquiring and constructive manner is one of the most important features of potential researchers. Although such individuals may be considered strange, difficult or over-critical by their colleagues, there is no doubt that they are a vital part of the development of research.

Asking the research question (phase (i)) will almost certainly overlap with the next two phases of the process – that is, searching and reviewing and evaluating the literature – in the following way. Before having formally identified the research question, and before having undertaken a systematic search and review of the literature, published materials are likely to be read in order to help to decide exactly what to research. Figure 6.2 demonstrates this relationship.

It can be seen that formulation of the research question comes between a general and relatively unstructured literature search and review (from which it is partly derived) and a more structured and specific search and review (to which it gives direction).

Searching the literature

The relationship between the literature search and other early stages of the research process has been outlined earlier. Its relationship between other stages throughout the research is also important and considerable in that it is related to all stages and continues throughout. Although the intensive and formal search will occur at the early stages of the work, literature continues to be published

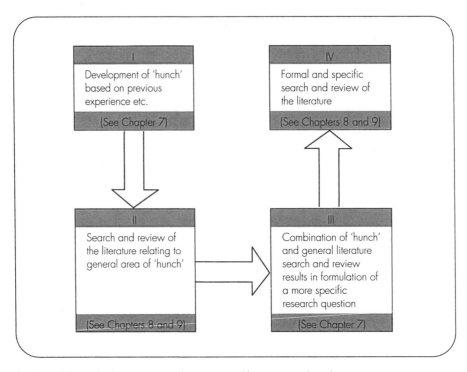

Fig. 6.2 Relationship between research question and literature search and review.

throughout the time it takes to undertake the study. Similarly, some aspects of the literature may be of particular relevance to the latter part of the study – for example, to data analysis.

Chapter 8 describes and discusses the means of, and facilities available for, searching the literature, and shows that a knowledge of this aspect of the research process can make the difference between finding a wealth of appropriate literature and wrongly concluding that 'nothing has been published relating to the subject'. As with all aspects of research, there are rules and guidelines which will make the task easier. There are also an increasingly large range of facilities, aids, organizations and resource people who can be of assistance. 'Practice will make perfect' if the potential researcher is motivated to learn and is willing to invest time and effort.

Reviewing and evaluating the literature

The literature review, although described in a different chapter from that dealing with searching the literature, is closely related to the search in that both occur virtually simultaneously. Indeed, the review of material found early in the search often gives direction to subsequent parts of the search. However, because the search and review require very different skills, these two closely related phases are dealt with in two chapters rather than one. The major feature of the literature *review*, and one which differentiates it from the literature *search*, is that the review consists of a critical evaluation of the literature obtained as a result of the search.

The value of acquiring the skills required to undertake a literature search and review is by no means restricted to their use in the research process. These skills are also central to the notion of professionalism in that all nurses and midwives require to be familiar with the literature in their subject area. Without skills in literature search and review it is difficult, if not impossible, to have a firm understanding of the literature.

Preparing a research proposal

Figure 6.1 places 'Preparing a research proposal' towards the beginning *and* at the end of the outline of phases of the research process; and this is done for the following reasons. The researcher uses a knowledge of the entire research process in constructing a research proposal. The proposal, when constructed, will include some detail of all phases of the research process. Finally, having constructed a research plan which is contained in the proposal, the researcher then implements that plan and thereby carries out the piece of research. It is necessary to prepare a proposal before undertaking a piece of research, but it is only after the first-time researcher has become familiar with the research process that a proposal can be prepared. Thus, first learn the theory relating to the research process, prepare a practical research proposal, then, if submision of the research proposal is suc-cessful, carry out the research.

In Chapter 10 general and specific guidelines are available to those who are undertaking a research study and have to prepare a proposal. Whatever the local regulations relating to gaining permission, failure to prepare and present the proposal to the appropriate persons and committees may cause long delays or, still worse, damage an otherwise excellent research project.

Gaining access to the research site

The research site refers to the place where research data are collected, or to the group from/about which data are to be collected. It can vary in size from a community nurse's case load or all the babies born in a maternity unit in a seven-day period, to the number of trained nursed in a sample of hospitals in a large city. In some instances the researcher will be part of the organization in which the data are to be collected, and may consequently find entry to the research site relatively easy. When the nature of the study is more complex and involved, entry into facilities which are not part of the organization in which the researcher is employed, or associated with, may be considerably more difficult. In the absence of guidelines to the means of gaining entry, this part of the process can present considerable difficulty. Surprisingly, it is a topic which receives very little attention in discussions of the research process, or in many research reports. It is intended that Chapter 11 will provide a number of suggestions which will minimize this potential difficulty.

Research design

A considerable range of research designs are available, with Chapters 12 to 22 dealing with a *selection* of those which are in relatively common use. The research design is not to be confused with the data-collection method(s) that are used in a study. The research design is used to describe the overall research approach that is to be used; the data collection method(s) describe the means by which data for a study will be collected. Thus, the data-collection method is part of the research design.

Many data-collection methods, such as interview or observation, can be used as part of a number of different research designs. For example, interviews or observation might be used as part of quantitative, qualitative, experimental, action, descriptive or evaluation research.

Decisions regarding research design precede the selection of data-collection method. First, the design is selected on the grounds that it is the most suitable to answer the research question, and the most suitable data-collection method is then selected.

Although some research designs are mutually exclusive in that they cannot occur simultaneously, others are less so. For example, experimental and descriptive designs are quite different. An experimental design will include *descriptions* of phenomena before variables are changed and/or introduced as part of the experiment. However, a descriptive research design will not include such a change to, or introduction of, variables. Another example of 'overlap' is the relationship between designs for action research and those for qualitative and quantitative research. For example, action research may include qualitative or quantitative design, or both.

Grounded theory is both a form of research design *and* a data-collection method; discussion of it is equally appropriate in this section ('Research design') *and* the following ('Data collection'). Grounded theory is presented in this section as an example of qualitative research design, although it is also a method of collecting qualitative data.

Data collection

The choice of one or more data-collection instruments, followed by actual collection of data, is a phase which offers considerable scope and choice.

Researchers have a wide range of means of collecting data available to them, and need to consider which of these are best suited to their needs. If the researcher wishes to collect respondents' opinions, an interview or questionnaire may be chosen. Alternatively, if she wishes to establish what a particular work group does, observation, or the critical incident technique may be used. The purpose of this book is not to present the entire range of data-collection techniques that are available, but to introduce six commonly used techniques in Chapters 23 to 28, and provide references to suitable publications where more may be learned about the use of each. It is important to realize that, when using an existing method of collecting data, you must judge whether or not it is exactly suitable to your needs and, if not, adapt it to meet personal requirements. Finally, bear in mind that no method of collecting data is perfect; each has its own limitations and strengths. The job of the researcher in this respect is to select or adapt a method which is as near perfect as possible, and to discuss fully the strengths and weaknesses of this chosen method.

Data handling

Having collected data, they need to be handled in a way which will enable the aims and objectives of the research to be met. The major elements of data handling are storage, analysis and presentation. Although these three topics have considerable overlap, they do require different skills and considerations.

Data storage

Having collected research data, they are stored in a manner that will allow easy access. If very small quantities of data are collected, for example ten questionnaires, then no special storage techniques may be required. However, if larger quantities of data are collected, for example 1000 questionnaires, some form of storage which will assist counting and sorting must be used.

At present, nurses, midwives and others store large amounts of data in the form of information about patient care, features of clinical practice, management and education. However, the researcher often finds difficulty in retrieving the data in order to examine some aspects of patient care or clinical activity, management or education. This difficulty relates to the means by which information is stored – on charts, graphs and in books – these being the storage techniques with which all nurses and midwives are familiar. Although increasing use is being made of non-manual means of storage (computing systems, for example), manual methods are still widely used for much information. Chapter 29 describes data-storage techniques which are commonly used by researchers and which enable easy retrieval and analysis.

Data analysis

Chapters 30 and 31 describe two approaches to quantitative analysis: the use and manipulation of numbers to respectively describe and make inferences from the data. These chapters introduce two types of data analysis: descriptive and inferential statistics. They are not designed to teach you how to understand fully the statistical techniques but to help you to understand what statistics are, what they can and cannot do, and how to further knowledge of the subject. In dealing with data analysis, the researcher, as in all phases of the research process, recognizes and takes full account of personal limitations and seeks expert assistance at an early stage.

Data can be analysed by other than statistical techniques; they can also be analysed by means of the researcher's thought processes and the subsequent use of words to describe and discuss the data – that is, by using qualitative analysis. Indeed, many important pieces of nursing research have used qualitative rather than quantitative (statistical) data analysis. Chapter 32 deals with qualitative analysis of data and demonstrates how conclusions from the data can be derived without necessarily applying either descriptive or inferential statistical techniques. However, as with other phases of the research process, the application of quantitative or qualitative data analysis techniques are not necessarily mutually exclusive. For example, in some circumstances, it may be necessary to apply quantitative techniques to qualitative data.

Data presentation

The presentation of data following its analysis, and as part of writing a research report, offers a variety of techniques from which to choose. Choice will obviously depend on the nature of the data and what one hopes to achieve with its presentation. While the use of words is a crucial part of data presentation, and one with which nurses and midwives are familiar, alternative forms of presentation can add considerably to its impact and meaning.

Reporting research

Reporting research, including the preparation of a written report, is a feature of all pieces of successfully completed research. There can be no doubt that this phase of the process presents real challenges. However, there is also no doubt that, with the help of an experienced supervisor, the beginner can develop the skills required to report research successfully.

While the structure and form of many research reports is often similar, it is not always so. There is no blueprint for all reports, the structure of each being determined by the research design used. The word 'report' in this book refers to any means used to present the research findings to others. Examples include the preparation of a research-based thesis and writing articles. Throughout this book, the need for full, continuous and complete documentation in relation to all phases of the research process is shown to be essential. Beginners frequently assume (wrongly) that report writing begins at the stage of the research process entitled 'Reporting research'. In reality, nothing could be further from the truth in that the written report will include material documented during all phases of the process. This documentation, appropriate supervision and systematic application of the phases of the research process will not, of course, guarantee success. However, it will maximize that possibility.

Ethical issues in research

Although Fig. 6.1 concludes with reference to ethical issues in research, that does not imply that the subject is of less importance than the others or that it occurs as an afterthought. Ethical issues are an integral part of all phases of the research process, as well as to the use and application of research. All phases of the research process, therefore, include a full consideration of appropriate ethical issues.

PART II

The research process

Although the phases of the research process are presented in sequential and separate chapters, it is essential to see these as being interrelated and, in some circumstances, occurring in a differing sequence. In preparing these chapters, decisions were made about what to include and exclude. Although all major steps in the process are included, not all research designs, or all possible means of collecting, storing or handling data, are discussed. However, those topics chosen for inclusion are in relatively common use in most research studies.

The four major sections of the research process are 'Preparatory work' (see Chapters 7 to 11), 'Research design' (see Chapters 12 to 22), 'Data collection' (see Chapters 23 to 28), and 'Data handling' (see Chapters 29 to 34).

In this Fourth Edition, the opportunity has been taken to revise and update all chapters, and to extend the text by including a number of additional subjects. In particular, chapters dealing with validity and reliability, single case study design, longitudinal design, and the research, education, management and practice interface have been added.

An understanding of the elements of the research process does not, in itself, equip the beginner to undertake a research study. All beginners must undertake further extensive reading, and subsequently work under the supervision of others who have appropriate research skills.

A: Preparatory work

As with all complex activity – and research is no exception – it is necessary to do a considerable amount of preparatory work prior to undertaking the main task. Time so invested will maximize the possibility of the research being of high quality. The preparatory work described in this section also includes making decisions regarding all of the topics dealt with in Chapters 12 to 35. Thus, a knowledge of the subjects dealt with in those chapters is necessary before the preparatory work can be completed and decisions can be made regarding research design, data collection, and data handling.

This preparatory stage of the research study is more time consuming than is often realized; it might use as much as one-third of a total 'time budget'.

The elements of preparatory work, although presented in sequence and separately, are closely related. 'Asking the research question', for example (see Chapter 7), is a basis for, and an integral part of, all other aspects of preparatory work, and of the research process generally.

The research question gives direction to the search and review of the literature (see Chapters 8 and 9) which in turn influence the developing research question.

Once the research question has been finalized, and the preliminary literature search and review has been undertaken, all aspects of the proposed study are encapsulated in the form of a research proposal (see Chapter 10). The proposal has a number of functions, one of which is to obtain funding, obtain permission to collect data, and gain access to the research site (see Chapter 11).

CHAPTER 7

Asking the research question

Desmond F.S. Cormack and David C. Benton

Excitement and wonder are emotions that are commonly experienced by those who undertake a piece of research. However, we have observed that these emotions are often replaced with feelings of uncertainty when the inexperienced researcher tends to ask a research question. This uncertainty can be easily rectified if a number of guiding principles are followed.

In this chapter, it is intended to identify and address those issues which often cause inexperienced researchers concern when attempting to formulate a research question. This initial stage of the research process can not only be difficult, but is crucial to the success of the remaining parts of the study.

The process of asking a research question is very rarely a once and for all event. It is highly unlikely that you will suddenly scream 'Eureka' and be satisfied with the first question that comes into your head. More often the process entails days, weeks or even months of thought and effort to refine and sharpen the question that you will eventually feel happy and confident to research. The development of the research question can best be seen as a process of systematic refinement and can be schematically represented by Fig. 7.1.

It has been our experience that attempting to ask a research question generates a large number of associated queries to which the neophyte researcher often finds difficulty in obtaining answers. Those questions most frequently expressed about asking the research question will be identified, and, by providing solutions, this chapter will assist in the process of asking your research question.

What is a research question?

This may seem a rather obvious question, but is often asked by those who are embarking upon the research process for the first time. It is perhaps important for us to make explicit at this point that we are using the term 'research question' as shorthand for 'research question/statement/topic/subject/hypothesis/problem/issue'.

A research question occurs in one of two forms: it is either an interrogative or a declarative statement. A research question in the interrogative format is a

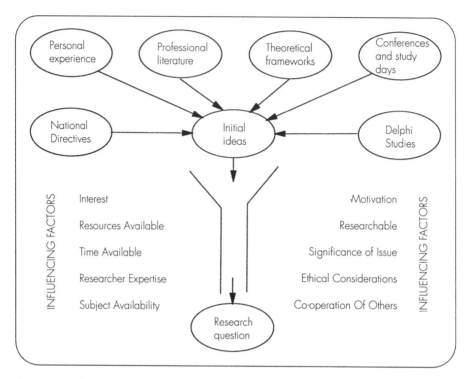

Fig. 7.1 Developments of a research question.

statement, in question form, which identifies a gap in knowledge: for example, 'What is the relationship between the provision of post-registration education and the retention of staff?' A declarative research question is a statement that defines the purpose of the study by declaring the intention to investigate a particular event, phenomenon or situation: for example, 'The purpose of this research is to investigate the relationship between the provision of post-registration education and the retention of staff.' The research question (or questions) is often translated into the aims of a study. However, the question comes first.

A 'good' research question, in the case of experimental research, is one that is short, sharp, specific and clearly states or implies a relationship between two or more variables. In the above example, the variables are post-registration courses and staff retention. The variables identified must be capable of observation and measurement. Furthermore, the phrasing of the question should be free from value judgements and bias, since it is the prime objective of any research study to investigate the problem identified from a scientific and objective stance. However, in the case of qualitative or descriptive studies, specific variables will not be identified but clarity should still be sought – for example, 'An ethnographic study of the role of newly qualified midwives'.

Do I need a research question?

Research is a scientific and logical process of investigation and requires that you follow a particular direction of enquiry. Unless you have a clearly defined research question, you will be unable to progress your study in a planned and efficient manner.

In essence, the research question identifies and describes a gap in nursing or in midwifery's knowledge base which the research study seeks to fill. It helps to focus thoughts and efforts, assisting in developing a framework which will guide you through the entire research process. You cannot undertake a research study without identifying a research question.

Most research studies will have one specific, or primary, research question but some may have a number of secondary or subsidiary questions. Secondary questions must relate to the primary question. For example, the primary research question, 'What is the relationship between the provision of post-registration education and the retention of staff?' may have the following secondary questions:

- Which post-registration courses are available?
- Who provides the funding for post-registration courses?

How do I find a research question?

Inexperienced researchers often find difficulty in identifying the research question. Nevertheless, you will find that no sooner have you thought of one topic to investigate and another will come to mind. This experience is often confusing, since with so many valuable topics to investigate, how can you decide which is the most important? In addition, you may be unfamiliar with the existing literature – a fact that often compounds uncertainty and confusion. If this is not bad enough, lack of familiarity with the research process may also cause additional perplexity. However, do not let all the initial uncertainty put you off. If you are interested and motivated towards conducting research, you will identify, in time, a specific topic which you will find suitable for investigation. To assist you in identifying a research question, you may wish to consider a number of sources which will help to identify a gap in the existing knowledge base.

Your own experience

Turn to your own experience. How often have you questioned, either in your mind or with your colleagues, a situation, treatment or outcome, wondering what has happened, why it should be that way or how you can improve it? In seeking to identify a research question various sources can be consulted or used to stimulate ideas (see Fig. 7.2).

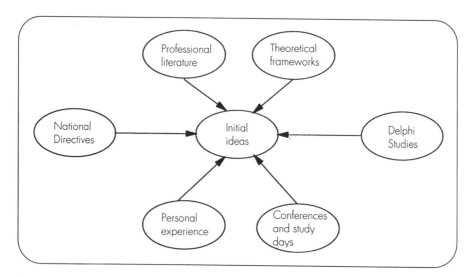

Fig. 7.2 Getting ideas for a research question.

Professional literature

Professional literature often triggers further research. You may note the findings of a study and consider whether such an approach can be applied in your own area of practice or to the particular client group you work with. The deliberate use of methodology already reported, but used in a different setting and with another subject group, is termed replication. Such an approach is extremely valuable since far too few nursing studies have been conducted with more than one client group or in different locations. It is perhaps appropriate to note at this point that the research question does not have to be novel to be worth while. However, if you choose to repeat a study that has already been carried out, it is important that you examine the previous study carefully and avoid any methodological or conceptual flaws.

Alternatively, if you read a number of research reports about a topic, you may notice inconsistencies in findings which can stimulate further research. You may wonder why the results obtained with one group, or at one location, or using a particular method, are different from those reported elsewhere.

Yet another means by which research questions can be derived from literature is when a gap in the existing knowledge base is observed. For example, as new problems arise or new illnesses are discovered nurses and midwives may enjoin the analysis of how the problem might best be addressed.

Theoretical frameworks

In the past 40 years, a number of theoretical frameworks have been proposed: Peplau's (1952) interpersonal relations model, Roy's (1980) adaption model and

Rogers' (1970) unitary man model, to name but three. Each of these models can be used as the basis for the development of a research question. The model can be tested to determine whether it can predict the outcome of treatment. To date, few studies have been developed to test the available theoretical models and, as yet, most remain inadequately validated.

Conferences and study days

When you attend a conference or a study day it is often the discussion that occurs during coffee and meal breaks that proves to be the most valuable element of the day. Such interactions can result in the discovery of a wide variety of means of treating a particular client, often prompting thoughts which can be developed into a research question.

National directives and Delphi studies

From time to time the Government or a national body will identify specific topics which they feel require investigation. Such topics are usually of major national concern and have significant implications for the health of the nation.

Another means of identifying topics of concern to a large number of individuals is the use of a Delphi survey. A Delphi survey is a technique where subjects are asked to respond to a series of questionnaires. The first questionnaire usually attempts to elicit views on a specific topic. Subsequent questionnaires feed back the original comments made by the subjects who are then asked to rank their statements in order of importance. This approach may yield a number of topics that can then form the basis for further investigation.

How can I decide which question to study?

Often you will have a number of ideas which you may wish to investigate. The tentative questions identified may be related, or may be on completely different subject areas. The problem is how to decide which one of a number of topics to investigate first. There are a number of guiding principles to assist you in making your choice.

Interest and motivation

The research process can simultaneously be exciting, stimulating, arduous and depressing. When things are going well, nothing seems to be too much of a problem, but there are those times when you will confront difficulties. Unless the research question focuses on a problem about which you feel strongly, it is likely that during difficult times you will be unable to sustain enthusiasm for the study.

Any research questions considered for investigation must therefore be of sufficient interest to keep you motivated through the 'bad' as well as the 'good' times.

A researchable question

Not all questions are amenable to investigation. Any question which poses a philosophical or ethical question is not directly answerable by research. For example, 'Is it ethical for foetal tissue be used for cerebral implantation?' poses an ethical question, and although it is possible to debate this issue, no amount of research will give you an answer. The question is not researchable.

It is often possible to change the focus of the question which addresses an ethical or philosophical dilemma to one that is researchable: 'Does the implantation of foetal tissue alleviate symptoms of Parkinson's Disease?', for example. Although it is possible to answer this question by research, it does not address the original ethical question; it may, however, provide evidence which will influence your viewpoint on the issue.

Problem significance

Any problems selected should be of significance to the client group you care for and/or to the knowledge base of nursing or midwifery. The significance of a problem can best be judged by assessing the question's worth in terms of a number of criteria. First, does the question address a problem which affects large numbers of patients? Second, will the outcome of the research significantly improve the quality of life of individuals or groups? Third, does the question address a nursing or midwifery problem? Finally, will the results be suitable for use in a (non-research) practice environment?

Feasibility

Many potentially interesting and researchable questions have to be discarded because they are not feasible. If you are to assess the feasibility of a research question, you must consider a number of issues. These would include time available, resources available, researcher expertise, ethical considerations, subject availability, and co-operation of others.

Time available

If you are undertaking a piece of research for the first time, it is likely that you will have difficulty in trying to assess how much work is involved and how long it will take. You can, however, make a more accurate assessment of the feasibility of undertaking a particular study by drawing up a detailed timetable. It is also important to note that, for certain elements of a study, you will be able to arrange a schedule to suit your own pace, but alas some will be determined by those individuals or agencies providing support and information. A good starting point for attempting to assess the length of time the study will take is to use a framework for phases in the research process (see Chapter 6). Each phase in the process can be broken down into as much detail as possible, then time allocated appropriately. The total length of time required can then be calculated and an appropriate decision taken – that is, proceed with the study, or try to negotiate time from your employer, or redefine the study in such a way as to 'effect' the time available, or reject the study as being unfeasible. Remember, if you have a detailed breakdown of time required, you are in a stronger position to argue for the appropriate study time.

If you are aware of anyone who has conducted some research, seek her advice. Valuable information about how long literature searches will take and more importantly how long it will take to locate and access literature, can be obtained from librarians.

If approval from an ethics committee is required, studies may often be delayed for considerable periods of time. It is not uncommon for such a committee to meet on a bi-monthly or even quarterly basis. If delays are to be avoided, it is important that you make contact with the committee at an early stage.

Resources available

Closely associated with the requirements for sufficient time, is the need for appropriate and adequate resources. The resource requirements for any study can vary considerably. A study undertaken as part of a course may need only nominal resources, whereas some research will require vast quantities of both material and money.

When attempting to assess feasibility, it is important to identify clearly all the resources you will require to enable you to complete the study. Obviously the design of your study will influence the amount of resources required. By starting with a detailed timetable, you are less likely to omit items. Always consider literature search charges, photocopying, telephone, postage, computer access, and any specialized equipment, travel costs, office space (often a premium), document typing and report production. The more detailed the list you can produce, the better prepared you are to assess the feasibility of the study.

Researcher expertise

It is important that you examine closely the level of expertise required to undertake and successfully complete the study you have identified. Unless such an assessment is undertaken, it is likely that you will end up attempting a study which you are unqualified to carry out. A timetable of events can be particularly useful. If there are a few elements about which you have little or even no knowledge, you can seek assistance and support at an early stage. With appropriate advice and supervision, what would have been unfeasible can become possible.

Ethical consideration

When assessing the feasibility of a particular study, you should always consider the ethics of undertaking the research. Research should cause no harm or distress and it is important that any proposals should be reviewed by an unbiased individual or a group. If patients are involved, or if your research involves any invasive procedure, it is normal practice to seek the approval of the District's or Health Board's ethics committee. Research that does not have the potential to advance our knowledge should not take place. Similarly, any piece of work that does not offer subject's confidentiality and anonymity, should on most occasions be considered inappropriate. Only if a study can be shown to be ethically acceptable should it be considered feasible (see Chapter 5).

Subject availability

If you intend to investigate a very rare phenomenon, it is likely that either you will be unable to recruit enough subjects to your study, or you will have to travel considerable distances to do so. Consequently, it is important to identify and assess the availability of subjects, for without subjects you have no study. Furthermore, it is important to recognize that potential subjects may not be as enthusiastic about the research study as you are. It is likely that some may refuse to participate and this is a point well worth consideration.

Co-operation of others

When you plan a study, identify those individuals and groups who will come in contact with your work. It is always worth investing time, at an early stage, gaining their support. Any individuals who will be directly involved should be contacted personally and given the opportunity to discuss issues of concern. Only after obtaining the co-operation of all those involved in the study should it be undertaken. More specific information on the closely associated issues of gaining access to research sites is provided in Chapter 11.

How can the research question best be described?

Research questions, despite being short, clear and specific, will still require to be explained in some detail to those who read the final report. In addition to being implicit in the title of the study, an explanation of the rationale for undertaking the study should appear very early in any publication. The fact that a gap exists in the knowledge base, and that the research question has relevance to nursing or midwifery, should be clearly established and stated.

A common difficulty experienced by novice and expert researchers alike is the imprecise nature of language. Words often have more than one meaning and, hence, if your research question is to be described in absolute terms there is a need to offer precise definitions of any words, terms, or procedures central to your research. The normal definition which is given in the dictionary is frequently inadequate. It is therefore necessary to state the operational definition of terms, that is, the definition given to words by the researcher – that is, by you. For example, a dictionary might define a patient as 'a person who is receiving medical care', whereas you may choose to operationally define the term patients as 'any male, who is hospitalized in a surgical ward, who has undergone surgery in the previous 24 hours, and who is aged between 16 and 65 years'.

Does the research question influence the research process?

It should be evident that the research question has total influence on all aspects of the research process. Having asked the research question, all others aspects of the study are designed to answer it. For example, the question determines the scope and content of the literature review. A methodological approach will be selected that is capable of answering the question. All collected data will be destined for analysis and this will provide results. The results will present an answer to the question which, when compared and contrasted with previous research, will determine any recommendations. The research question is the thread which unifies the entire study.

Relating the research question to the research process

It is common for inexperienced researchers to have difficulty in defining the exact relationship between the research question and other components of the study.

How do the title of the study and the research question relate?

The research question should be formulated first and subsequently the title of the study should be derived from it. Often there is little difference between the two. A suitable and appropriate title for the research question posed earlier might be:

'A study of the relationship between the provision of post-registration education and the retention of staff.'

Is the aim of the study the same as the research question?

Although they are not identical in expression, they are identical in meaning. Some researchers decide to pose a number of questions which the research seeks to answer. Others convert the question to a series of aims which, when achieved, provide a solution to the research question. In the example used in this chapter, the question may generate the following aim:

'To describe the relationship between the provision of post-registration education and the retention of staff.'

Is the research question the same as a hypothesis?

Despite the fact that a hypothesis can be derived from a research question, if that question seeks to establish whether or not there is a relationship between two or more variables, the research question and the hypothesis are not the same. The hypothesis for the study suggested above might state:

'The retension of staff is increased by the provision of post-registration education.'

It is not always possible to derive a hypothesis for a research question. The hypothesis can only be stated for those studies suitable for investigation at the outset by quantitative methods, and which predict a relationship between two variables. For example, if the research question had asked, 'Which factors influence staff's decision to remain with a Health Authority for more than five years?', then a hypothesis could not be formulated until the factors had been identified.

How does a research question relate to literature review?

It has been suggested that the research literature itself may stimulate the formulation of a research question. Irrespective of whether the question was, or was not, stimulated by a publication, the literature review should cover two main domains which support the question's formulation. First, the question should be derived from a specific theoretical perspective so as to ensure that any findings can be appropriately integrated into the knowledge base. Second, the literature review should identify any previous research carried out and provide an objective critique of the work. It is common for the literature review to move from a general description of the topic to a more focused evaluation. The move from the general to the specific is a means of identifying surrounding issues in order to place the research question in context.

The literature review should be considered fundamental to the development of any research question. The literature presented to the reader should cogently argue that there is a need for the study to take place and that the findings will have potential significance to nursing or midwifery, or those cared for.

Can the original research question be changed?

Having conducted preliminary work, it is not uncommon for the research question to be modified or even abandoned completely. If it is to be modified, this is done prior to the specific literature review. The research question cannot be changed or modified at a subsequent stage. If this is done, the research process must be restarted.

A change or modification may take place following a pilot study if the pilot study indicates that such a change is necessary. In that case, the pilot study is repeated until the research question is found to be appropriate. Furthermore, it is not uncommon for researchers to be tempted to add secondary questions at the pilot study stage. However, this temptation should be avoided if possible. Any addition will result in extra work and may require further resources which may not be available. If the research question is to be modified or secondary questions added, a full assessment of the implications of such a change must to be made.

Conclusions

The process of asking the research question is, in part, simply the logical application of a number of guidelines. However, those questions which identify a significant issue are often the result of inspired curiosity. All professional nurses and midwives who take a critical and questioning view of clinical practice, management and education have the ability to identify such issues and generate a research question. This chapter has summarized the common sources of research ideas and considered the process by which those initial ideas are moulded into a final research question by the influence of various factors. Asking the research question is central to the entire research process. Once you have identified a research question, you are well on the way to completing the study. It is now up to you to decide whether you wish to pursue the opportunity.

References

Peplau, H. (1952) *Interpersonal Relations in Nursing*. New York: Putman.

Rogers, M.E. (1970) *An Introduction to the Theoretical Basis of Nursing*. Philadelphia: F.A. Davis Company.

Roy, C. (1980) The Roy adaption model. In J.P. Riehl & C. Roy (eds), *Conceptual Models for Nursing Practice*, 2nd edn. New York: Appleton Century Crofts.

Further reading

Belman, L. (1997) R&D priorities. *Nursing Times* **93**: 19, 39.

Benner, J. (1997) Researching health care topics on the Internet. *Nursing* **27** (9): 28–9.

Weekes, D.P. (1992) Developing a research question: where to start? *Journal of Pediatric Oncological Nursing* **9** (4): 187–91.

Wootton, J.C. (1997) Directory of databases for research into alternative and complementary medicine. *Journal of Alternative and Complementary Medicine* **3** (2): 179–90.

Wootton, J.C. (1997) Directory of databases for research into alternative and complementary medicine: an update. *Journal of Alternative and Complementary Medicine* **3** (4): 401–3.

CHAPTER 8

Searching the literature

David C. Benton and Desmond F.S. Cormack

The ability to conduct a literature search is essential to any type of research. Indeed, it has been argued that the skills associated with literature searching should be considered a fundamental skill requirement of all professional nurses. Whether from a research or a professional perspective, the ability to conduct a literature search is essential if nurses are to question their practice, management or education in a structured and meaningful way.

Without reference to the past, we are unable to learn from mistakes. The techniques discussed in this chapter help to empower the reader with skills that enable the discovery, location, and unlocking of the wealth of material which constitutes our profession's knowledge base.

The research literature

Every day we come into contact with a wide variety of research literature, the volume of which seems to be constantly increasing. By research literature we mean any form of information, either paper or electronic, that relates to nursing research, irrespective of source, format or quality. Chapter 9 deals with how to review and evaluate the quality of literature.

Research literature can originate from many sources such as individuals, groups, academic institutions, professional organizations, voluntary departments or manufacturers and suppliers of products. Clearly, the volume of material available is unmanageable unless you are selective in the material you consult. Depending on the research topic, certain types of literature may be of greater value than others to the enquiring nurse. Research literature can come in many forms, each of which has particular characteristics which, if known, can assist you in deciding the likely value of the material prior to obtaining access. Figure 8.1, for example, lists common formats used to convey information to the nursing profession.

Journals

Journals are frequently used by researchers who wish to obtain information on a specific topic. However, not all journals publish original research. Journals such

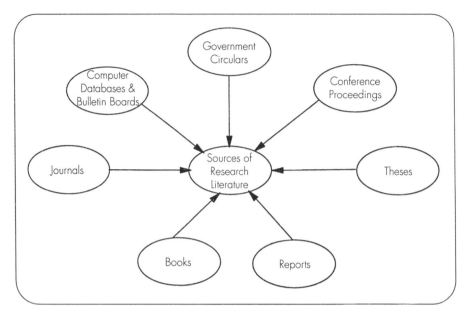

Fig. 8.1 Sources of literature used in conveying research information.

as the *Journal of Advanced Nursing, Nursing Research* and the *Western Journal of Nursing Research*, which publish original material, are termed primary journals. Invariably, papers published by these journals are refereed – that is, all papers are examined by an independent external expert prior to publication – which tends to ensure that only papers of the highest quality are published.

Secondary journals form another valuable source of information and although they do not usually publish original papers they do serve an important function. Articles published in secondary journals could be described as a means of providing a 'taster' of the full paper and often consist of a brief synopsis of research published in a primary journal. These articles are usually written in less technical terms in order to appeal to a wider audience; hence, secondary journals are an ideal means of ensuring that a piece of work is disseminated more widely than would be possible otherwise.

There are a number of specific types of secondary journal. First, there is the limited circulation journals which are distributed free to members of an organization or specialist interest. *Reflections* is an example of a limited circulation journal which is distributed to all Sigma Theta Tau members – an international nursing honour society. It contains brief, often opinion-based, articles specific to Sigma Theta Tau members or gives snippets of information about work specific members are undertaking. Second, there are review journals, which provide information on preselected topics. Articles are frequently written by subject experts who, in the course of the article, will debate the findings of a particular piece of research. *Advances in Nursing Science* is an example of such a journal.

Third, there are professional journals, for example *Health Visitor*, which are aimed to cater for the needs of the practitioner as opposed to the academic sector. This type of secondary journal will often focus on the aspects of utilization of research rather than on pure findings.

Although we have drawn a clear division between primary and secondary journals, the reality is somewhat different. Secondary journals, for instance, will often publish original work – something that can confuse informed researchers and mislead them into discounting an article prematurely simply as a result of its apparently poor 'pedigree'.

Books

Books are a major source of information for researchers. Unlike journal articles, which are limited by space, material published in book form usually has the opportunity to develop arguments in more detail, provide a more extensive literature review, and generally provide a more substantive treatment of the subject. However, books take longer to get into print and although the main objective is to provide information they are also published to make money for a publishing company, two factors which may detract from their academic value.

Another point to consider is whether a book has single or multiple authors, for this can sometimes lead to variations in the quality of individual chapters and problems with the flow and development of arguments. It is fair to say, however, that this should be the exception rather than the rule, if the book has been checked by an experienced editor.

Reports

Many research studies are published in report form and unfortunately, as a consequence, only reach a limited audience. Authors can take steps to avoid this by submitting their work to abstracting services such as *Nursing Research Abstracts*. Some health authorities also endeavour to increase the availability of reports produced by encouraging authors to submit copies of their work to a local collection. Despite such undertakings, reports are notoriously difficult to obtain, can be of extremely variable quality and come in all manners of shapes and format. Nevertheless it is often useful to obtain original reports as opposed to journal articles since the report will often give fine details which, by necessity of space limitation, are frequently omitted from the published work. It is common to find included within the appendices of reports, copies of data-collection instruments, or other such valuable materials.

Theses

Theses, sometimes referred to as dissertations, are usually the product of higher academic study. Accordingly they can be a veritable goldmine of information since they include in-depth literature reviews, detailed methods sections, as well as findings and learned debate. Usually no more than three or four copies of theses are produced and this can cause difficulties for those who wish to read them. However, most universities send copies of all doctoral and master of philosophy theses to the British Lending Library where they are microfilmed and can then be made available on request. In addition, those nurses who live within travelling distance of London can consult the Steinberg collection at the RCN library. This collection contains copies of a large number of theses and dissertations, either written by nurses or of interest to the nursing profession.

Conference proceedings

It is not always possible to attend a conference in person, and although we would argue that there is no real substitute for being there and getting involved in the debate, conference proceedings can provide a valuable source of information. Papers appearing in conference proceedings usually consist of the latest, most up-to-date, state-of-the-art material. Papers are often rewritten in light of comments made by the audience and are then submitted for publication in primary journals. Conference proceedings can thus provide researchers with access to materials at an early stage. Although for the more prestigious conference proceedings, papers often go through a rigorous review procedure, this is not always the case, and material gleaned from such sources can occasionally be of variable quality.

Government circulars

The Department of Health issues a wide variety of documents each year, many of which can be of interest to the nurse researcher. However, the distribution and access to these documents is often limited in the first instance to senior officers of a health authority. Researchers who think that the Department of Health may have published material on a specific topic can peruse the current edition of *The Hospital and Health Services Year Book* (Institute of Health Service Management, 1998) which, among other things, lists all current Government circulars.

Computer databases and electronic bulletin boards

With the advent of relatively inexpensive computer equipment, increasing amounts of information are being held on computer databases. You can often obtain the most up-to-date information from this type of source. Unfortunately use of these systems is often expensive – you require the correct equipment and you usually have to use a telephone line – and the organization running the service can charge quite high fees for the privilege of access. Another disadvantage of these systems is that the amount of information stored on any one item is often limited to essential details and a brief abstract. A relatively recent development is the electronic bulletin board which enables researchers or anyone with the right equipment to 'post' material to an electronic board which can then be read by others. Researchers from across the world can therefore exchange or stimulate ideas with like-minded colleagues who have the correct computer equipment.

Choosing a library

Irrespective of your topic of interest, it is highly unlikely that you will have all the literature you require immediately to hand. For most of us, it is necessary to use a library as the main source of our research literature, whether it be in journal, book or any of the formats previously discussed.

Not all libraries are the same and some offer far more in the way of services than others, and the researcher should make a point of exploring all local libraries to discover their strengths and weaknesses. Some will allow access to all their facilities but some, such as those attached to universities and colleges, may restrict users who are neither students nor staff of the institution to reading rights only. There are a number of features which are particularly useful and will make the task of literature searching far easier. Many of these will depend on the size of the library.

First, if the library is large, it may have subject specialist librarians who will be able to greatly assist you in a search for material. Conversely, in smaller specialist libraries, such as those attached to colleges of nursing or health studies institutions, it is usual for the librarian to have extensive knowledge of health care literature. If you are to make the most efficient use of your time, endeavour to contact the librarian at the onset of the search and engage that person's assistance. Librarians are specialist in literature storage and its retrieval; seek their advice and save time.

Second, it is important to familiarize yourself with the cataloguing system of the library. Unless you know how materials are catalogued, you will be unable to retrieve them. Again, seek the assistance of the librarian and read any guides that may be available. Most libraries publish a short guide that will show the layout of the stock and tell how it is catalogued. Recently, some libraries have started to employ the use of personal stereos for this purpose and these can be hired or borrowed. These walk you round through a guided tour of the layout and give instructions on how to find material.

There are a number of methods of cataloguing materials, but the two most commonly used for health care literature are the *Dewey Decimal Classification Scheme* and the *National Library of Medicine Classification Scheme*. The Dewey Decimal Classification Scheme uses a series of numeric digits to break down subjects from the general to the specific. The National Library of Medicine Classification Scheme uses a combination of letters and numbers. Although manual card index systems are still quite common, larger libraries are now tending to install computer systems for cataloguing their material. Whichever approach is being used, become familiar with the system so as to maximize the chances of finding the material you wish to find when conducting a literature search.

Third, some libraries offer a more comprehensive range of textbooks and journals than others. If a library is to be of value, then a wide variety of stock that covers both major and minor nursing specialities is required. Textbooks should be up to date, but, perhaps more important for a researcher, the journal holdings should be extensive and ideally should have had subscribers for as long a period as possible. Back issues of journals are a valuable source of literature, and since nursing research often addresses diverse health care themes, access to nursing, medical, general sciences, social sciences, education and professional journals allied to medicine, is desirable.

Fourth, a range of reference texts, including indices, research abstracts and bibliographies, is essential. These may be available in a variety of forms; for example, they may exist as books, or they may be accessible by means of on-line or compact disk-based computer systems.

Fifth, even the most comprehensive library will not stock everything that its subscribers could possibly want. Accordingly, access to an inter-library loan service is very important for a researcher who is attempting to achieve an in-depth coverage of a topic. Inter-library loan requests can be expensive, but a good library will often offer a subsidized (or even free) service which is prompt to respond to reasonable requests.

Sixth, most researchers will require access to photocopying facilities which are reasonably priced. However, it is essential that copyright laws are not infringed; these limit the use that can be made of copies and the amount of material that can be reproduced from any one book or journal.

Seventh, microfiche or microfilm readers can be useful, particularly if you require access to theses. In addition, some libraries stock microfilm of back issues of their journals to save space; if this is the case, some means of obtaining a printed copy of an individual article should be available.

Finally, some libraries will have a special reference collection which can be of great assistance to a researcher. The Royal College of Nursing, for example, holds the Steinberg collection which includes copies of many master and doctoral theses relating to nursing and conducted both in the United Kingdom and overseas. Appendix 8.1 at the end of this chapter gives details of material available from the Royal College of Nursing and other national libraries.

How to search the literature

Anyone who has attempted to look for literature related to a particular subject, quickly discovers that there is usually a wealth of material available. Of course, not all literature provides exactly what you require, hence it is necessary, systematically, to identify only those items which relate directly to the subject under study. A literature search can be defined as the process of systematically identifying published materials which meet set predetermined criteria. For example, the subject of the search might be: 'Worldwide literature, published between 1990 and 2000, relating to the role of the community psychiatric nurse treating patients with medical diagnosis of paranoid schizophrenia.' Literature searching, which is a critical component of any research study, can be conducted either manually or with the aid of computer technology.

You will often need to consult the literature at various stages of the research process. First, it will assist in the definition of the topic to be studied. Second, it will provide substantive material for both the theoretical and methodological frameworks. Third, it will enable you to contrast findings with previously reported studies. The ability to search the literature efficiently and accurately is clearly central to the development, conduct and completion of any research study. Without a specific strategy, a literature search will not only prove time-consuming, but will also yield an incomplete coverage of the topic. Try to have a rough idea of an area of interest before you walk into a library. If you simply browse along the shelves you may or may not, depending on the size of the library, find some material on your topic of interest. Such an approach is clearly unacceptable for it will waste valuable time and is no way of ensuring that all the material available on the subject will be found. Although serendipity is a wonderful and even joyous experience, it is neither scientific nor time-efficient and for these reasons make use of tools such as the subject index, the author catalogue, classification catalogue, indexes, abstracts and bibliographies.

Subject index, author and classification catalogues

All libraries will have author and classification catalogues as well as a subject index of their book stock to enable material of interest to be found. Author catalogues are simply a listing of all stock organized in alphabetical order by author. Joint authors, series entries as well as the chairpersons of Government committees, are usually included. Classification catalogues list all stock as they appear on the shelves in the library. The order of the stock is determined by the particular classification system in use. By examining the classification catalogue you can identify all books on a particular subject stocked by the library, irrespective of whether they are out on loan. The subject index, for those who are not fully conversant with the classification system, can be considered as a key to enable access to the library's book stock. All major (and minor) subjects are listed along with the corresponding classification code thus enabling researchers to go to the appropriate part of the classification catalogue and identify the material held. For libraries that still use manual systems, the index and catalogues often consist of a series of card indexes. If, however, a computerized system is in use, material is stored in a relational database. The term 'relational', although a computer jargon term, effectively emphasizes the fact that although the material in the catalogues and index are separate, they are closely related.

Both journal holdings and audio-visual material are usually catalogued and indexed separately from book stock. Audio-visual catalogues are usually indexed in the same manner as books. However, access to journal articles is usually obtained, in the first instance, by indexes, abstract and bibliographies.

Indexes, abstracts and bibliographies

The stock held by any one library will be limited by a number of factors such as the needs of the population the library serves, the means by which and by whom new stock is added to the collection, the budget and the physical space available. The examination of stock held locally on any one topic will, on most occasions, result in the identification of only a small part of the literature available on the topic. What is required is some means of knowing what material is available, not just locally but nationally and internationally if a complete and detailed literature search is required. Examination of indexing, abstracting and bibliographic tools can all be used to achieve far greater coverage of the topic.

Indexes

Indexes are used to list all material published in a specified list of journals. The material is indexed by subject heading(s) and by author(s). Indexes are generally produced monthly, bimonthly or quarterly and cumulated annually. There is a wide selection of indexes available, but not all extensively cover nursing journals. For example, *Index Medicus*, although listing well over 3000 journals, includes only 25 nursing titles, whereas the *Cumulative Index to Nursing and Allied Health Literature* covers just over 300, the predominant number of which are nursing and allied health periodicals. The *International Nursing Index* and, despite its name *Nursing Bibliography*, are two further examples of indexes commonly available in this country. The choice of index or indexes that should be consulted to achieve optimum coverage of the literature available will be dependent on the specific topic. There is a degree of duplication between the various indexes, hence, if time is at a premium, and it usually is, go to the librarian for advice as to which indexes are likely to be the most appropriate.

The amount of detail given in an index about a particular article is limited to that likely to be found in any reference, that is:

- name of author(s) [but not always all of them]
- year of publication
- title of article
- name of journal

- volume and part numbers
- page numbers of article.

The drawbacks of such a brief description are obvious, and what sounds like a valuable reference often turns out to be of only peripheral or no value.

Abstracts

The major drawback with indexes is that no detailed information about the content of an article is given. Only by retrieving the article, sometimes by means of an inter-library loan, can you be sure of the content. Abstracting journals, however, circumvent this problem since, in addition to all the general reference data, a short abstract is also given which gives a succinct synopsis of the article. The quality of the abstract given can, however, vary considerably from a simple outline to a detailed summary of the entire study, giving all the major points.

As with indexes, there are a wide selection of abstracting journals available, all of which have different criteria for material inclusion. Perhaps the best-known abstracting journal in the United Kingdom to deal with nursing research is *Nursing Research Abstracts*; valuable material, however, can often be obtained from those sources that have a wider coverage. These include *Hospital Abstracts, Health Service Abstracts, Social Service Abstracts* and *Excerpta Medica.*

Bibliographies

Bibliographies can be a useful starting point for any researcher. They are, essentially, a reference list of books, periodical articles and reports on some particular subject. A number of national libraries, professional organizations, and many of the libraries in colleges of nursing produce such bibliographies. For example, the Royal College of Nursing has published a bibliography of nursing literature in two series, and the Scottish Health Service Centre library regularly publishes specialist bibliographies. Furthermore, the Royal College of Midwives, the Health Visitors Association and, in addition, many colleges of nursing, produce a 'current awareness service'. This is a particular type of bibliography that regularly covers a (usually preset) number of topics listing all the articles, reports or newly published books on the topic since the publication of the previous current awareness bulletin.

Manual or computerized searching

Until the advent of relatively inexpensive compact personal computers, most libraries had only manual systems for accessing literature. Researchers would have to thumb through card after card of the subject index, classification, or author catalogues, until they found the material they sought. This could take considerable time and effort, particularly since there is no way of knowing from a card system whether a book is available or out on loan.

Modern computer-controlled library stock management systems hold their information on a database. A database can be thought of as a form of electronic card index system which is extremely efficient and flexible in the manner in which information can be stored and retrieved. Not only will a database hold all the usual information about a book, it will also record whether the book is in stock, out on loan, or reserved for a subscriber. Users of such systems can, by the use of a limited number of commands, search the library catalogue for books on a subject or subjects, ascertain whether they are in stock, print a list of the books on the topics and request that those out on loan be reserved on their return to the library, all without leaving the computer terminal.

Similarly, indexes, abstracts and bibliographies are now available via computer systems. Until recently, the only way to access the databases containing this information was via the telephone line (on-line searching). Databases were located some distance from the library and were maintained by commercial companies (hosts). Although a number of databases are maintained in the United Kingdom, the most popular and largest host organizations are located in Europe and the USA. However, the introduction of compact disk read-only memory (CD-ROM) technology, has meant that the entire database for major indexes such as Medline or CINHAL can be stored on a single 4.5 inch compact disk.

The storage capacity of a compact disk is truly phenomenal since the equivalent information contained in the books on 20 feet of library shelves or the entire twelve volumes of the original Oxford English Dictionary can be held on one single-sided disk.

Both on-line and CD-ROM systems are more expensive than their manual counterparts. Libraries have to pay a subscription to use the database as well as possess the appropriate computer equipment and, in the case of an on-line system, have to pay telephone line rental and connect charges in addition to a payment for all data accessed. These additional costs have resulted in most libraries not allowing individuals to use on-line systems themselves. Instead, you explain the search that is required to the librarian who then conducts the search on your behalf. Databases held on CD-ROM are, however, usually accessible to the researcher since there is no telephone, connect or access charge. On-line databases are nevertheless more up to date (by a month or two) than either the CD-ROM or manual base systems and if this is an important consideration then the additional cost may be justified.

On-line and CD-ROM searching has a number of distinct advantages over manual systems. Specifically, they can save you a tremendous amount of time, are far more flexible in the manner in which literature can be retrieved and can produce printed lists of references on request. Conversely, there are a few minor disadvantages: for example, cost and the fact that users do require a minimal degree of computer literacy; keyboard skills; and the knowledge of the commands, are also required.

Conducting a search

Conducting a literature search, if given detailed thought, is relatively straightforward. The process should be systematic and unhurried if optimum results are to be obtained.

The first step in the process is to think around the research topic. Authors may use different terms for your topic of interest. If you are to retrieve material successfully, time is needed to consider all key words and their synonyms or associated terms that can be used to describe the topic to be researched. To achieve this, a number of approaches can be used. For example, it is often helpful to 'brainstorm' your thoughts and commit them to paper; all thoughts should be noted and none dismissed prematurely. Having done this, consult a good thesaurus and write down all synonyms. Now try to group them together and form logical links between the topics.

Next, decide whether to conduct a manual or a computer search. If a computer system is available, then a considerable amount of time can be saved; a computer will also allow you to use search strategies based upon what are known as logical operators. The two most common logical operators are 'AND' and 'OR'. By use of 'AND' and 'OR' you can search for a combination of key words simultaneously. For example, if you were interested in finding material on the treatment of alcohol abuse, a search using the word treatment would yield many references as would a search using alcohol abuse. However, by stipulating that you are requiring material that refers to both treatment AND alcohol abuse, you could obtain a smaller but more specific result. Use of the logical operator 'OR' will yield a result that includes all those references that include either treatment OR alcohol abuse (or both).

Irrespective of whether a computer or manual search is to be conducted, great care should be taken on deciding which catalogues, indexes, abstracting journals and bibliographies should be consulted. An appropriate choice may result in fewer references being found.

Throughout the literature search, the help and assistance of a subject specialist librarian, or an experienced researcher, can be invaluable as both can often help to focus thinking, offer advice, and assist in the selection of appropriate sources. Having selected the sources, it is then necessary to examine the subject and key word headings – those used by the index, for example – to enable you to finalize the search strategy. Computer systems will allow entries to be searched word on word, and often this rules out references that are inappropriate to the research topic. The use of key word fields will increase the number of usable references. Bear in mind that the more specifically defined and exacting your search criteria, the fewer references you will retrieve. Figure 8.2 illustrates how a seemingly unmanageable number of references and research can be searched to produce a useful bibliography. The search was conducted using a CD-ROM based product, a version of the ERIC (Education Resources Information Centre) database. As currently seen, the commands issued (in block capitals) are easy to use and simple to recall.

Command	References found
FIND Research	101 222
FIND Utilization	4 839
FIND Nursing	1 661
FIND Research AND Utilization AND Nursing	41

Fig. 8.2   Sample dialogue of CD-ROM literature search.

The complete list of 41 references, including abstracts, can be reviewed on screen before deciding whether to widen or restrict the search further and to print the entire list, or only a selected portion, for future use.

Literature searching is a simple process, but it does take time. Even when computer technology is used it is not always possible to be absolutely sure of a reference being exactly what is required, and only once an article is read can you be sure of its value and significance to the study. The process of accessing articles is invariably the most time consuming. Often articles are not available locally and it is necessary to request them on inter-library loan. The process of requesting an inter-library loan for material can add considerably to the time required to conduct the literature search. However, when the literature search and retrieval are complete, it is then necessary to read and critically appraise the articles obtained. These and subsequent steps, such as the coherent synthesis of material, are dealt with in the following chapter (Chapter 9).

References

Institute of Health Services Management (1998) *The Hospital and Health Services Year Book 1998* (ed. by N.W. Chaplin). London: The Institute of Health Services Management.

Further reading

Hunt, D.L. *et al.* (1998) Searching the medical literature for the best evidence to solve clinical questions. *Annals of Oncology* 9 (4): 377–83.

Rowlands, J. *et al.* (1995) ABC of medical computing. Online searching. *British Medical Journal* 311 (7003): 500–4

Wilkinson, J. *et al.* (1995) How to conduct a literature review. *Nursing Standard* 10 (9): 28–30.

Appendix 8.1: List of national libraries

Department of Health
Wellington House
135–155 Waterloo Road
London SE1 8UG
Tel. 0171-972-2000
Ext. 24204

Open to all NHS employees but
appointment is required. Holds an
extensive international collection of
material relating to health services.
Photocopying available.

Health Education Authority
Hamilton House
Mabledon Place
London WC1H 9TX
Tel. 0171-383-3833

Open to the public. Wide selection of
photocopying and selective literature
searching service available.

King's Fund Centre
Library
11–13 Cavendish Square
London W1M 0AN
Tel. 0171-307-2400

Open to the public without appointment.
Extensive collection of material on health
care, equipment and practice.
Photocopying and literature search service.

Northern Ireland Health & Social Services
Library
Queen's University
Institute of Clinical Sciences
Grosvenor Road
Belfast BT12 6BJ
Tel. 0123-232-2043

Open to students and staff of Queen's
University and all health and social services
staff throughout Northern Ireland.
Comprehensive collection of material on all
aspects of health and social services.

Royal College of Midwives
Library
15 Mansfield Street
London W1M 0BE
Tel. 0171-580-6523

Open to RCM members, and members of
the public on request to the librarian.
Extensive collection of material on
midwifery and computer search services
available.

Royal College of Nursing
Library
20 Cavendish Square
London W1M 0AB
Tel. 0171-409-3333 Ext 3610

Open to RCN members (non-members
should contact the librarian). Holds the
Steinberg collection of nursing research and
material on nursing and allied health
literature. Photocopoying and literature
search available.

Development Group (Scottish Office)
Centre Library
Crewe Road South
Edinburgh EH4 2LF
Tel. 0131-332-2335

Open to all Scottish health service
employees. Comprehensive collection of
material relating to all areas of health and
practice.

Welsh National School of Medicine
Library
University of Wales
School of Medicine
Heathpark
Cardiff CF4 4XN
Tel. 0122-274-7747

Open to all students and staff of the
university and for reference to all nurses.
Collects material mainly on medicine,
dentistry and nursing.

Wellcome Institute for the History of
    Medicine
Library
183 Euston Road
London NW1 2BP
Tel. 0171-611-8888

Open to the public for research and
reference only. Collection of material
relating to the history of medicine and
allied subjects.

The Health Promotion Library Scotland
Health Information Division commissioned
    within HEBS
The Priory, Canaan Lane
Edinburgh
Tel. 0131-536-5593

Provides a wide range of material on health
promotion. Holds a wide range of reports
commissioned within Scotland. Good
Information Technology resources to
conduct searches, etc.

CHAPTER 9

Reviewing and evaluating the literature

David C. Benton and Desmond F.S. Cormack

Reviewing and evaluating the literature is central to the research process. However, many neophyte researchers have some difficulty in mastering the skills required to systematically read, critically appraise, then synthesize their views into a coherent, structured, and logical review of the literature. Unfortunately, not all published articles are of the same quality or scientific integrity, and all research papers have both strengths and weaknesses. By being able to identify these strengths and weaknesses, the researcher is able to make sound judgements regarding the adequacy, appropriateness and reliability of the material presented, the validity of the conclusions drawn and the applicability of the recommendations made.

Although this chapter cannot hope to teach these skills fully, it does set out to identify a number of points on how they can best be developed. While it is important to be able to appraise and make critical judgements on the content of a single article to enable the researcher to assess the worth of the material under consideration, it is the integration of the literature base into a well-structured, tightly argued and succinctly written review that challenges most of us. However, the researcher should not underestimate the importance of conducting a critical and systematic review of individual articles for it is these that form the basic building blocks of a scholarly evaluation of the literature.

A place to read

How often have you sat down to read an article only to be interrupted by the telephone or a request for assistance? Although this may be acceptable when reading material for pleasure, such interruptions can cause the researcher to waste a great deal of time reading and re-reading the same article unproductively. If you are going to critique a research paper find a quiet, comfortable, well-lit spot with plenty of room to spread out the material. Try to choose an area which you can, over time, associate as the place where you go to work on your research study. Ensure, at the outset, that you have at hand adequate supplies of pencils, highlighting pens, and papers for taking notes. One final point:

set yourself a time limit or, better still, decide to complete certain tasks before you stop for a break.

Identifying the structure of a research publication

Most research publications, whether qualitative or quantitative, follow a recognized structure. A knowledge of the structure of a research report gives clues as to where to look for certain facts or details and thus enables the researcher to scan an article rapidly in order to assess whether the article is of value and worth the investment of time in detailed reading.

The process of scanning an article should be systematic and thorough. Examine a full page at a time with a left to right movement of the eyes while simultaneously 'panning' down the page. Inspect the start of each paragraph for clues to its content. Pick out headings, enlarged, bold, underlined or italic print as well as perusing all illustrations, graphs and tables. For books, monographs, theses, or longer research reports, use the contents list or index for initial clues as to the content. Always stop and read any phrases that signal conclusions or recommendations. For example, 'it has been demonstrated...', 'the outcome of the investigations is...', 'it is suggested...', 'in conclusion...', 'therefore...', 'hence...', and 'it is recommended...'.

Certain types of article, for example the research report, consistently follow a standard format. By being aware of the format you can turn in the first instance to those parts of the report that are most likely to yield valuable information. Furthermore, by being aware of the form and function of the various parts of a research article, readers are in a position to evaluate the worth of the material presented. The left-hand column of Fig. 9.1 details the possible component parts of a research paper.

Having scanned an article and concluded that it is worthy of more detailed review, each of the areas identified in Fig. 9.1 can be critically examined. To enable the researcher to assess the worth of a particular research paper, a series of questions should be asked. The format used in Fig. 9.1 is designed to assist in identifying the strengths and weaknesses of the paper being assessed. As a general point the greater the number of 'No' and 'Don't know' responses checked the more ambiguity there will be and hence the greater care that will need to be taken in drawing any conclusions from the paper.

Recording of critical evaluation

Once the detailed appraisal of an article is complete, it is essential that all relevant information gleaned is recorded in a manner that will facilitate recall at a later date. Without such documentation, it would be necessary to read, re-read and perhaps even search for articles time and time again.

The most common method of storing references is the alphabetical card index system. For example, 10 cm by 15 cm (4 in by 6 in) filing cards may be used, one for each reference. The cards may then be stored alphabetically, usually under the first letter of the author's surname. The card should contain the formal reference to the publication (name of author(s), year of publication, title of article, name of journal, volume and part numbers as well as page numbers of the article). It is also useful to include the location of where the article can be found or obtained – for example, University Library, City Library, personal copy, etc. In addition, a brief summary of the article can be noted on the back of the card.

By using the international classification of disease coding system, literature can be indexed in such a way to facilitate recall on a disease-oriented basis. While this may provide a well-established, international classification framework, we would suggest that the use of subject classification systems used by such indexes as the *Cumulative Index of Nursing and Allied Health Literature* or *The International Nursing Index* is more applicable to those conducting nursing research. In addition, using one of the nursing index classification systems has the advantage that references identified from such sources will already be classified. The use of existing subject classification will accordingly save the researcher time and will also ensure that personally held references will be consistent with their internationally classified source. With the advent of inexpensive and powerful personal computers, the reference material can be stored by means of database software packages (Cormack & Benton, 1990). The database package enables references to be recalled in a fast, efficient and flexible manner. References can be searched simultaneously on a number of criteria, and those identified can be displayed on a screen or printed for subsequent use. Irrespective of the type of approach chosen to store the information, it is necessary to ensure that a minimum amount of data in addition to the critique are recorded. For example, in the case of journal articles, it is necessary to record the author(s), publication date, article title, journal title, volume and part number and page numbers. In the case of books, additional information such as book title, editor(s), publication place and publisher is required. In the case of a card-based system the information needed to access the article can be recorded on the front of the card and the critique written on the back. In the case of a computer-based system, two screens can be used, with the first equating to the front of the card and the second to the back.

Writing a literature review

It has already been stated that the ability to critique an individual article is essential to the writing of a literature review. However, it is the manner in which these individual reviews are integrated that often presents the greatest challenge to both the experienced and inexperienced researcher.

Heading	Questions to be asked	Yes	No	Don't know
Title	• Is the title concise? • Is the title informative? • Does the title clearly indicate the content? • Does the title clearly indicate the research approach used?			
Author(s)	• Does the author(s) have appropriate academic qualifications? • Does the author(s) have appropriate professional qualifications and experience?			
Abstract	• Is there an abstract included? • Does the abstract identify the research problem? • Does the abstract state the hypotheses (if appropriate)? • Does the abstract outline the methodology? • Does the abstract give details of the sample subjects? • Does the abstract report major findings?			
Introduction	• Is the problem clearly identified? • Is a rationale for the study stated? • Are limitations of the study clearly stated?			
Literature review	• Is the literature review up-to-date? • Does the literature review identify the underlying theoretical framework(s)? • Does the literature review present a balanced evaluation of material both supporting and challenging the position being proposed? • Does the literature clearly identify the need for the research proposed? • Are important references omitted?			
The hypothesis	• Does the study use an experimental approach? • Is the hypothesis capable of testing? • Is the hypothesis unambiguous?			
Operational definitions	• Are all terms used in the research question/ problem clearly defined?			
Methodology	• Does the methodology section clearly state the research approach to be used? • Is the method appropriate to the research problem? • Are the strengths and weaknesses of the approach chosen stated?			
Subjects	• Are the subjects clearly identified?			

Contd

Heading	Questions to be asked	Yes	No	Don't know
Sample selection	• Is the sample selection approach congruent with the method to be used? • Is the approach to sample selection clearly stated? • Is the sample size clearly stated?			
Data collection	• Are any data collection procedures adequately described? • Has the validity and reliability of any instruments or questionnaires been clearly stated?			
Ethical considerations	• If the study involves human subjects has the study ethical committee approval? • Is informed consent sought? • Is confidentiality assured? • Is anonymity guaranteed?			
Results	• Are results presented clearly? • Are the results internally consistent? • Is sufficient detail given to enable the reader to judge how much confidence can be placed in the findings? • Does graphic material enhance clarity of the results being presented?			
Data analysis	• Is the approach appropriate to the type of data collected? • Is any statistical analysis correctly performed? • Is there sufficient analysis to determine whether 'significant differences' are not attributable to variations in other relevant variables? • Is complete information (test value, df, and p) reported?			
Discussion	• Is the discussion balanced? • Does the discussion draw upon previous research? • Are the weaknesses of the study acknowledged? • Are clinical implications discussed?			
Conclusions	• Are conclusions supported by the results obtained? • Are the implications of the study identified?			
Recommendations	• Do the recommendations suggest further areas for research? • Do the recommendations identify how any weaknesses in the study design could be avoided in future research?			

Fig. 9.1 Questions to be asked of various sections of a research report.

A review of the literature should be written objectively, with criticism based on factual material and supported by appropriate evidence and argument. In addition, any review should be balanced with both the positive and negative aspects of material being discussed. Furthermore, the implications of any flaws identified in previous work must be highlighted. A good literature review will provide far more than the critical appraisal of a series of articles, it should create a structure upon which further research can be based. Gaps in the knowledge base will be identified, as well as strengths and weaknesses of the previous work. The issue of structure is central to the production of a sound review and warrants further detailed discussion.

Structure of a literature review

Having spent hours, days or even months reviewing individual articles, it is essential that equal emphasis be placed on how these individual appraisals will be woven into a structured, coherent review. Just as with all other component parts of the research process, unless this activity is planned, then time and effort are likely to be wasted. By spending some time on the development of an outline, the researcher will have a guiding framework for the production of the review. Figure 9.2 identifies the component parts of such an outline.

As can be seen from Fig. 9.2, the literature review should start with an intro-

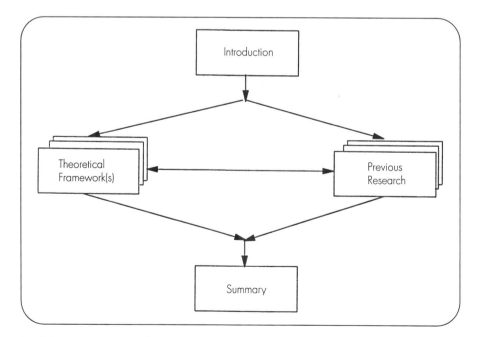

Fig. 9.2   Literature review outline.

duction. This introduction should contain some reference to the sources consulted as well as an indication of the amount of previous work published. The rationale for any constraints should be clearly stated. For example, in the case of a review of the literature on HIV and AIDS it would be reasonable to limit the search from 1980 onwards since before that time there is little literature available. In addition, the introduction should (briefly) describe the structure and purpose of the review in order to guide the reader and help to place all the evidence in context.

The main body of the review will consist of the critique of previous work addressing both theoretical and prior research dimensions. The author should paraphrase previous work whenever possible. Direct quotes can be used to emphasize central issues, but when these are taken out of context of a document, their significance may be lost, or worse still, they may be interpreted differently by the reader. Furthermore, long quotes may interrupt the flow in the development of an argument.

Figure 9.2 attempts to convey that, when reviewing the literature on any topic, a number of competing theoretical frameworks may exist, as well as any number of previous research articles that provide conflicting research results. A well-organized review will clearly present the various theoretical perspectives identified, detail strengths and weaknesses of each, and compare similarities and differences between them. Research findings should be related to the appropriate framework and any anomalies explored and explained (if possible) in terms of the theoretical models available. Any gaps in the research or inconsistencies should be clearly identified. Articles central to the development of arguments should be dealt with in depth. Researchers may choose to set out, in summary form, an illustration of the major findings along with any strengths and weaknesses of the individual articles reviewed (see Fig. 9.3). Such an illustration can assist in identifying common findings or discrepancies in the results as well as providing an opportunity to collate, in an easily accessible form, both strengths and weaknesses in the existing literature. A summary under each of the headings can be made if the quantity of literature being considered is not too extensive. Such summaries can then be readily expanded in the main body of the literature review.

Unless the literature is analysed in detail, and the interrelationships between previous publications identified, the quality of the review will be poor. Inadequate analysis and synthesis of literature results in a review that may only present a series of disjointed paragraphs that echo the findings of previous studies. By planning the review, a logical, structured and coherent argument for further research, or an appraisal of the current state of knowledge, can be presented.

The review should conclude with a summary of the synthesized findings of the previous work which should clearly describe the extent of the current knowledge base. Gaps in the knowledge base or inconsistencies both in terms of the research results and in the theoretical frameworks should be restated succinctly, thus forming the rationale for conducting further research.

Author(s) and date	Methodology issues	Results	Recommendations
Brown, A. (2000)	Qualitative; poor sampling method	Inconclusive	Implement practice change
Green, A. (1999)	Quantitative; random control trial; small sample size	Inconclusive	Replicate with larger sample
Red, A. (2000)	Qualitative; grounded theory study	Categories seem saturated; theory seems saturated	Test predictive power of theory
Summary			
Range of authors, but all recent publications	Variety of research approaches but some weaknesses in design	Theory has been developed but no conclusive quantitative results reported	Further research required before practice change is advised

Fig. 9.3   Previously published literature (fictitious).

Presentational issues

When the researcher is considering a number of research papers, it is essential that the material is presented in a way that facilitates understanding. Great care should be taken to use the most appropriate referencing system to ensure that the flow of any argument is not disrupted. It is, however, often the case that researchers are restricted by the requirements of the journal or institution for which they are preparing the work. Nevertheless, if you have a choice be conscious of the impact that a poorly referenced review can have on the reader. We would argue that either the Harvard or the Vancouver (numerical) method of reference citation significantly adds to the clarity of the argument.

Harvard system

This is perhaps the most widely used system for citing references within scientific publications. In essence it requires that the research cites the surname of the author followed by the date of publication of the work being cited from within the text. It is usual that both are included within parentheses unless the author's name forms an integral part of the sentence. For example, two fictitious references are cited to illustrate the format that is normally used:

> *Research methods are being increasingly taught as part of the pre-registration curricula (Black, 1999). However, Brown (2000) has argued that this is not enough and specialist post-basic courses need also to be offered.*

As can be seen from the above example, full reference details are not included within the text as this would interrupt the flow of the sentence. Cited material is detailed in a section headed 'References' at the end of the article. All cited material is listed in alphabetical order. If two articles are cited from the same author then they are placed in chronological order. If, however, two articles are cited by the same author and published in the same year, then it is necessary to add 'a' or 'b' within the year descriptor. For example:

Brown, J. (2000a) The first paper cited in the text. *Journal of Tomorrow's Science* **99** (1): 23--32.
Brown, J. (2000b) The second paper cited in the text. *Journal of Tomorrow's Science* **99** (3): 145–63.

When using the Harvard system and there are multiple authors it is usual to cite only two in the text. Three or more are cited by use of the first author's name followed by *et al*. So Brown & Black (1999) would appear but in the case of Brown, Black & White (2000) only Brown *et al*. (2000) would appear. Although each journal may have different rules about giving the details of multiple authors it is usual to give the names and initials of all authors in the reference list.

Vancouver or numerical citation system

The other citation system in common use is the Vancouver or numerical system in which a number (e.g. (1)) appears in the text. At the end of the article all cited material appears in the order referenced.

In the case of books, and when the researcher is referring to a particular section of the cited work, a page number may also be added (1, p. 22).

Irrespective of which system is used, book and journal sources are treated similarly when being cited in the text. However, slight differences do appear in the reference list.

In the case of *journal* references it is usual to give the author's surname and initial(s) followed by the date, the article title and the journal title, followed by both the volume and part numbers as well as the page numbers. The journal title appears in italics. For example *Nursing Research, Journal of Advanced Nursing* or *Nursing Management*. When a *book* is cited, slightly different information appears in the reference list. In this case the author's surname and initial(s), date of publication, title of the book, place of publication and publisher. For example, Black, D. (1999) *The Basis of Life*. London, Fast & Accurate Publishers Ltd. In this case it is the book title that is printed in italics. For further information on more complex material, such as unpublished reports, further details can be found in specific texts on publication (Cormack, 1994).

Identifying the anatomy of a published review

To conclude this chapter, and to reinforce the various points made, we shall give a brief analysis of a published text, 'Learning to care: A review of the literature', by Smith (1985), which uses the Harvard reference citation system.

First, the title of the work clearly informs the reader of its content. Specifically, it states that the article is a literature review and that the topic is learning to care. The author is identified as being a senior nurse (research) and is both academically and professionally well qualified.

Second, an abstract is provided. Although it has no title, it is enclosed in a box at the start of the article, and separated from the main text. It clearly outlines the content of the article, identifying that the author intends to review the literature and the relationship between the provision of care and learning to nurse. Furthermore, it is identified that the principal means of evaluating this relationship is by examining the quality of care, and this is identified by the use of reference to dependency studies, quality assurance instruments and the nursing process.

Third, the introduction informs the reader of the extent and nature of the literature review conducted, as well as providing a succinct statement on the purpose of the article.

Fourth, major headings are used throughout the publication and these conform to the principal elements reported in the abstract. This consistency assists the reader in comprehending the logical progression of the arguments presented. Various themes are well integrated throughout the article with the relevance of the material being frequently stated in terms of the relationship between learning to nurse and the giving of patient care.

Fifth, throughout the article, the author does not simply report the findings of previous studies, but examines the material in terms of content, method, theoretical perspective. In short, a comparative analysis both in terms of theory and research has been undertaken, resulting in a review that compares and contrasts the findings of previous work.

Finally, although the author does not include a heading in the article, a summary is presented. This final paragraph draws together all the various threads presented, but, unfortunately, an additional element is also introduced. The introduction of Donabedian's (1966) 'structure, process, outcome' model at this late stage without the inclusion of appropriate debate, detracts from what is otherwise a well-written critique of the literature.

The article by Smith (1985) demonstrates many of the points that have been discussed in this chapter. Writing a critical review of the literature is a skill that requires to be learned. If you are to become a nurse researcher, or if you are to practise from a research base, it is essential that you are able, proficiently, to conduct a critical review of the literature; learning from the past you can change the future and increase the quality of care delivered.

References

Cormack, D.F.S. (1994) *Writing for Health Care Professions.* London: Blackwell Scientific Publications.

Cormack, D.F.S & Benton, D.C. (1990) Reading the professional literature. In D.F.S. Cormack (ed.) *Developing Your Career In Nursing*. London: Chapman & Hall.

Donabedian, A. (1966) Evaluating the quality of medical care. *Millbank Memorial Fund Quarterly* **44** (2): 166–206.

Smith, P. (1985) Learning to care: a review of the literature. *Nurse Education Today* **5** (5): 178–82.

Further reading

Eysenck, H.J. (1995) Meta-analysis of best-evidence synthesis? *Journal of Evaluative Clinical Practice* **1** (1): 29–36.

Crombie, I.K. (1996) *The Pocket Guide to Critical Appraisal*. London: BMJ Publishing Group.

Cook, D.J. (1997) Systematic reviews: synthesis of best evidence for clinical decisions. *Annals of Internal Medicine* **126** (5): 376–80.

Droogan, J. & Song, F. (1996) The process and importance of systematic reviews. *Nurse Researcher* **4** (1): 15–26.

CHAPTER 10

Preparing a research proposal

Senga Bond

Research proposals may be written for a number of reasons: to obtain funding, to present to a higher degrees committee in a university, for ethical approval or as an academic exercise as part of a research course. This chapter focuses on the first of these since this depends on being able to achieve the other reasons.

Preparing a research proposal will be addressed in two ways. First to provide beginning researchers with some straightforward guidance about possible structure and content. The second is to suggest some ways of making a proposal more appealing and thus more likely to be funded.

The most important function of research proposals is to make explicit a reasoned argument about the need for the proposed study on practical and theoretical grounds and how it will be carried out. The very act of writing a proposal assists in identifying the strengths and weaknesses of a study. This is achieved through the process of setting down a clear statement of the question that the study proposes to answer, the methods that will be used to find the answer and the resources required to do it. Information should also be provided about how the study findings will be disseminated and any products likely to arise. The particular form that a proposal takes will depend on the requirements of the funding organization and some produce special forms giving guidance about the different sections within which information should be provided. It is essential that these directions are followed. This chapter offers general guidance about preparing a proposal which may be amended to suit the requirements of a particular case.

Typical content of a research proposal

It is useful to have a checklist of the main topics to be included. Such a list would contain the following:

1. Title of project
2. Summary
3. Justification for the study
4. Related research

5. Aims and objectives
6. Plan of investigation
7. Ethical considerations
8. Products arising from the project
9. Dissemination
10. Resources
11. Budget
12. Curriculum vitae

Let us consider each of these headings in turn and give some pointers to the kind of information within each one.

Title of project

Research projects become known by their title, so it is important to make the title explicit and relatively brief while describing the proposed study. Sometimes studies change in direction during their evolution while the subject matter remains essentially the same. An experiment may collapse or the nature of the variables being considered in a survey may be altered on the basis of pilot work. The title should be able to override these changes while still conveying the essence of the study. The use of words like 'evaluation' and 'survey' in titles are helpful in alerting readers to the approach the study will take. It is more informative to call a study 'An evaluation of counselling for patients who have had a mastectomy' than to call it 'Caring for mastectomy patients' even if the design or counselling methods change over time.

Summary

In practice this is usually written after the main body of the proposal has been put together since it requires to be succinct yet state clearly the objectives of the study and how it will be carried out. It should contain only the most relevant information. The space allocated to it or word length specified means that every word is important and it is an art to describe a major project in a paragraph.

Because it appears early, the summary again alerts the reader to what to expect in the subsequent text. The summary is an important indication of the quality of the remainder of the proposal and so it requires careful consideration and probably several drafts to ensure all of the main points are included.

Justification for the study

The statement of the problem which opens the main body of the proposal must convince the reader that the proposed study is important. It must introduce the research questions and put them into a context which indicates the importance of the problem, its size, costs and consequences. It should identify how the proposed study will add to previous work and build on theory. In nursing studies there are likely to be practical implications of the research so that, as well as having value in contributing to knowledge, its utility value needs to be stressed. There may be methodological gains, for example in developing a new research instrument, which would have future applications, as well as gains in education or practice.

In developing the problem statement the researcher needs to keep a careful balance between putting forward claims for the study which are either too grandiose or too general or that the study is no more than the whim of the researcher based on some closely held belief. Novices often express research as setting out to prove something – for example, that parents prefer booked home visits from health visitors – rather than as an open question of their response to different systems of visiting, or a formal hypothesis of preference. There is also a tendency to be over-ambitious when enthusiasm for the topic overrides their judgement about delivering the project. A key piece of advice therefore is *to focus on the manageable*.

When writing this section it is sometimes helpful to type in a bold face a succinct statement of the problem to draw the reviewer's attention and to foreshadow the remainder of the proposal.

Related research

Next, it is important for the researcher to demonstrate her command of the current state of the field and how this study would move it forward. To achieve this, the key studies which provide the basis for the proposed project should be included. Indicate in language for non-specialists how they are relevant to the proposed study and how this study moves beyond them. This review should relate both to substantive concerns and methods, and be provided in sufficient detail to inform the reader of its relevance. It may also be useful to include knowledge of studies underway as a reflection of the author's competence in keeping abreast of developments, as well as point out how they differ from the study being proposed.

At this point the theoretical aspects of the study and the firmness of the theoretical base should be described. This information can be extremely influential in demonstrating the researcher's grasp of complex issues and in showing that the study has more than practical implications.

The development of the literature base is a major feature of the research process described in Chapters 6 and 9 and it is equally an important feature of the research proposal. If the literature search and the literature section of the proposal is an afterthought, it will shine through by virtue of its unrelatedness to the remainder of the proposal.

Aims and objectives

Any reviewer of proposals likes to see clear, specific and concrete objectives which are achievable. List and number them in order of importance in a clear sequence, taking only a sentence or two for each.

The remainder of the proposal will be judged in relation to what you have told the reader about what this study aims to do. To achieve this, avoid vague terminology and generalities; define criteria as specifically as possible. Do not leave it up to the reader to have to do the guesswork about what the objectives are or their order of priority.

The objectives of the study may take the form of questions when research is exploratory or a survey where specific facts are being sought. It may be possible to state objectives in the form of testable hypotheses where there is a basis for predicting results. It is more enlightening, as well as more convincing, if hypotheses are stated whenever possible. However, these need to be precise, with relationships clearly specified.

Plan of investigation

This section could be called *Plan of Investigation, Procedure or Method* and is likely to be the section most carefully read by funding and ethical committees. Up to this point, the researcher has been able to present a picture of the positive implications of the research and what it hopes to achieve. It is when procedures are spelled out that those reading the proposal gauge the researcher's capacity to undertake and complete the proposed work.

The specific format of this section will depend on the methods adopted. Different emphases will be required depending on whether the study takes a survey, an experimental, or field study approach. Irrespective of method there are several important matters to convey and these are best written in discrete sections.

Method/design

The design to be adopted and the precise methods and techniques to be used should be clear. Simple descriptions are more readily available for particular types of experiment and for survey research than for other types of research, and can be specified in advance. Equally it is straightforward to indicate whether the study is prospective or retrospective, cross-sectional or longitudinal. For exploratory studies, case studies or ethnographic research, the basic method should be made equally clear, and this section will often require appropriate adaptation when the application forms are set out as if for trials.

For experimental studies details will be required about which variables are controlled and how control is to be achieved. In some instances, there may be complete randomization while, in others, subjects may be matched on known relevant variables, or included in a factorial design. What is important here is showing awareness of relevant variables and how control can be realistically managed. In health services research, control of all variables is virtually impossible and the challenge is to make the best use of available situations and be sophisticated in designs which offer the closest approximation to experimental proof.

When compromises have to be made to facilitate experimental design in the 'real world' of patient care, then the reasons for such compromises should be made clear. For example, if patients are to be allowed some degree of choice of treatment or randomization is clustered by wards or general practices rather than individual patients, the reasons for doing so need to be made explicit. The general point is that often the reasons for not adhering to the 'gold standard' of the RCT expected by some funding bodies should be spelled out.

Specification of design in observation studies, survey research using case notes or other forms of data should make clear that this is the intended method.

Population and sample

The initial literature review will have indicated the nature of the population relevant to the study as well as giving a clue to the generalizability of the study findings. This section will include a clear statement of the population from which the study sample will be drawn, and details of the characteristics of the sample. When particular sampling techniques are used, for example stratified or cluster sampling as described in Chapter 22, this choice should be justified.

Evidence should be provided that the sample is available and can be recruited and that, where appropriate, a sampling frame exists. Clear criteria for inclusion and exclusion should be included, or variables by which individual subjects will be matched.

Critical also are questions of sample size, which will be dealt with in greater detail in Chapters 15 and 22. Reviewers will be looking for indications that the sample size will be big enough to detect differences or carry out other appropriate statistical manipulations to produce a clear answer. It is generally expected that proposals for experimental designs include power analysis, providing a statement of the expected and acceptable size of effects, at what degree of power, and the sample size required to detect them.

It is equally important to specify the sampling intended in field studies. Case studies or individuals will be selected on some criteria and sometimes these can be specified in advance, for example to include a gender, ethnic or occupational mix or other theoretically relevant variable. When these can only be specified on the basis of ongoing theory development, then this should be made clear.

Data collection

In this section, measures and procedures to be used for data collection are described. These should reflect back to the variables included, show that the measures to be used represent acceptable operational definitions of them, and that they have appropriate measurement or psychometric characteristics. In many topics of relevance to nursing research, well-validated scales exist and it would be foolish to develop a new scale. Where proposed measurements have been used in other relevant studies it is helpful to indicate this. When methods of measurements do not already exist and new methods are proposed, these are best described in detail as an appendix to the proposal. In some cases reviewers wish to see copies of instrumentation, test items, questionnaires or interview guides. It makes sense to find out if this is required. However, for some studies, a substantial part of the work entails such methodological developments.

While data-collection techniques may involve conventional methods like self-completion questionnaires and interviews, they may also involve invasive-biochemical or physical measures or assessment of observed behaviour. Only if novel techniques are involved should mention be made of the apparatus to be used to obtain these data and whether any special conditions are required for their use. If the data to be collected or the methods used to collect them are likely to be controversial, then plans indicating how problems would be dealt with should be included.

Pilot and development studies

Providing evidence that the above are based on findings of a pilot study increases the chances of impressing readers about the viability of the project. Indeed many proposals are submitted to enable pilot work to be carried out as a preliminary to a larger, definitive study. A pilot study will tell reviewers what steps will be taken to ensure that the proposed methods are workable, are acceptable to subjects and are manageable. The pilot study is worth specifying in some detail. For example, to conduct a postal sample survey from first principles, it would be necessary to go through several stages to arrive at a questionnaire before proceeding to a postal pilot study to gauge its acceptability and response rate. If an already validated instrument was to be used again, then obviously the amount of development and pilot work would be that much less. When new methods are to be used – for example, lap-top computers to collect interview data – or new scales have to be developed, then the development work will be much more time-consuming and important to the eventual quality of the study. It is always worth investing time and effort to ensure that the development, feasibility or pilot work for a study is thorough, and this should be stressed in the proposal. These may be presented as the first phases of a project.

Analysis

It is essential to have considered analysis in the development of any study, even though it may be some way from becoming actuality. It is most important to show that the methods of analysis are consistent with the objectives, design of the study and data. Again, in some respects this is easier to specify in advance for quantitative studies. It is less easy to describe details of the analytic procedures used in qualitative studies, especially if reviewers are unfamiliar with these techniques. In cases where complete specification is not possible, the stages of data analysis can be outlined indicating an appreciation of the kinds of methods likely to be used. If studies rely on multivariate or discriminant techniques or longitudinal analyses, then this should be specified even if it has to be at a general level. It should be indicated that sufficient statistical expertise is available to inform and, if necessary, carry out statistical analysis. Knowing what techniques to apply to the analysis of data is more important than indicating that a statistical package like SPSSx or Mini-Tab are to be used. Similarly, stating that a qualitative data software package like NUD*IST is to be used is no substitute for detailing analytic methods. Access to computers and appropriate software packages are taken as universally available, and it is therefore important to convince the reviewers that you know what analysis is appropriate and have the necessary personnel, hardware and software to achieve it.

Work plan

Details of the time scale and plan of work should be included to show the anticipated duration of each stage of the study. The complexity of the plan of work would reflect the complexity of the study. Providing a clear timetable with milestones to be achieved through the process of the study offers another opportunity to demonstrate that the proposal is realistic and achievable. Major milestones, such as having all data-collection tools ready, completion of patient recruitment and completion of data collection and analysis, should be included. When the study is more complex and different activities are happening simultaneously, then more sophisticated flowcharts or critical paths may be necessary to identify the anticipated progress of the work. Often a diagram says more than words.

Generally, the time taken to complete each part of a study is underestimated, particularly data collection which depends on a prospective series. The tendency is to be over-optimistic. This can also apply to the time it takes to negotiate entry to study sites and gain ethical approval to collect data. Formal project planning activities should be undertaken to determine the time scale required in relation to critical events. A clear and realistic time schedule is another indication of the researcher's competence and the likelihood of a successful project.

Ethical considerations

The reviewer of a research proposal will have been alerted to any ethical problems while reading the methods section. The proposal may be reviewed by a committee whose primary objective is to assess the scientific methods of a study, but they will not be unaware of ethical issues and they are likely to assess whether 'the ends justify the means'. Many grant-awarding bodies require a study to have approval from an ethics committee prior to any award being made.

A proposal viewed by an ethics committee, however, will take an entirely different perspective. Ethics committees consider the science of the proposal but will be giving most attention to the protection of human and animal subjects from undue distress. When submitting a proposal for ethical clearance, documentation about information for subjects and how written consent will be obtained and the forms used to collect data should be submitted. Ethical matters may also be relevant to describing the protection of subjects from any negative consequences of a study, and protection of staff can equally apply when they may be involved in handling noxious substances or administering procedures. How data will be stored and measures taken to protect the identities of subjects or participating institutions should be included through adherence to the requirements of the Data Protection Act.

Products arising from the project

The end product of most research studies is a final report to the funding or commissioning body or a thesis. However, products may also be new research instruments or methods of data collection as well as teaching or clinical aids. If the study is likely to yield a product of value, then ownership of the intellectual property rights and the patents to the product need to be made clear at the outset. This is especially so if an industrial company is involved. Also it may be appropriate to include costs for product development in a proposal.

Dissemination

Increasingly, attention is required to the dissemination of the results of research. Reports and published papers are taken for granted but they are not the only way to present results. Videos, presentations, etc., may be equally if not more relevant in some instances as a means of disseminating findings to particular audiences. It may be appropriate to make specific suggestions about how this is to be achieved, especially through executive summaries of findings targeted to specific audiences. Some grant-awarding bodies are more interested than others in dissemination over and above traditional publications.

Resources

It is important that the resources required to carry out the study are realistically appraised. Resources, whether human, material or financial, need to be specified.

Personnel

The person(s) who will direct the project, the principal investigator(s), should be clearly identified together with the amount of time intended to be devoted to the project. It may be that this is a proposal for a full-time commitment or for only a few hours in a week. Spell out the time implicated. Academic and clinical collaborators and relationships with them and their responsibility and commitment to the project should be included. Where a complex study is involved the right mix of expertise may be an important element. It must be clear how they have contributed to the proposal.

It is especially important for inexperienced researchers to obtain the support of established research workers. In this respect it can be useful to show that active consultation has taken place in the development of a proposal. Indicate the kind and amount of assistance offered by those experienced in research or particular technical competence associated with data processing, analysis, costings and so on.

Other resources

Describing particular services or back-up facilities can strengthen a proposal. Good computer and library facilities fall into this category, as do sufficient space and secretarial support. Where established networks are integral to a project or co-operation has been obtained from particular agencies or institutions, some indication of this, like letters of agreement, may be included as a helpful appendix.

Budget

Preparing a research budget requires as much skill as preparing other parts of the proposal. It is amazing, when a maximum amount of money is specified in calls for proposals, how many are costed at just that amount! Part of the skill in budgeting lies in locating other people who know the prices of commodities – staff salaries as well as equipment and other consumables. However, knowing the details of data collection and processing makes costing much easier – how many hours it takes to collect data, how much travel time and mileage, how much data processing will be required. Preparing a budget means translating the time scale and plan of work into financial terms.

Novice writers have a tendency to want to skimp the budget, earnestly believing that if a project costs less it improves the chance of being funded. Undercutting the budget simply reflects inexperience. Sharp-eyed critics will quickly notice where there has been undue trimming and what is feasible in the costs quoted. Equally, where excesses are included, like a new computer for a short project, or large travel budgets, they will be cut. Sometimes budgets can be a matter of negotiation if they are thought to be too high by virtue of over-elaborate sampling or extended time scales. However, to be caught short of cash and time can be disastrous and funding bodies do not take kindly to requests for extensions of time or increased budgets. In preparing a budget, use a checklist to include main headings such as:

- Research staff salaries
- Secretarial staff salaries
- Data-collection costs, for example purchase of equipment and other materials, printing, travelling expenses, stationery and postage
- Data-processing costs
- Book purchases/library costs
- Conference attendance
- Product development
- Dissemination
- Overheads

It is sometimes useful to separate costs into capital costs, to include the purchase of necessary equipment, and recurrent costs. It is useful to check whether your library will expect a fee for inter-library loans and special book purchases. Some organizations, especially universities, ask for overheads. Check out whether this is so and the current rate. Parent organizations also wish to check a budget statement before it is submitted and salaries, etc., usually have to be counter-signed by someone with specific expertise in this matter. An appropriate budget is always a matter of careful specification rather than just pulling some notional figure out of the air.

Curriculum vitae

Attach an appropriate curriculum vitae for all principal investigators. This is not always essential but is usually asked for and it does no harm to include one. Its contents should be appropriate and include details of:

- Name
- Age
- Qualifications
- Education
- Work experience
- Research experience
- Recent relevant publications

One or two pages is usually sufficient to show whether the applicant has the appropriate experience and performance record to conduct the study.

Final review

Research proposals usually go through several drafts. Indeed, there would be a major cause for concern if they did not! There are a number of things to be achieved in reviewing proposals, not least is to consider its physical presentation. Nicely spaced typescript with a major effort on legibility, lucidity and clarity of presentation are all important. The use of small type should be avoided. While readers of a proposal will not be consciously evaluating it on how it is presented, nevertheless the relatively small amount of time it takes to ensure a pleasant layout which is easily followed will be time well spent. Using devices like a bold typeface, underlining, spacing, using diagrams, flowcharts and tables are useful to attract the reader's eye. These devices are often more useful in presenting details than reams of text.

It is also useful to ask others with experience of successfully submitting proposals to check over your efforts. Most people are pleased to assist, as long as there is evidence that you have made proper attempts to produce a good piece of work and adequate time is allowed.

Some general comments

This chapter has discussed developing the research proposal primarily from the point of view of having it approved for funding. It should also have demonstrated the need to write down a clear statement of proposed research in the form of a protocol to assist the researchers themselves. Matters of making explicit a proposed time schedule and proper project management techniques can be fundamental to the successful execution of a project. However, in the development phase of a study proposal it is even more helpful to gain the advice and assistance of experienced researchers who have themselves submitted successful proposals. The gains to be made from the experience of others in such matters are invaluable.

Some funding bodies offer the opportunity to submit an outline proposal for approval before submitting a full proposal. This permits a degree of negotiation about the focus, content, methods and so on.

Different funding bodies considering a proposal will be looking at quite different things, and it is important to identify their primary concerns and give those concerns special consideration. Check whether the funding body has any special focus in terms of the subject matter, whether there is any specific geographical area or limits to funding. (In Chapter 4 some sources of research funding were identified.) Check if the funding body has any particular requirements in the manner in which a proposal is presented, and this may involve no more than a telephone call to the appropriate secretary. Some organizations have a checklist or a particular form on which proposals must be made, and it is wise to adhere strictly to notes of guidance. Other organizations regard the form of the proposal as a measure of the worth of the researcher and offer no guidance on preparing a proposal.

It is also helpful to know how proposals are reviewed. Sometimes they are sent to external referees with particular expertise for comment, while others are dealt with completely 'in house'. As well as scientific referees, there may also be 'customer' referees who are looking for the utility of the research in practical or policy terms, rather than the quality of the science. Knowledge of the membership of a review committee can be useful in anticipating areas to which special attention or orientation should be given. When a committee of mixed expertise reviews proposals, all its members should be able to understand the nature of the study. At times there could be a problem of orientation – when biological or physical scientists are asked to review a proposal with a social science orientation. In instances like this, it is important to avoid excessive jargon while maintaining appropriate specificity.

There is skill in achieving a balance between identifying every single possibility and spelling out every detail and providing sufficient detail to convince reviewers that the applicant has the ability to complete a worthwhile study. To some extent the degree of specificity is related to the state of knowledge in a particular field and to the extent to which the study is exploratory or explanatory. Writers of proposals have to rely on their judgement to some extent but, as a general principle, it is better to include more information than to leave out something that others may regard as important. However, the reviewing panel will be abreast of standard methods and these do not have to be detailed.

The length of the proposal can be of some concern. Sometimes maximum length and number of pages is specified. If lengthy details of specific steps are required then these can be included as appendices to avoid crowding too much into the main text and losing the crispness of the presentation. The purpose of appendices is to provide additional supportive information for reviewers who do not feel that the main text is sufficiently detailed, but should not require to be read to obtain a clear impression of the study.

This book is intended primarily for people who are new to research and this chapter may be used to assist those who have never developed a proposal – or a successful one! Some funding bodies are keen to support new research workers but are not likely to want to risk large sums of money or invest in potentially unmanageable studies. It is wise, then, to begin in a relatively small way or to ask for only funding for the pilot work or first stage of the project. This safeguards both the funding body and the research worker should something go drastically wrong. It would be better still to have an experienced researcher as a co-applicant.

Finally, do not be dismayed if a first attempt is rejected. One can always learn from it. Unfortunately, not all grant-awarding bodies provide information detailing why a proposal is rejected and this is singularly unhelpful to the recipient of the rejection slip. However, increasingly, referees' comments are given to applicants. In some cases grant bodies may refer the project – that is, suggest that the researcher re-work it under guidance. In some cases it is almost as if referral is the rule and few proposals are accepted the first time round. It is always helpful to obtain copies of proposals that have been funded by the body to which you are applying. This does not imply slavish adherence to that particular format but it does give some indication of the type of proposal more likely to be welcomed and, hence, succeed in being funded.

There are several books, chapters in research texts and other publications devoted to offering advice about writing research proposals and some are listed below. These offer useful suggestions and go beyond this introductory chapter.

Further reading

Burns, N. & Grove, S.K. (1997) *The Practice of Nursing Research*, 3rd edn. Philadelphia: W.B. Saunders.

Fraser, J. (1995) *Professional Proposal Writing*. London: Gower.

Grant, D. (1998) How to get a grant funded. *British Medical Journal* 317, 1647–8.

Hodgson, C. (1989) Tips on writing successful grant proposals. *Nurse Practitioner* 14 (2), 44–9.

Locke, L.F., Spirduso, W.W. & Silverman, S.J. (1993) *Proposals that Work*, 3 edn. London: Sage.

Ogden, T.E. & Goldberg, I.A. (1995) *Research Proposals: A Guide to Success*. New York: Raven Press.

Polit, D.F. & Hungler, B.P. (1998) *Nursing Research: Principles and Methods*, 6 edn. Philadelphia: Lippincott.

Ries, J.B. & Leukefeld, C.G. (1995) *Applying for Research Funding*, Thousand Oaks, California: Sage Publications.

Sandelowski, M., Davis, D.H. & Harris, B.G. (1989) Artful research: writing the proposal for research in the naturalist paradigm. *Research in Nursing and Health* 12 (2), 77–84.

CHAPTER 11

Gaining access to the research site

David C. Benton and Desmond F.S. Cormack

Having identified a research question, conducted a systematic review of the literature and decided upon a research design, a further critical step that novice researchers often find difficult is gaining access to the research site. If research is to be conducted which requires access to either human subjects or confidential individual-based patient information, then careful negotiations will need to take place if delays in this important step are to be avoided.

The process of negotiating access to the research site is often complex and challenging and will inevitably bring the researcher into contact with a wide range of individuals and groups. This experience can be rather daunting for the novice researcher but should be viewed as a learning experience since it is an integral part of conducting a research study. Even an apparently straightforward study often involves negotiating access with a wide range of individuals and groups.

Since the introduction of the National Health Service (NHS) reforms, the issue of research access has become even more complex in some respects. The introduction of a market ethos has resulted in some researchers experiencing a degree of difficulty in negotiation access. Not only are the managers of NHS Trusts conscious of the need to protect the interests of often vulnerable research subjects, but they may also be concerned, if such research produces adverse findings, that their market position might be compromised if data relating to quality of care are handled in an insensitive way. However, the change of government, although maintaining the separation between those who buy care and those who provide it, has heralded a shift in culture towards one of partnership and collaboration. Despite this, researchers can still find gaining access a confusing and stressful process. It is therefore essential that the researcher is clear on how to proceed in gaining access to the research site.

The research site

In this chapter the research site is the term used to describe a wide variety of settings within which research may take place. It may be a hospital, a community-based service, a private or voluntary sector institution, an individual's home or, in the case of population-based research, a street corner where individual members of the public may be approached. To a certain extent the research question may need to be modified in light of the discussions and negotiations that inevitably will take place in pursuing access with the various gatekeepers to the research sites. Within this discussion, the gatekeepers are those individuals who can either facilitate or block access of the researcher in conducting the study. It is therefore critical that the researcher should initiate discussion to gain access at an early stage.

For a novice researcher it is often worth while considering discussing with peers their experiences in gaining access. Such discussion can often provide opportunities to rehearse the approach that may be taken. Also the assistance of an experienced researcher in reviewing a novice researcher's proposal may highlight issues that, from the gatekeeper's perspective, may have problems or, from an external perspective, may require clarification. This, therefore, will ensure that you have had an opportunity to consider such issues in a safe environment in order to formulate an appropriately detailed response to any points likely to be raised.

It is important to note that in negotiating access it is acknowledged that the gatekeeper can only give the researcher permission to *ask* potential subjects to participate. Negotiated access does not guarantee that the research subjects will agree to participate in the study.

Research where negotiated access is not required

If data are already published then no permission or negotiation needs to take place to gain access to the material. For example, library-based historical research is an example of a research design that does not require the researcher to gain formal access to the research site. This, of course, is only the case if the research materials are in the public domain.

Frequently, specialist collections of material may require the permission of the librarian – particularly if they are of key historical value and/or are original source material which may be damaged by excessive handling. If this is the case, the researcher may need to convince the owner/librarian that her skill in handling delicate original data sources is sufficiently adequate and will not cause any damage.

Some researchers believe that collecting non-invasive data from the general public does not require special permission. To a certain extent this is true, however a researcher who approaches members of the public may fall foul of the law since she may be reported as causing a nuisance. It is always advisable for researchers to alert the local constabulary of their intentions to conduct data collection. This is particularly the case if the data are to be collected on a busy street where the process may cause obstructions or delays in the flow of pedestrians.

Accessing the gatekeepers

There are a range of gatekeepers who can facilitate or inhibit the researcher's access to a research site. Gatekeepers generally fall into one of two camps: professional or organizational.

Organizational gatekeeper

Conducting research within any health care institution or setting requires that the management of the organization is aware of the activity taking place. This is essential so that the potential cumulative impact of different studies can be appropriately monitored. A key gatekeeper is therefore the chief executive officer (CEO) or the general manager of the organization. It is unlikely that the CEO will deal with the request directly since most organizations will have a named individual who has been appointed to take the lead on research and development. In large organizations this individual is likely to be called the research and development director. In smaller organizations the responsibilities may be discharged by a senior member of the organization's team – possibly the nurse or medical director. The names of senior officials of NHS institutions and independent sector providers can be obtained from an up-to-date version of *The Hospitals and Health Services Year Book* (Institute of Health Service Management, 1998). However, in light of the rapid changeover of staff, it is always advisable to telephone the organization to validate the information gleaned from such texts. It is normal practice that such individuals should be approached in writing in the first instance. The researcher should give brief details of the study to be conducted, the likely impact for the organization and a request to meet with either the CEO or his nominated deputy. Contacting the CEO is a critical step, particularly if the study to be conducted requires access to case records. In the UK a case record is the property of the Secretary of State for Health. However, safe custody is delegated to the CEO of the Trust. Indeed, with the advent of the increased development of electronic data records and their associated portability, access to personal material for non-clinical purposes is being closely controlled.

Professional gatekeepers

If the researcher is seeking access to a particular patient group, then there may well be a number of professional gatekeepers who will require convincing that the researcher is both capable and competent to undertake the study. As multidisciplinary working becomes the norm rather than the exception, then the range of professional gatekeepers is expanding considerably. It is therefore always best for the researcher to attempt to identify who might be involved in the care and treatment of the subjects/patients she intends to recruit into the study. By doing this a list can be generated of those individuals who may have a view on any research that is proposed to be conducted with 'their' patient. In the past it was generally acceptable to approach the head of a particular professional group to seek approval for access. However, with the fragmentation of hierarchical lines of management this is no longer always appropriate. It is therefore essential that the researcher is clear about how the various professional groups work within a potential research site. Only then can an appropriate approach be made to, perhaps, the professional head of nursing, medicine or any other allied profession. Many research studies have run into difficulty because of failure to approach the right people at the right time.

Having identified the professional gatekeepers, again a written response should be made with the offer of following this up with a face-to-face meeting.

Whether approaching organizational or professional gatekeepers, it is essential that the researcher is well prepared for this encounter. The researcher should take to the meeting an adequate number of copies of the research proposal. The initial contact with the gatekeepers can have a profound effect on how easy or difficult access to the research site will be. It is therefore advisable that the researcher be clear before the meeting about the ground that will be covered. Ideally, an opening explanation of the study will have been prepared. This will stress the significance of the work, the commitment that will be required from the organization providing research access and, perhaps most significantly, what they will gain from the study. At the very least, be prepared to offer a copy of the research results and come back and present the findings to the senior managers of the organization and/or those individuals who have been involved in the process. If the initial contact is managed well, then a commitment may be obtained from the senior officers to give support in gaining access lower down the organization. A letter of introduction may significantly influence the co-operation of others within the organization. It is, however, important that such a letter should not be used as a mechanism to coerce people into agreement, but it certainly can assist in providing additional authority to the researcher since, hopefully, it will make reference to the importance of the work and the commitment of senior management.

It is also important at this early stage to establish how ethics committee approval can be sought. The Department of Health published a new guide to the establishment of research ethics committees and, on the whole, these are now functioning well throughout the country (Department of Health, 1991). A more recent publication on standards relating to the functioning of these committees has been produced (National Health Service Training Directorate, 1994). Access to both the guidance on the operation of committees and the standards of functioning can be a useful additional aid to the novice researcher seeking to negotiate access.

Access and power relationships

In the previous section, we have alluded to the fact that a letter of support from the chief executive officer or professional head can influence the participation and agreement of others in provision of access to research subjects. The problem of coercion becomes more acute if there is a line relationship between the researcher and the subjects, or there is a care dependency relationship. For example, the authors are aware that nurse educationalists often use student nurses as the subjects for research study. If the research is conducted with their own students, then often students may feel that they have no option but to co-operate in the study. Similarly, nurse teachers may feel unable to refuse a head of department access to the teacher's own students since a clear hierarchical power relationship is present.

The primary concern for all should be the well-being of their patient or those they care for. This tenet is enshrined within the document issued by the United Kingdom Central Council for Nursing, Midwifery and Health Visiting on exercising accountability (UKCC, 1989). A researcher who is a nurse and also wishes to conduct research within her own hospital or institution must be careful that both the research subject granting permission, and the manager/professional head approving access, must be clear of their role and not be swayed by personal knowledge of the researcher. It is therefore essential that adequate external advice is available to the researcher in ensuring that the decisions that are being taken regarding access within an institution in which the researcher is known, are comparable to those that would be taken if the researcher was proposing to do the study in an institution elsewhere.

Ethics committee approval

All research conducted within the auspices of the National Health Service and involving human subjects or personal information relating to them requires the approval of the local ethics committee. The responsibility for establishing an ethics committee lies with the Health Authority, not the hospital or institution. Clear guidance has been developed by the Department of Health (1991) on how these committees should be constituted and run. This guidance was initiated since, in the past, many researchers found that ethics committees, if they existed, met on an infrequent basis and the decision-making process was often unclear. More recently, an additional set of documents on the standards by which ethics committees should be assessed has been developed. Ethics committees are encouraged to comply with these standards and to audit themselves against them. Access to the guidelines for the establishment of ethics committees, and for the standards of their functioning, can be a useful and informative source for novice researchers wishing to navigate their way through the process of successfully gaining ethics committee approval. It is important to make contact with the ethics committee at an early stage to ascertain whether or not there is a specific protocol that requires to be followed in making an ethics committee application. For example, it is not uncommon for the format of the protocol to be specified in detail. The researcher will sometimes be presented with a computer disk with a draft format that needs to be completed. In addition to a pro-forma, extensive guidance explaining the type of response required for each section is often provided. Clearly, early access to such material is essential if delays are to be avoided.

Historically, research ethics committees tended to be most familiar with randomized control trials, for example, assessing the effectiveness of new therapeutic agents. Thankfully, most ethics committees now have considerable experience with the full range of research designs. However, it is often in the researcher's best interest to identify who among the membership of the ethics committee has a particular interest or understanding of the approach being proposed. Initial contact with this individual may assist in ensuring that all necessary information is presented to the committee.

In those health districts that have a large number of teaching establishments, a model of devolved responsibility is often in operation. This is where individual members of the committee will be given the responsibility of screening protocols and contacting the researcher at an early stage, conducting a detailed ethical review and presenting the work at the committee for debate. Obviously, it is in the researcher's interest to ascertain if such a model is in place since the member with devolved responsibility for the intended study may provide useful guidance at an early stage.

Although it is unlikely that a neophyte researcher will attempt a multi-centre research project as her first study, there are a number of issues relating to access that are peculiar to this sort of design. Historically, researchers who wished to gather data from subjects located across several organizations would need to apply to each individual ethics committee and try to negotiate approval with each one individually. Each ethics committee might ask for minor changes which would then need to be approved by all other committees. This approach was most unsatisfactory since, at best, it delayed approval and, at worst, often resulted in one ethics committee requesting changes that another would not agree with. To remedy this situation a system has been established where a researcher who wishes to undertake multi-centre studies can gain approval from a single regionally based ethics committee. In England each NHS region has its own committee, while Scotland, Wales and Northern Ireland have one each.

Litigation and insurance

The recent increases in the number of cases of litigation against researchers and the host organizations within which they operate has led to ethics committees being particularly conscientious in ensuring that the researcher and the organization have adequate insurance (Mander, 1992). Drug companies will provide insurance cover, sufficient to deal with any claims, for harm caused by the particular drug that is being tested. However, this does not usually cover errors in administration. If, for example, the researcher were to administer the wrong dose of drug, then it is likely that the researcher rather than the company would be liable. This is a particularly complex field and it is the responsibility of the ethics committee to ensure that all research is adequately insured. It is therefore essential that the researcher discusses with the chairman of the ethics committee the type of insurance that her particular study will require, and the proof necessary to be presented as part of the application process.

Informed consent

Another area that often causes novice researchers some particular difficulties is that of informed consent. For research subjects to be able to make an informed choice they need adequate information, in a language that is readily understandable to them, giving details of what will happen to them and any associated risks. In the past many researchers were reluctant to provide such information since they would argue that to do so might influence the outcome of the research. Such an argument is no longer defensible and any researcher seeking to hide information from a subject will not be given research approval by the ethics committee.

Confidentiality and anonymity

Assurances regarding subject confidentiality and anonymity will also require to be addressed. It is often possible to offer people anonymity provided that the subjects are drawn from a large enough pool and that the reporting of results is done in a way that does not localize the information to a particular hospital department or ward. Researchers must therefore be careful when writing-up their studies not to breach confidentiality or anonymity.

Numbers of subjects and their selection

Another area which the research ethics committees are particularly concerned with is the number of subjects to be approached and how they are selected. The researcher will need considerable clarity over this point if her study is to gain ethics committee approval. Clearly dependent on the research design, the number of subjects and the method of sampling may vary considerably. You should, therefore, be prepared to defend both the size of the sample and the method of sampling against challenges from the committee. Clarity over the advantages and disadvantages of the various approaches that could be used to select the sample for the particular study being proposed is a worthwhile preparatory step.

Since the publication of guidance on the establishment of local research ethics committees, all committees must report on an annual basis the research that has been approved by the committee (Department of Health, 1991). This list can obviously provide the researcher with much useful information since it can identify work already going on in the field that may interact with the researcher's own planned study. Furthermore, it can also provide a ready-made network of individuals with an interest in the researcher's field. This information is in the public domain and therefore it is legitimate for a novice researcher to approach researchers already conducting work in the field. Early contact with such individuals can often provide valuable insights into how access to the research site can best be facilitated.

Approaching subjects

Having successfully navigated the gatekeepers, both professional and organizational, and gained the approval of the local ethics committee, research subjects still need to be approached. The method of selection will have been detailed as part of the research protocol, as will the information that will be provided to ensure informed consent. However, the manner in which subjects are approached can have a significant influence on whether they agree or refuse to participate. A quiet, polite, unhurried and assertive approach is often the most successful. Sufficient time must be set aside to ensure that the potential subjects have adequate opportunity to ask any questions. Impatience or tactlessness not only result in research subjects declining to participate but may also result in the professional organizational gatekeepers withdrawing access as reports of such behaviour are fed back. Generally speaking, subjects are usually more than willing to participate provided the researcher takes the time to explain what the study is about and gives the individuals the respect they deserve. After all, without the good will of research subjects, researchers would be very limited in the type of study they could conduct.

Conclusions

Gaining access to a research site can be time-consuming. However, if the researcher identifies the necessary gatekeepers at an early stage, approaches them in a systematic way, and seeks the support of peers in the process, access to the research site is a relatively straightforward step.

Like many things in this life, having successfully negotiated access to a research site for the first time, the second and subsequent occasions become far easier. This is not simply because the researcher is aware of who needs to be contacted, but also a track record has been established. Accordingly, researchers need to pay particular attention to any promises made in relation to the feedback of research results to ensure that access on a subsequent occasion is not denied.

References

Department of Health (1991) *Local Research Ethics Committees*. London: HMSO.

Institute of Health Service Management (1998) *The Hospitals and Health Services Year Book*. London: Institute of Health Service Management.

Mander, R. (1992) Seeking approval for research access: the gatekeeper's role in facilitating a study of the care of the relinquishing mother. *Journal of Advanced Nursing* **17** (11): 1460–4.

National Health Service Training Directorate (1994) *Using Standards for Local Research Ethics Committees*. Bristol: National Health Services Training Directorate.

UKCC (1989) *Exercising Accountability: Advisory Document*. London: United Kingdom Central Council for Nursing, Midwifery and Health Visiting.

Further reading

Morse, J.M. (1992) Re: The role of nursing research committees. *Nursing Research* **41** (6): 374–7.

O'Carroll, D. and McMahon, A. (1998) Research and development co-ordinating centre. *Nursing Standard* **12** (38): 32–3.

Traynor, M. and Rafferty, A.M. (1997) Policy for research in nursing: a new centre. *Nursing Standard* **11** (21): 32–3.

B: Research design

The research design represents the major methodological thrust of the study, being the distinctive and specific research approach which is best suited to answering the research question(s). As will be seen in Chapters 12 to 22, the major research designs – which are not always entirely mutually exclusive – each have individual advantages which make them appropriate in particular circumstances.

Selection of the research design is influenced both by the research question and the aim and objectives of the research. Selection of a research design is always preceded by clearly identifying the purpose of the research. In selecting an appropriate design, it is useful to have a general knowledge of a variety of designs and thereby be able to consider a range of possibilities, eliminate those which are not appropriate, and select the one which is best suited to your particular study. As with many aspects of the research process, it is rarely possible to achieve perfection. In selecting a research design, bear in mind that whichever one is chosen, it will be imperfect and have some limitations with regard to your particular needs. However, careful consideration of research designs will enable selection of the one which has the 'best fit' for your particular study.

The chapters in this section are intended to give readers of research reports an insight into a few selected research designs. They are also intended to give researchers, working under supervision, an introduction to the major research methodologies, and to provide the basis for selecting a specific design which can then be studied in detail by making use of the references provided at the end of each chapter.

CHAPTER 12

Qualitative research

Sam Porter

The first questions to be asked in relation to qualitative methods are: 'What is it?' and 'What makes it different from other forms of research?' The short answer to these questions is that the uniqueness of qualitative research lies in the fact that it does not focus primarily upon the identification and explanation of facts, but upon the illumination of people's interpretations of those facts. As a consequence, qualitative research is an appropriate mode of enquiry when researchers wish to study the understandings and motivations of the research subjects. These rather sweeping statements require clarification. The conventional way of providing this is to contrast qualitative with quantitative approaches. Numerous divisions can be set up between the two methods.

Contrasting qualitative and quantitative methods

The first difference that can be noted between the two approaches is the focus of their analysis. While the focus of quantitative research is primarily upon *numbers*, often aggregated into statistics, qualitative research concentrates on *words*, either in the form of speech or writing. In addition to their focus of analysis, each approach is associated with a number of assumptions. Quantitative methods are often associated with the aim of identifying and explaining causal relationships between events. Thus, by noting that apples always fell to the ground when loosened from a tree, Newton was identifying a causal relationship. By propounding his law of gravity, he explained the relationship.

Qualitative researchers often argue that this sort of explanation is inappropriate when the subject matter of research is the actions of human beings. Apples have no choice but to fall to the ground; humans often do have a choice about the sort of behaviour they display. As a consequence, it is argued that research into human behaviour should focus on the motivations that people have for doing the sorts of things they do. In short, qualitative research is often associated with the search for reasons rather than causes. This in turn means that, in contrast to quantitative methods whose aim is often to *explain* why something happens, qualitative approaches seek to *understand* the interpretations and motivations of people.

While quantitative researchers often aspire to *objectivity* – the assumption that facts can and should be presented in a manner untainted by the feelings, opinions or bias of the researcher or researched – qualitative researchers emphasize the importance of *subjectivity* – the assumption that the sole foundation of factual knowledge is private experience.

Belief in the significance of subjective factors in qualitative research is not limited to the subjectivities of the researched. Qualitative analysts often assert the need for researchers to reveal the values, interests and influences associated with their own subjective experiences. This process is termed *reflexivity* (Hammersley & Atkinson, 1995). Good research involves reflexivity at several levels. First, researchers should identify the theoretical framework they are operating within, along with the values and commitments they adhere to. Second, they should reflect upon how personal factors specific to their own biographies may affect the research. Finally, researchers should describe and reflect upon the import of the methods used in their research and the context within which it is conducted.

To signal their reflexivity, qualitative researchers often use the first person active to describe themselves, rather than the traditional third person passive ('I noted …' instead of 'it was noted by the researcher …'). In line with this qualitative tradition, I shall use the first person to refer to myself in both this chapter and Chapter 32.

Artificial divisions

Having set up a number of divisions between qualitative and quantitative methods, I should warn readers that neither style of research fits neatly into these categories. The purpose of this contrast was to give a flavour of the ideas underlying different approaches to research, rather than to make definitive statements about them. Indeed, I am acutely aware that, in contradiction to what I said above about reasons and causes, my own research (Porter, 1993a) provides an example of the use of qualitative methods to elucidate causal relations. One of the most encouraging aspects of recent advances in research has been the willingness of researchers to overcome divisions through the incorporation of that which is best from both traditions into their research designs.

The theoretical foundations of qualitative research

As with any system of investigation, qualitative research is founded upon a number of wider assumptions, which can be classified according to four levels of understanding. These levels are ontology, epistemology, methodology and methods. What is meant by these rather daunting philosophical terms, will be explained below. However, before examining the four levels, two points need to be underlined. First, it needs to be emphasized that the following is only one (albeit common) version of the assumptions underlying the use of qualitative methods; alternative groundings can be constructed. Second, these are assumptions and are therefore open to debate and disagreement. Despite being presented here in the form of a catechism, they should not be taken as gospel.

Level 1: Ontology

Ontology concerns questions about what exists.

Question: What is the subject matter of qualitative research?
Answer: Social reality.

Question: What is the nature of social reality?
Answer: Social reality involves the meaningful actions and interactions of individuals.

Qualitative research has been much influenced by a branch of philosophy known as *phenomenology*. The basic premise of phenomenology is that the nature of the outside world, independent of our thoughts about it, can never be known. All that can be known is how people perceive and interpret that reality. After all, how do we know anything, except through the use of our senses and mental faculties? Thus for phenomenology, the aim of knowledge is not to uncover the nature of the external world, but to understand how we come to know the world as we do. One of the consequences of this position is that reality is not a fixed entity. It changes and develops according to people's experiences, and the social context within which they find themselves.

The significance of social context is crucial because it is through our social interactions with others – parents, teachers, friends and health care professionals, to name but a few – that our understandings and preconceptions about the nature of reality are formed. This is not just a one-way process, in that through our interactions with each other, we help create the social world around us. It is for this reason that it was stated above that social reality only exists as meaningful social interaction between individuals.

As a qualification it should be noted that, for some qualitative researchers, acceptance of the importance of social context implies that phenomenological understanding is not enough. They argue that social reality is more than individuals' understandings; it also consists of the social structures that enable and constrain the actions and interpretations of individuals (Porter, 1993a). Nevertheless, it remains true to say that phenomenology is the bedrock of most qualitative research.

Application of phenomenology to nursing leads qualitative researchers to concentrate on people's experiences of being ill. As Benner & Wrubel (1989) put it: 'Illness as a human experience of loss or dysfunction has a reality all its own.' This line of reasoning entails a rejection of the traditional medical model of the ontology of illness, which equates the reality of illness with physical manifestations of disease or disablement. The focus of the medical model is seen as unacceptably narrow, in that the reality of sickness cannot be reduced to the biochemical processes of the disease from which a person is suffering. Proper understanding must include the person's subjective experience and understanding of the illness, and the social context within which that experience and understanding occur.

The significance of this revision of the ontology of illness should not be underestimated. Jerrett (1994), in her phenomenological study of the experiences of parents with chronically ill children, makes the point well when she argues that: 'their subjective experience is fundamentally important not just because it involves a personal reassessment of objective reality, but because lived experience is reality'.

Level 2: Epistemology

Epistemology concerns questions about what we can know about what exists.

Question: What counts as knowledge of social reality?
Answer: Our knowledge of social reality equates with our understanding of the meanings and motives which guide the actions and interactions of individuals.

The connection here between epistemology and ontology is clear. If social reality consists of the experiences and understandings of people, then knowledge of reality will be knowledge of those experiences and understandings. An example of the application of this sort of epistemological assumption to nursing research can be seen in Melia's (1982) pioneering qualitative study of student nursing. For Melia, the reality of student nursing lay in the students' own constructions of their nursing world. Therefore, the interest of the research 'lay in obtaining the student nurses' view of nursing, in other words to allow the students to "tell it as it is"'. For Melia, 'telling it as it is' involved gaining knowledge of the experiences, understandings and motives of the subjects that she was researching.

Gaining such knowledge is not as simple as it first might seem. A thorny question that has long troubled phenomenological researchers is whether or not it is actually possible to get inside people's minds in order to fully understand their experiences. One problem here is that, in a completed research report, the understandings of the subjects have been filtered through the understandings of the researcher, and it is very difficult to tell the degree of distortion that has occurred in the process. As Melia (1982) observes, the part played by the qualitative researcher in the production of data is crucial.

The epistemological claims of qualitative research are cautious; for many qualitative researchers absolute knowledge of reality is simply not possible – knowledge of social reality will always be coloured by the interpretations of the researcher (Porter, 1993b).

Level 3: Methodology

Methodology concerns questions about the manner in which we can gain knowledge about what exists.

Question: How can we know about the nature of social reality?
Answer: Social reality can be discovered by looking at it through the perspective of the individuals living in it.

Question: How can such a perspective be gained?
Answer: This perspective can be gained by using methods which illuminate the meanings and motives of subjects.

Qualitative researchers are required to interpret as accurately as possible the experiences, meanings and motives of subjects, from the perspectives of those subjects. Accuracy in the reproduction of subjects' perspectives largely depends upon the researcher's knowledge of and familiarity with the social setting being studied. Gaining this familiarity takes a considerable period of time, spent either as a participant observer or an interviewer. The qualitative researcher needs to immerse herself as fully as possible in the lives or work of the people she is studying.

However, irrespective of the degree of involvement, the influence of the researcher's own perspective will remain, and it is necessary to construct a methodology which takes account of this. Here lies the importance of reflexivity. By openly examining and reporting on how their own experiences and understandings have impinged upon the nature of research, researchers open up their influence upon the research to the scrutiny of readers, who can then make their own judgements about the authenticity and persuasiveness of the findings.

Thus Melia (1982), in a reflexive account of her research, outlined for the reader the degree of knowledge that she had of the social world of the student nurses in her study. She pointed out that, having trained and practised as a nurse, she had a degree of familiarity with the setting, with the jargon used and with hospital ways in general. However, she was careful to point out gaps in her knowledge of the specific social world that she was examining. She noted that her experience of training was not the conventional three-year programme in which her subjects were studying, and that she had trained in a different institution to that in which they were training.

It can be seen how Melia's reflexive account gives her readers the opportunity to judge the degree of knowledge that she had about the world of her research subjects, and thus about the accuracy of her reproduction of their perspectives. In the absence of statistical tests for reliability and validity, this sort of reflexivity is crucial to qualitative research if it is to be persuasive.

Level 4: Methods

Methods are the techniques used to collect evidence about what exists.

Question: What are the best ways to gather information about the meanings and motives of individuals?

Answer: Those methods which:

(1) enable researchers to become involved in the social world of the subjects they are studying – an involvement that can give researchers direct experience of the meanings and motives of subjects;

(2) give subjects the opportunity to describe and explain, in their own words, the meanings and motives which provide the basis for their actions and interactions.

A number of methods have been devised by qualitative researchers to gather data, either by involving themselves in the subjects' social world or by allowing subjects to describe their understandings on their own terms. These methods include in-depth interviews, oral history, participant observation and conversation analysis.

In-depth interviews

The most common qualitative method used in nursing research is the in-depth interview. Other terms for this form of interviewing are 'unstructured' (if there is no prior format for the interview), 'semi-structured' (if there is some format, but the interview is allowed to expand beyond the bounds of that format), 'informal' or 'ethnographic'. The rationale for in-depth interviewing is to give subjects the opportunity to describe their experiences in their own words.

In-depth interviewing can be used either as a free-standing method of enquiry or in conjunction with participant observation. When combined with participant observation, the information supplied by interviewees can explain and put into context that which the observer has seen during observation.

In in-depth interviews, the researcher starts out with only a general plan about the direction the conversation will take. Qualitative researchers tend to avoid questionnaires or heavily structured interview formats for two reasons. First, it is argued that informal interviews provide a more natural setting. If people are allowed to chat freely about their lives in a non-threatening environment, they will tend to be more forthcoming. Second, it is contended that the way questions are constructed in structured interviews and questionnaires tends to reinforce the questioner's assumptions. This leads to two dangers. First, interviewees may feel pressurized into agreeing with what they perceive as the researcher's pre-conceptions about the 'right' answer. Second, there is a danger that the researcher will be entirely off the mark, asking the wrong questions about the problem being investigated. If there is no opportunity for interviewees to have an input outside the confines of a predetermined structure, then such errors may go unnoticed by the researcher. It is argued that in-depth interviews can overcome these problems because they involve less influence on the part of the interviewer and more influence on the part of the interviewee.

Many examples of this method could be chosen. One is Wuest & Stern's (1991) study of families of children with persistent middle ear problems. Wuest & Stern interviewed ten such families in order to learn about the factors that influenced family interaction. They discovered that one of the main concerns of family members was how to manage the day-to-day practicalities of family life. The interviews revealed that families felt that they were not getting adequate support from health professionals to help them to cope with their situation. Wuest & Stern concluded that nurses have the potential to become a major resource for families with chronically ill children by providing this service.

Oral history

A variant of the in-depth interview is known as *oral history*. This is used if the social setting the researcher wants to find out about existed in the past, thus making it impossible for the researcher to become directly involved in it. As in in-depth interviews, subjects in oral histories are given the opportunity to describe and explain their past experiences in their own words.

A good example of the use of this method in nursing research is Keddy *et al*.'s (1986) examination of the relationship between nurses and doctors that pertained in Canada in the 1920s and 1930s. To gain information about what it was like to be nursing in this era, Keddy *et al*. (1986) taped 34 semi-structured interviews with older nurses, asking them to recall past events and experiences from their work histories. One of the main themes that emerged from these interviews was the significance of nurses' relationships with doctors in this era – a relationship in which doctors enjoyed almost absolute authority.

Participant observation

Participant observation is the classic qualitative method. As its name implies, it involves researchers participating in the daily life of their research subjects, while at the same time observing the actions and interpretations of subjects going about their day-to-day business. The aim of this qualitative method is to attain an *insider's* view of the group under study. This is gained both by the researcher's direct experience, and by the information given to the researcher during conversations with members of the group under study.

The recording of data gained from participant observation may be done through audio- or video-taping. However, the most common method of data recording is the use of fieldnotes. As the name suggests, these are observations written manually into a notebook by the researcher. They involve detailed descriptions of social situations and interactions that occur in the 'field' of research, *field* being the term used for the location where data are gathered.

Participant observation has a long history. However, it was not until the early twentieth century that it was developed as a method of scientific enquiry by

European anthropologists such as Malinowski (1922), who used it to study non-western cultures, and by the 'Chicago School' of sociology, who used it to examine subcultures closer to home.

Despite being a well-established method of social research, there are limitations to its use in nursing research, especially when the proposed subjects of research are health care clients. This is largely due to the practicalities of research – it is very difficult for a healthy researcher to participate in the social world of those who are ill. Given that the primary focus of qualitative nursing research is upon this group, the possibilities of participant observation, in contrast to those of in-depth interviewing, are somewhat limited. However, qualitative nursing researchers can participate in the social world of clinical nurses. One example of this approach is my own work into the influence of gender upon nurses' professional relationships with medical colleagues (Porter, 1992). The data for that study were gathered during three months of participant observation conducted in an intensive care unit. By working in the unit as a staff nurse, I was able to immerse myself in the occupational lives of my research subjects.

First, I looked to see if there were any differences in the quality of interaction depending on the sex of those involved. I found that while the gender of a nurse had little effect upon the quality of interaction between nurse and doctor, the gender of a doctor had quite a strong effect, with female doctors often being more egalitarian in their dealings with nurses than their male counterparts. Examination of nurses' attitudes to gender issues showed that they resented doctors' expectations for them to act as handmaidens, and regarded it as perfectly valid to respond to medical pomposity in an assertive manner. However, while nurses were prepared to criticize doctors who were openly chauvinistic, they did not extend their critique to medicine as a whole, seeing sexism as an individual phenomenon rather than an institutional ethos.

It can be seen from this example that participant observation can be used both to discover the nature of interaction in a social setting, and to illuminate the understandings and motives of those involved in the interactions.

Conversation analysis

A more formal method of observation of social interaction is used in the technique of conversation analysis. The aim here is to study how people talk to each other in everyday settings. Emphasis lies in how conversations are technically constructed to accomplish ordered conversational interaction. Because even the smallest nuances in conversations are important in this type of research, the use of a tape recorder is essential. Even better is a video recorder, which also records gestures and facial expressions, thus giving a fuller picture of the processes of communication.

In this form of research, the researcher usually takes on a passive role, allowing research subjects to carry on normal day-to-day conversational activities, and recording them while they do so. The recordings of conversations are then transcribed using a specialized annotation, in which, for example, the lengths of pauses are timed to a tenth of a second, and interruptions and overlaps of speech are marked. What is said is recorded phonetically, rather than being translated into standard English. While this sort of detailed analysis of mundane encounters may seem trivial, conversation analysts assert its importance on the basis that talk is the building block of all social interaction and that, conversely, broader social processes permeate down to conversational interaction.

A pertinent example of the use of conversation analysis can be found in Brewer *et al.*'s (1991) study of the conversations of children with severe learning difficulties. By studying the group dynamics of conversations, Brewer and colleagues discovered that, contrary to popular images that regard children with learning difficulties as communicatively incompetent, these children possessed considerable conversational skills. One child was seen as highly adept at orchestrating encounters with others, skilfully organizing, structuring and controlling conversations. However, the other children were far from incompetent as co-conversationalists, and were capable of appropriate responses and turn-taking. By methodically breaking down the talk of children with severe learning difficulties into the basic component parts of verbal interaction, Brewer *et al.* (1991) demonstrated the organized nature of their conversations, thus providing a useful challenge to our preconceptions.

The functions of qualitative research in nursing

As has been seen, the purpose of much qualitative research is to describe the meanings and motives of an identified group of people as faithfully as possible. The focus can be on patients, as in Johnson's (1994) study of how overweight people restructure their perspectives during the process of dieting; on relatives, as in Jerrett's (1994) study of parents with chronically ill children; or even on nurses, as in Melia's (1982) influential study of the lives of student nurses.

However, qualitative research is not always descriptive. It can also be used to test theories. An example of this approach can be found in May's (1992) examination of the degree to which Foucault's (1973) notion of the 'clinical gaze', which characterizes the relationship between doctors and patients as entailing medical surveillance, can be applied to the nurse–patient relationship.

Qualitative research can also be useful in policy evaluation. An example of this approach can be found in Mason's (1994) comparative study of community maternal and child health policies in Jamaica and Northern Ireland.

Conclusions

The increasing significance of qualitative research in nursing is indicated by the fact that in the first edition of this book it did not merit a chapter of its own. It now merits several, and there is good reason to believe that its importance will continue to grow. The change in nursing philosophy, away from a mechanistic approach to patients towards a more holistic perspective on care, leads to more emphasis being put upon the wants, needs and fears of patients. This change in emphasis inevitably entails the adoption of research methodologies which allow for the elucidation of those wants, needs and fears.

The shift towards qualitative research has been accelerated by the increasing influence upon nursing academics of feminist research concerns, which also place personal experience at the centre of the research agendum. Hagell (1989) makes this point very clearly:

'Nursing, as a discipline, has a distinct knowledge base which is not grounded in empirico-analytical science and its methodology but which stems from the lived experience of nurses as women and as nurses involved in caring relationships with their clients.'

Given the convergence of nursing concerns and qualitative ideas about the importance of people's experience, there are good reasons to believe that qualitative methods will enjoy an increasingly prominent place in nursing research. Indeed, it could even be that the use of qualitative research will come to distinguish nursing knowledge from the sort of knowledge that other, more mechanistically oriented, health professionals aspire to.

References

Benner, P. & Wrubel, J. (1989) *The Primacy of Caring*. Menlo Park, California: Addison-Wesley.

Brewer, J.D., McBride, G. & Yearley, S. (1991) Orchestrating an encounter: a note on the talk of mentally handicapped children. *Sociology of Health and Illness* **13**: 58–67.

Foucault, M. (1973) *The Birth of the Clinic*. London: Tavistock.

Hagell, E. (1989) Nursing knowledge: women's knowledge. A sociological perspective. *Journal of Advanced Nursing* **14**: 226–33.

Hammersley, M. & Atkinson, P. (1995) *Ethnography: Principles in Practice*, 2nd edn. London: Routledge.

Jerrett, M. (1994) Parents' experience of coming to know the care of a chronically ill child. *Journal of Advanced Nursing* **19**: 1050–6.

Johnson, R. (1994) Restructuring: an emerging theory on the process of losing weight. In J.P. Smith (ed.) *Models, Theories and Concepts*. Oxford: Blackwell Scientific Publications: pp. 31–46.

Keddy, B., Jones Gillis, M., Jacobs, P., Burton, H. & Rogers, M. (1986) The doctor–nurse relationship: an historical perspective. *Journal of Advanced Nursing* 7: 327–35.

Malinowski, E. (1922) *Argonauts of the Western Pacific*. New York: Dutton.

Mason, C. (1994) Maternal and child health needs in Northern Ireland and Jamaica: official and lay perspectives. *Qualitative Health Research* 4: 74–93.

May, C. (1992) Individual care? Power and subjectivity in therapeutic relationships. *Sociology* 26: 589–602.

Melia, K. (1982) 'Tell it as it is' – qualitative methodology and nursing research: understanding the student nurse's world. *Journal of Advanced Nursing* 7: 327–35.

Porter, S. (1992) Women in a women's job: the gendered experience of nurses. *Sociology of Health and Illness* 14: 510–27.

Porter, S. (1993a) Critical realist ethnography: the case of racism and professionalism in a medical setting. *Sociology* 27: 591–609.

Porter, S. (1993b) Nursing research conventions: objectivity or obfuscation? *Journal of Advanced Nursing* 18: 137–43.

Wuest, J. & Stern, P. (1991) Empowerment and primary health care: the challenge for nurses. *Qualitative Health Research* 1: 80–99.

Further reading

For readers wishing to study qualitative research in more depth, the following large text is probably the most useful source:

Denzin, N.K. & Lincoln, Y.S. (1994) *Handbook of Qualitative Inquiry*. London: Sage.

This volume has subsequently been reprinted in three paperback volumes:

Denzin, N.K. & Lincoln, Y.S. (1998) *The Landscape of Qualitative Research*. London: Sage.

Denzin, N.K. & Lincoln, Y.S. (1998) *Strategies of Qualitative Inquiry*. London: Sage.

Denzin, N.K. & Lincoln, Y.S. (1998) *Collecting and Interpreting Qualitative Materials*. London: Sage.

For more specific applications of qualitative research to nursing:

Holloway, I. & Wheeler, S. (eds) (1996) *Qualitative Research for Nurses*. Oxford: Blackwell Science.

CHAPTER 13

Grounded theory

David C. Benton

A casual review of any scholarly journal that publishes nursing and midwifery research will reveal a wide range of methods used by researchers encompassing both quantitative and qualitative approaches. However, a similar review of the same journal ten years ago would yield a quite different picture. In the past ten years, it has been observed that there has been a noticeable increase in the number of published studies which use qualitative techniques. This increase can be attributed to the fact that nurses now feel confident enough as researchers to select the most appropriate methods to meet the needs of the topic under study. It can be argued that any method which facilitates the discovery of variables associated with the provision of care can contribute to the development of nursing knowledge and the associated theory base. Furthermore, inductive approaches to the development of theory can be readily employed by those who wish to undertake research and to practise related topics.

One means of inductive theory generation which has been consistently utilized by nurses since its development by Glaser & Strauss (1967), is that of the *grounded theory* method. This method has been used by researchers to develop inductive theories on topics as diverse as couple communication patterns, quality of care from the patients' perspective and competence validation and cognitive flexibility. There is a need for nurses and midwives to develop their own theories of health care – theories which have been developed directly from the everyday practice of members of the profession. Since grounded theory entails the development of theory from data that have been methodically obtained from the real-life setting, it is ideally suited to the needs of those who wish to investigate topics about which little is known.

Many aspects of nursing and midwifery are qualitative in nature and, as yet, under-researched. This fact, along with the need to develop a knowledge base, has resulted in the utilization of the grounded theory method. It is the intention of this chapter to clearly identify the processes involved in undertaking a grounded theory study and provide guidance which will assist you, should you wish to conduct research using this method.

The grounded theory method

The grounded theory method is ideally suited to the investigation of those topics about which there is little prior knowledge. The method developed by Glaser & Strauss (1967) requires that you approach data collection without a preconceived framework. Without an open-minded approach, there is a danger that significant material will be ignored since data that are seen as not fitting the existing model may be disregarded. The use of the grounded theory approach will enable you to develop theories based on the reality of the topic under study. This process will encourage you to explore data in order to discover the basic social and psychological processes operating within the area of enquiry.

Unlike quantitative methods, the grounded theory approach does not proceed in a linear fashion. Grounded theory is typified by the concurrent activities of data collection, organization, and analysis. This process continues until a theory is developed which is of sufficient detail and at a sufficient level of abstraction to explain the variation in the data observed. The process by which the grounded theory is generated is known as the constant comparative method – a method by which every element of data is compared with every other element.

Data sources and methods of collection

Data are commonly generated through field observations or by examination of documentary evidence. Field observation is a process where data are generated by observation, interview or video- or audio-taping. This entails close interpersonal contact with the subjects of the study. To help you to understand the role you play in this process, it is advisable to keep a daily journal or diary. Thoughts, impressions, or emotional reactions experienced, can all be recorded and may assist in understanding the material gathered.

Data collection initially starts with an attempt to examine the wider issues surrounding the topic under study. Only when you have established the wider context should more focused investigation begin.

Interviews and observation are two techniques frequently used to generate data for a study utilizing the grounded theory method. These techniques are not unique to grounded theory and are described in detail in Chapters 24 and 26 respectively. Nevertheless, data obtained from these sources can be confusing at first. However, since organization and analysis of the data begin at an early stage, this should enable you to identify areas which can be clarified in subsequent interviews or observations.

Theoretical sampling

Theoretical sampling is the term used to describe the manner in which data sources are identified and selected for inclusion in a study and is integrally linked with the constant comparative method of data analysis. Initial decisions about sampling are based upon general understanding of the area under investigation. This initial decision is the only decision that you can pre-plan, since the selection of all other data sources is controlled by the emerging theory. Unlike other forms of research, such as the experimental or survey design, you are unable to identify the size and characteristics of the sample at the outset of the study. In a grounded theory design, you are only able to identify the sample, retrospectively, once the theory has been generated.

Individuals, groups, or situations, are selected to provide comparison data. Theoretical sampling can either attempt to minimize or maximize the differences between the comparisons being made. By minimizing differences, you can collect data which can assist you in identifying the basic properties of categories and the specific conditions under which they exist. Furthermore, minimizing differences can also assist you in identifying those fundamental ways in which categories vary. Maximizing differences between data sources increases the chance of identifying different properties of the categories and finding those properties which are most stable.

Reliability and validity of data

Quantitative researchers have sometimes suggested that there is a tendency to ignore the issues of reliability and validity or to consider them irrelevant, when undertaking research based in the qualitative paradigm.

If research is to be of value, then it must address the issues of reliability and validity. Glaser & Strauss (1967) have argued that reliability is established by taking findings back to those respondents who provided the original data from which you generated the theory. Respondents can then confirm or refute the theory developed. If this process is used on an ongoing basis, then it is similar to the test/retest approach that is used in quantitative research to establish reliability.

Validity of the theory can be established on the same basis as that advocated for reliability. By taking developing theory back to the original informants, you can receive feedback which can be used to establish validity.

Grounded theory addresses the issues of reliability and validity. More general issues concerning reliability and validity as applied to qualitative research were addressed in Chapter 3 where reliability and validity relating to quantitative research was fully discussed. However, by using independent experts, it is possible to examine various aspects of the process of developing grounded theory for reliability and validity. It is suggested that not only can the method provide data on the reliability and validity of a study, but it is also capable of identifying investigative bias and conceptual clarity.

Data recording

The grounded theory approach is dependent upon the accuracy of the source data; thus, data recording is a vital step in the entire process. Data are most frequently recorded by use of audio-tape or/and written notes. Alternatively, you may choose to use video-tape which, in addition to a verbal record, can also provide data on non-verbal behaviour. If audio-tape is used then it is necessary to add non-verbal data at the stage of transcription. Transcription is the process where the audio record is typed ready for coding and analysis.

The choice of audio, video or written data recording will be dependent upon a number of issues. The recording and transcription of audio- or video-tape requires access to equipment and possibly secretarial resources. Written methods of recording are less expensive, but the data may not be as accurate or complete unless you are able to use shorthand. Consequently, since completeness and accuracy are important, and if adequate resources are available, tape should be used. However, dependent on the location and preferences of the respondents, it may not be possible or appropriate to use recording devices. Informants may refuse to participate if tape is used, or they may be working in areas where background noise could result in a poor quality recording, incapable of transcription.

If you are unable to use any form of data-recording technique during the interview or observation, then it is important that a permanent record is made as soon after the event as possible. Go to a quiet place and either write or dictate notes, identifying and recording as much detail as possible.

Whichever approach is used, it is important that certain information always appears on the data record. First, the name of the interviewer/observer and the date, time and place where the interview/observation occurred. Second, the individual, group or subject being interviewed/observed. For clarity, all pages should be typed with double spacing and ample margins. Ideally, the interviewer data should appear on one side of the page and the interviewee data on the other. All pages should also be numbered and referenced to ensure that data do not go missing or appear out of context. Figure 13.1 illustrates an example of how a transcribed interview should appear. Please note that the name and source of data would not normally appear on published material: in this case, all identifying characteristics are fictitious.

Explaining terminology

There are a number of terms that have particular meaning when applied to the grounded theory approach. These include substantive codes, categories and

Interview:	John Brown, Director of Quality
Date and Time	10/08/1999 10:30 AM
Location	Rural Health Authority
Researcher	Mary Smith Page 3 of 28

Interviewer
What were your hopes for the post?

Interviewee
While there might have been more lofty aims to do with integrating research into practice and all that sort of thing, it was much more about safeguarding nursing. It was about getting influence, I felt that nursing had lost influence when general management came in. Because of the kind of research that was put forward I got the feeling that general managers didn't value what was being done. To get any sort of credibility there was a need to take the initiative by getting it right. Playing the game by their rules.

Fig. 13.1   Excerpt from interview illustrating a suitable layout.

properties, theoretical constructs, core categories, and saturation. An understanding of the meaning of these terms and the relationship between them is vital if you are to undertake a study using a grounded theory design.

Substantive codes

When data are collected, you require to examine the various incidents in order to label those items or words which you feel contribute to the comprehension of the underlying processes. Coding of the actual substance of the data is referred to as *substantive coding*. At this early stage of coding, individual words or short phrases are highlighted in the text and codes are written in the margin. To ensure detailed theoretical coverage, each sentence and incident should be coded into as many substantive codes as possible – a process known as *open coding*. This may result in some data being coded into more than one substantive code. This process can be supported by the use of computer technology and software, but this will be discussed elsewhere (see Chapter 33).

Categories and properties

Glaser & Strauss (1967) suggest that categories can be thought of as analogous to variables in quantitative research. Categories are produced when a number of substantive codes are condensed into a higher level of abstraction. Categories are commonly used to describe a class of individuals, events, situations or phenomena that have certain characteristics in common. To have meaning, a category must be capable of being uniquely defined. For example, when examining data about the help-seeking behaviour of alcohol abusers, the category 'support person behaviour' might emerge, which could refer to 'nurses', 'doctors', 'psychologists', 'social workers', 'family', and 'friends' who exhibited certain characteristics.

In grounded theory, the characteristics of a category are referred to as the 'properties' of the category. By studying the properties exhibited in different occurrences of the category throughout the text, similarities and differences can be identified, thus refining the definition of a specific category or, conversely, leading to the generation of new ones. Furthermore, such an examination will allow you to identify the situations or conditions under which the categories occur.

Theoretical constructs

Having identified the substantive codes and then derived categories, there is a need to interweave the component parts into a coherent entity which has meaning both to you as a researcher and to those who contributed to the data. Theoretical constructs are the means by which the various categories are linked. However, it is important not to attempt to develop theoretical constructs at too early a stage as there is a danger that vital codes, categories and properties will not yet have been discovered.

One means of identifying theoretical constructs is by asking questions of the categories so as to attempt to move categories from lower to higher levels of abstraction. Specifically: 'What is the category conveying?' Alternatively, you can hypothesize about the relationships that may exist and test them back in the field.

By posing a series of seven questions, it is easier to identify relationships among categories. Six questions should address cause, context, contingency, consequence, co-variance and conditions. Figure 13.2 illustrates how these questions can be posed in general terms, and, in addition, a supplementary question is identified that can assist in theoretical construct formation.

1　'What is/are the cause(s) of behaviour manifest in a particular category?'
2　'Under what context does the category manifest itself?'
3　'Is the category contingent upon any circumstances?'
4　'What are the consequences of the existence of this category?'
5　'Does a change in this category result in a change in another category – do two or more categories co-vary one with another?'
6　'What are the conditions for the existence of this category?'
7　'How do cause, context, contingency, consequence, co-variance, and conditions interrelate?'

Fig. 13.2　Questions to assist the development of theoretical constructs.

Core categories

By linking categories together, one, and occasionally more, core categories will evolve. When you generate a theory, the core category should be at its centre and should be capable of explaining much of the variation in behaviour discovered in the data. Most other categories and their properties should relate to the core category, integrating in such a way as to produce a theory that is capable of explaining the maximum amount of variation in behaviour.

A number of criteria can be used to assist in the identification of the core category in study data. Figure 13.3 summarizes criteria for a core category.

1 It is central to the theory.
2 It is capable of accounting for a large percentage of variation in the pattern of behaviour.
3 It must appear frequently in the data.
4 It is clearly related to the majority of other categories.
5 It takes longer to define the precise nature of the core category and its properties than other less central ones.
6 A core category has clear implications for more general theory.
7 As the core category is developed and its properties discovered, theory formation as a whole will move forward.

Fig. 13.3 Criteria for a core category.

Saturation

A category is said to be *saturated* when examination of the data reveals no further properties and the categories are completely developed. In other words, examination of data yields only recurrences of material that has already been discovered, coded, and integrated. If, despite attempting to identify new data from diverse sources, nothing new is found, then at this stage a category can be termed *saturated*. This implicitly implies that a category developed by studying only one data source cannot be considered saturated. Glaser & Strauss (1967) suggest that single sources can at best yield only a few categories and some of their properties. If you therefore intend to undertake a piece of research which uses the grounded theory method, you will require access to diverse data sources if you are to achieve saturation of categories.

Constant comparative method

The constant comparative method lies at the heart of the grounded theory approach and is the principal method of data analysis used in theory generation. This method of analysis entails the comparison of incidents with incidents, allowing the generation of categories. Incidents are then compared with categories – a strategy which allows you to identify the properties of the categories (see Fig. 13.4). In the early stages of category development, the comparisons of incidents with categories will generate anomalies, and it is at this point that you should stop coding and record a memorandum on your thoughts on the matter (such memos are discussed in detail later in this chapter). This process then progresses to the comparison of category with category, category with construct, and construct with construct. Comparison of similar incidents will assist you in defining the basic properties of categories; it will also help you to identify the context under which the category exists or operates. Specific differences between incidents aids the clarification of boundaries and the relationship or links that exist between categories.

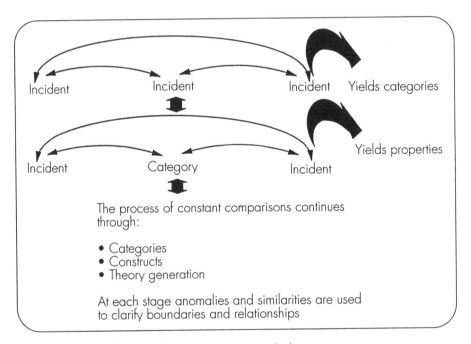

Fig. 13.4   Schematic illustration of constant comparative method.

As the process proceeds, you will eventually discover that you are no longer identifying new properties of categories and that the relationships between categories begin to crystallize – saturation has been reached. No longer are you discovering major anomalies in your categories, and modifications are more in terms of clarifying the relationships which link the categories and constructs together. When you have reached this stage, it is likely that you will be able to write a theory that is dense and capable of describing the basic social processes involved in the area under study. However, it is important to compare the various categories for underlying similarities which will allow you to reduce any duplication of properties or categories before you write the theory.

Memo writing

When undertaking grounded theory research memo writing is a method by which you facilitate and record the analytical process. Memo writing is at the very centre of the grounded theory method. By recording thoughts, questions and hypotheses in a permanent form, you will find it easier to track the development of categories, properties, theoretical constructs, the core category and ultimately the theory. However, memo writing is much more than simple note taking.

Memo writing should start soon after the first data have been gathered and you have started to code and analyse the content. At first, memos may be rather superficial in nature, but they will become more abstract as increasing amounts of codes, categories, and properties are discovered. The memos should be thought of as a tool to assist you in exploring the developing categories and the relationship between them. Memos are written by you and are intended for you. Unfortunately, this process can be time consuming and monotonous, but it is essential to the development of the theory.

For clarity, memos should be recorded on separate cards and not on the data source. Index cards are ideal, facilitate cross-referencing, are inexpensive and are easy to store. Furthermore, when recording memos it is important that, in addition to the memo, certain other information is noted to allow you to identify what prompted your thoughts, views, questions, or hypotheses. For example, the memo should be dated, titled by the categories to which it refers, and give reference to the point that initiated your thinking. Figure 13.5 illustrates these points and gives an example of a memo written at an early stage of analysis based on the data contained in Fig. 13.1.

12.05.99	Professional Empowerment
Source	John Brown Interview 10.05.99 Page 3

A number of words and phrases seem to link together. These include getting influence, credibility, taking the initiative. I wonder how other professions see nursing research. Is nursing research seen as a way of winning back power lost as a result of organizational change?

Fig. 13.5 Index card illustrating memo writing.

Figure 13.5 illustrates that memos need not be long. However, it is important that they are recorded immediately, when thoughts are still clear. Hence always keep some index cards near at hand and record memos as and when thoughts occur. You often find that this can be at unexpected times and not just when you are working with data.

Sorting

Having accumulated a large number of memos, it is then necessary to sort them to facilitate the development of your theory. Initial memos, which focus on substantive codes, can be sorted to enable you to identify categories and their properties within the data. When adequate numbers of memos relating to categories have been written and are sorted, it is likely that a core category and basic social processes can be identified. Hence, sorting is seen as a means of achieving higher levels of abstraction.

When sorting, it is advisable to start by ordering memo cards by category. All memos relating to one category can then be compared for the existence of consistency. When reading through the sorted memos, frequent cross-referencing to other categories may indicate that it is possible to reduce these into one category at a higher level of abstraction. Any anomalies discovered may suggest the need to develop another category or at least gather further data to explain the differences.

Using literature

When conducting research which attempts to test existing theory, literature is used to place the research in context, describe its significance, identify variables and address issues of method, instrumentation, subjects and setting. Literature is consulted prior to the study in order to identify the hypothesis under examination. Although previous published research may be used to compare or contrast findings in the 'discussion' section, the literature is predominantly accessed, reviewed, and critiqued prior to commencement of the study. However, a research study that uses a grounded theory design uses literature in a significantly different way. First, an initial literature search can provide evidence that little is known about the subject under study, thus supporting the need for research and, more specifically, the appropriateness of a grounded theory approach. Second, an in-depth critique of literature prior to data collection and analysis should not be undertaken since this may provide you with a framework which includes categories that are inappropriate or incomplete. Third, literature should be treated simply as another data source – that is, it should be examined, coded, analysed and have memos written about it. Finally, access to literature should be ongoing. Concepts reported in published material can be examined at various stages throughout the duration of the study compared with those developed in your theory. Such an approach is particularly useful when addressing issues of reliability, validity and generalization. The existing literature can thus be used to support the developing theory.

Theory writing

Theory writing is an integral part of the grounded theory method and can be thought of as a natural extension of the memo-writing process. As categories are discovered and saturated, and theoretical constructs are proposed and evaluated, memos will concurrently become more abstract. By examining these abstract memos, a developing theory can be identified. Hence, writing the theory is not a deliberate and separate act, but an ongoing process. Nevertheless, when writing the theory, a number of points must be considered.

First, the theory should describe the underlying basic social psychological process which accounts for the majority of variation in the data gathered.

Second, you will have been working with the data for a considerable period of time. What seems perfectly clear to you may not be as easily comprehended by colleagues. To a certain extent, this is guarded against by constantly taking your developing theory back to those who are providing data. However, peer review is a useful way of checking that the theory is understandable and not open to misinterpretation.

Third, is the theory dense? It is essential that you examine your theory and assure yourself that all categories are saturated and connected via constructs in a meaningful way. Furthermore, it is necessary that conditions under which categories exist or operate are well defined, described, and supported by sufficient evidence from the data.

Fourth, the theory presented must be linked to existing knowledge. If you have used existing literature and documentary sources during the process of theory development, this should not present a problem. However, if discrepancies between the existing literature and the newly developed theory remain, they must be explored and explained.

Finally, a well-written grounded theory must be testable – that is, hypotheses (sometimes referred to as propositions) should be clearly stated. By stating hypotheses, you will provide direction for subsequent investigation. However, more importantly to those who provided the data, hypotheses should offer new insight into the practice, situation or event under study.

Conclusions

The grounded theory approach is a means of identifying the basic social psychological processes involved in the situation under study and, as a result, can be considered as a powerful means of developing nursing's knowledge base. By using this method, a theory evolves from nursing practice, and, consequently, it is likely that it is directly relevant to the clinician, thus offering greater understanding of everyday care. In conclusion, if you believe, as does the author, that understanding is necessary for the provision of high-quality care, then research using the grounded theory approach has much to offer the nursing profession.

References

Glaser, B.J. (1978) *Theoretical Sensitivity*. Mill Valley, CA: Sociology Press.
Glaser, B.J. & Strauss, A.L. (1967) *The Discovery of Grounded Theory*. New York: Aldine Publishing.

Further reading

Artinian, B.M. (1998) Grounded theory research: its value for nursing. *Nursing Science Quarterly* **11** (1): 5–6.
Green, J. (1998) Commentary: grounded theory and the constant comparative method. *British Medical Journal* **316** (7137): 1064–5.
Keddy, B., Sims, S.L. & Sterm, P.N. (1996) Grounded theory as feminist research methodology. *Journal of Advanced Nursing*, **23** (3): 448–53.
Sheldon, L. (1998) Grounded theory: issues for research in nursing. *Nursing Standard* **12** (52): 47–50.

CHAPTER 14

Quantitative research

Diana E. Carter

The quantitative approach emerged from the branch of philosophy known as logical positivism, which was founded on the belief that the world could be viewed as a machine, the task of science being to discover the laws by which the machine operated. Having discovered these laws and learned about them, the achievement of perfect predictability was seen as a natural follow-on. The means of understanding the world can be seen in the emphasis that is placed on the measurement and quantification of observable data, and quantitative research uses a systematic process of gathering and using numerical data to obtain information about the focus of interest.

Following a predetermined research design, objective and value-free collection of data in controlled settings is the underlying aim of this type of research and may go some way towards providing an explanation of cause and effect. Sometimes referred to as the traditional research process, it is regarded as being the acceptable method for developing a science.

Until quite recently a bipolar approach to research methods prevailed, with the proponents of quantitative research arguing that such an approach provides a more objective knowledge base to guide practice, while at the other end of the spectrum there were researchers who emphasized the advantages of the qualitative approach in the understanding of life experiences and their meanings. However, it is now recognized that each approach can make a valuable contribution to the investigation of phenomena significant to nursing, midwifery and health visiting. The research approach adopted depends on a number of factors including the nature of the phenomena to be investigated, the aim of the research, and the state of existing knowledge. Some studies may be exclusively quantitative or qualitative, while others may effectively combine these approaches.

If the collection of more numerically and measurable information is a priority, a quantitative approach is called for. This can be seen in the study of nurse educators' and student nurses' perceptions of effective clinical teaching behaviours, carried out by Li (1997). This study used a structured, self-administered questionnaire and incorporated a list of 48 effective clinical teaching behaviours which respondents were asked to rate according to their degree of perceived importance on a seven-point Likert rating scale. This allowed responses to be standardized and statistically analysed.

However, using different approaches in a single study can provide a much richer and deeper understanding of what is being investigated than would otherwise be the case. For example, the investigation of oncologists' and nurses' perspectives of the impact that breast cancer hormone treatment has on patients' quality of life (Working Group on Living with Advanced Breast Cancer Hormone Treatment, 1998) involved in-depth qualitative interviews with oncologists which was followed by a group discussion with a working group of issues arising from the interviews. This in turn generated a structured questionnaire which was used during telephone interviews with oncologists and nurses in the third phase of the study. Similarly, in their investigation of the effectiveness of tutorials in behavioural sciences for nurses, French *et al.* (1998) employed a between-methods triangulation research approach. This involves collecting different forms of data from the same subjects. French *et al.* combined quantitative measurement using a questionnaire and an inventory, and qualitative data collection using observation, personal journals and interviews. This facilitated a greater under-standing of the complexities of students' approaches to learning and the factors which affect satisfaction with tutorials than might otherwise have been achieved.

Reality and its measurement

From a quantitative point of view the world is seen as stable and predictable, and the researcher believes that 'truth' is absolute and there is one single reality that can be defined by careful measurement. Quantification (the use of numbers) in relation to, for example, amount, position, time and location, facilitates the description of both humans and the universe in such a way as to quantify their properties. To achieve such quantification requires precise measurement tools that will generate numerical data which can then be subjected to statistical analysis (see Chapters 30 and 31) in order to reduce and organize them and determine significant relationships. As with logical positivism, 'truth', according to the quantitative researcher, is to be discovered in common laws, principles and norms, and having discovered these it will then be possible to achieve the goal of quantitative research, which is generalizability. Generalization involves the application of trends or general tendencies (identified by studying a sample) to the population from which the research sample was drawn.

Reductionism

To discover reality, quantitative research systematically reduces or breaks down complex information or situations into their simpler component parts in order to gain an understanding of the whole. This is illustrated in a study by Koivula &

Paunonen (1998) which attempted to explain middle-aged Finnish men's smoking habits. In order to gain insight into respondents' attitudes and beliefs about smoking and related values the researchers identified four areas that they considered important: the health effects of smoking; positive effects of smoking; the place of tobacco in society and in the respondents' lives; and respondents' views on the opinion of others in their environment to smoking (Fig. 14.1). An attitude scale, consisting of statements about smoking, was developed with a number of items relating to each of these areas. Thus, the researchers broke the whole into parts that could be examined, as could the relationships among the parts in order to gain knowledge of the whole. The underlying assumption is that the whole is the sum of the parts and the parts organize the whole.

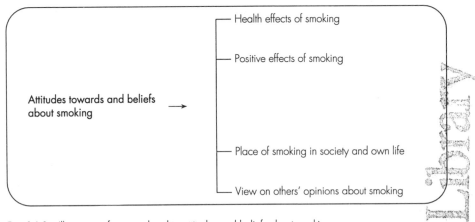

Fig. 14.1   Illustration of issues related to attitudes and beliefs about smoking.

Objectivity

In contrast to qualitative methods, which facilitate study designs where the researcher and subject are part of a two-way process in which understanding develops in the development of theory, the quantitative researcher objectively distinguishes self from the subjects of the investigation, believing that boundaries must exist between them in order to ensure objectivity. Objectivity is achieved by the researcher remaining detached from the study and endeavouring to avoid influencing the study (including the subjects) with his own perceptions and values. Avoiding researcher involvement will help to guard against biasing the study towards these perceptions and values. It is acknowledged that the qualitative researcher also strives to achieve objectivity, but some of the methods of data collection used (for example, participant observation) can, by their very nature, sometimes allow subjectivity to enter into the research situation. In quantitative research the position is held that subjectivity (for example, values and feelings) must not enter into the measurement of reality. Human behaviour is held to be objective, purposeful and, providing a valid and reliable tool is used, measurable.

Quantitative measurement

A prominent feature of the data collected using the quantitative approach is that they can be measured and quantified by statistical analysis. It should, however, be noted that qualitative methods (such as unstructured interviews and participant observation) may also provide data that can be quantified. Further information on quantitative analysis can be found in Chapters 30 and 31.

Types of quantitative research

Quantitative research includes descriptive, correlational, quasi-experimental and experimental research.

Descriptive research

As discussed in Chapter 18, the characteristics of individuals and groups such as nurses, patients and families may be the focus of descriptive research. This was the case in the study by Foxall *et al.* (1998) which included description of the health beliefs of women which might influence breast self-examination practices. Environments – for example, the environment in which nursing is carried out – situations and events such as specific nursing interventions, and systems of organization may also be described. For example, Adams & Bond (1997) used a self-completion ward profile to gather data describing ward characteristics and nursing practice and a previously developed and tested scale to describe nurses' perceptions of ward organizational features.

Descriptive research is a type of quantitative research which can also be used to determine the frequency with which a particular variable occurs, as seen in the study by Foxall *et al.* (1998) which described ethnic differences in breast self-examination practices where, for example, it was found that 43% of the African American nurses had examined their breasts 12 or more times during the previous year, 40% 5 to 11 times, and 17% four times or less.

Instruments used to obtain data in descriptive studies include questionnaires, interviews and observation.

Questionnaires

Questionnaires are designed to elicit information through the written responses of subjects. Although structured to the extent that each respondent will be faced with exactly the same questions in the same order, the degree of structure of individual items within the questionnaire can range from open-ended questions to closed (fixed alternative) questions. The decision about the type of question to ask will be determined to a large extent by the nature of the information required.

Gillespie & Curzio (1998) used closed questions to determine nurses' knowledge of blood pressure measurement. The closed questions were based on the British Hypertension Society's guidelines, which facilitated direct comparison of what nurses said they did with what the national guidelines recommend. In studies which use open-ended questions the researcher would need to develop categories and assign the open-ended responses to these so that tabulations could be made, as in the study of the beliefs of people with non-insulin-dependent diabetes by Dunning & Martin (1998). The relative strengths and weaknesses of open-ended and closed question are discussed in more detail in Chapter 25.

Interviews

Interviews involve the researcher interacting with the respondent to elicit the required information verbally. As with questionnaires, interviews can vary in the degree to which they are structured. However, quantitative research generally uses structured interviews in which an interview schedule ensures that each respondent will be asked exactly the same questions in the same order, although, once again, the degree of structure of individual items within the schedule can range from open-ended questions to closed (fixed alternative) questions. The data collected are handled in the same way as questionnaire data, with the number of responses in each category being tabulated. In their study of academic validation of prior and experiential learning, Clarke & Warr (1997) used a semi-structured interview schedule which included both closed and open-ended questions, the latter facilitating the respondents to express themselves in their own words. (Further discussion on interviews as a method of data collection can be found in Chapter 24.)

Observation

While observation is a commonly used method of data collection in qualitative research, quantitative research also uses observation techniques to produce numerical data. The observation techniques used employ previously developed mutually exclusive category systems so that the behaviour or events which are the focus of the observation can be organized and structured.

Observers may also make use of checklists and rating scales. Checklists are used to indicate whether or not a particular behaviour or event occurred and the number of times it was observed to occur, as in the observation study of nurses' interactions with mentally ill young people by Holyoake (1998). Rating scales allow the observer to rate the behaviour or event on a scale, thus providing more information than the dichotomous data from checklists, which simply indicate whether or not it occurred. (More information on observation is given in Chapter 26.)

Correlational research

Quantitative correlational research aims to systematically investigate and explain the nature of the relationship between variables in the real world. The quantifiable data from descriptive studies are frequently analysed in this way, as in the exploratory study by Barrett & Myrick (1998) in which data collected by means of a postal questionnaire were used to examine the relationship between the job satisfaction of preceptors and preceptees and its effect on preceptee clinical performance, preceptor/preceptee job satisfaction, and preceptee performance.

Experimental research and quasi-experimental research

Experimental research is the most appropriate for testing cause-and-effect relationships, and is considered to be the most powerful quantitative method because of its rigorous control of variables. Quasi-experimental studies are not quite so powerful in that they lack the intensity of control which is an inherent feature of experiments. This was acknowledged by Callaghan & Trapp (1998), whose quasi-experimental study of dressings for the prevention of nasal bridge pressure sores in patients receiving nasal intermittent positive pressure ventilation lacked randomization and a control group. (Experimental research is further discussed in Chapter 15.)

Control

Whatever type of quantitative research and data-collecting instruments you decide to use, if the findings are to reflect accurately the reality of the situation being studied your study requires to be designed in such a way as to maximize the amount of control over the research situation and variables. Through control, the influence of extraneous variables (variables which are not being studied but which could influence the results of the study by interfering with the actions of the ones being studied) is reduced.

Some of the mechanisms of control at the quantitative researcher's disposal shall now be discussed.

Sampling

When conducting research it is important to select a sample of subjects that is as representative as possible of the population being studied in terms of such variables as age, social class and educational level, because the characteristics of the participants in a study have been suggested to be the most common extraneous variables. If, for example, the study aimed to investigate the effect of a ward-based teaching programme on newly diagnosed diabetic patients' knowledge of their condition and its management, the age and educational level of subjects could function as extraneous variables. Both variables might be related to the outcome of interest, which in this case is the patients' knowledge of their condition and its management, in that they affect how much knowledge patients gain quite independently of the teaching programme. Thus their effects are extraneous.

Random sampling techniques will help to ensure the representativeness of the sample in that each member of the population will have an equal chance of being included in the study. (Chapter 22 gives more details of sampling techniques.)

Randomization

Randomization helps the researcher to control possible extraneous variables. Using the previous example of an investigation of the effects of a ward-based teaching programme on diabetic patients' knowledge of their condition, the researcher, having identified the population (patients with diabetes), would select a sample at random. This could be achieved, for example, by selecting every fourth patient from a computer-generated print-out of the population of diabetic patients. Thus, each member of the population has an equal chance of being selected, and if the sample is sufficiently large it will be representative of the population in terms of age and sex. It is often thought (erroneously so) that randomization is relevant only in respect of experimental research where subjects are randomly assigned to various treatment and control groups. However, it is also very relevant in relation to the data-collecting instruments used in non-experimental research. For example, to investigate patients' attitudes towards information given to them during their hospital stay, it might be decided to use a series of written statements with which subjects are asked to agree or disagree. Ideally, the researcher should ensure that the order of these statements is randomized so that, for example, there is no predetermined pattern in terms of positive and negative statements which could unwittingly interfere with subjects' responses.

The Hawthorne effect

If people are aware that they are participating in a study it is natural that they might alter their behaviour as a result, perhaps by modifying their responses to questionnaire items or by acting in a more friendly manner, knowing that they are being observed, in an attempt to present themselves in a better light. This psychological response is known as the Hawthorne effect and the quantitative researcher who is trying to measure reality needs to make every effort to minimize this. Holyoake (1998) attempted to do this by remaining discreetly on the fringe of activity when completing an observation checklist. Other strategies might involve the researcher in giving the subjects a simple explanation of the study but omitting to advise them of the actual relationships in which she is interested. In an experimental study, provided subjects' rights are not infringed, you could choose not to inform subjects whether they have been assigned to the treatment group or the control group.

Constancy of conditions

Ensuring that the study design is such that the conditions inherent in the research are the same for all participants is an important consideration for the researcher. Three aspects are briefly considered here: the research setting itself, control of input, and time factors.

The research setting

In the interest of achieving constancy, consideration needs to be given to the degree of control exerted over the actual research setting. For example, McLaughlin (1997) ensured that all subjects completed an attitudinal questionnaire on the first and last day of classes in mental health nursing and that they all received the same classroom teaching, thus ensuring that the same information was given to all the study subjects using the same medium and that the environmental conditions remained constant for both the attitudinal measuring (before and after the intervention) and the teaching itself. This facilitated measurement of the change that occurred in subjects' attitudes, as a result of which the researcher was able to conclude that classroom theory can alter student nurses' attitudes to the treatment of mentally ill people. Any discrepancy in terms of the research setting could have been reflected when the subjects' attitudes were measured at the post-teaching stage, in that if the environment had not held constant then the outcome (that is, the students' attitudes) may not be so much a reflection of the effect of the teaching intervention but more a reflection of the effects of the environmental conditions in which the attitude measurement and teaching were carried out.

Clearly, the more the research setting can be controlled, the more effective the researcher will be in reducing the influence of extraneous environmental variables, and the more accurate will be the examination of the cause-and-effect relationships of the variables studied.

Control of input

A lot of nursing research is concerned with measuring the effects of specific interventions and it is therefore important that control over these interventions is exercised. In the study described above (McLaughlin, 1997) all subjects received the same classroom theory. However, the pre- and post-classroom theory attitude measurements were followed by a period of clinical experience in a psychiatric placement after which the attitude questionnaire was completed for a third time. As the researcher acknowledged, the uncontrolled input (the students' contact not only with patients but also with their clinical supervisors) had variable impact on the resultant attitudes.

In some instances, the role of the subjects' families and friends may influence the situation the researcher is trying to control. Additionally, if knowledge levels are a focus of interest in a study, the intervention of, say, a teaching programme may stimulate the subjects to find out more about the topic themselves. Thus, if subjects' post-teaching intervention levels of knowledge are measured at a later date it would be difficult to determine whether any measured increase in knowledge was an effect of the teaching intervention or a reflection of additional information gleaned from other sources. This type of input is often very difficult to control.

Information given to the subjects about the study is within the researcher's control, and she should ensure that each subject receives identical information about, for example, the purpose of the study and the use that will be made of the data.

Time factors

Depending on the time of day, subjects may be more or less attentive to information being given. The time interval between an intervention and the measuring of the effects of this could also influence the findings. Similarly, subjects' responses to testing may also be influenced by whether this is carried out in the morning or the afternoon, and by the timing of data collection in relation to other events.

Conclusions

The quantitative–qualitative debate has waned in recent years and it is now generally accepted that both approaches have the potential to make valuable contributions to the development of nursing knowledge. Indeed, many studies combine qualitative and quantitative approaches to good effect, each approach serving to complement the other and each generating different kinds of knowledge that will be useful in practice.

References

Adams, A. & Bond, S. (1997) Clinical specialty and organizational features of acute hospital wards. *Journal of Advanced Nursing* **26** (6): 1158–67.

Barrett, C. & Myrick, F. (1998) Job satisfaction in preceptorship and its effect on the clinical performance of the preceptee. *Journal of Advanced Nursing* 27 (2): 364–71.

Callaghan, S. & Trapp, M. (1998) Evaluating two dressings for the prevention of nasal bridge pressure sore. *Professional Nurse* 13 (6): 361–4.

Clarke, J.B. & Warr, J. (1997) Academic validation of prior and experiential learning: evaluation of the process. *Journal of Advanced Nursing* 26 (6): 1235–42.

Dunning, P. & Martin, M. (1998) Beliefs about diabetes and diabetic complications. *Professional Nurse,* 13 (7): 429–34.

Foxall, M.J., Barron, C.R. & Houfek, J. (1998) Ethnic differences in breast self-examination practice and health beliefs. *Journal of Advanced Nursing* 27 (2): 419–28.

French, P., Callaghan, P., Dudley-Brown, S., Holroyd, E. & Sellick, K. (1998) The effectiveness of tutorials in behavioural sciences for nurses: an action learning project. *Nurse Education Today* 18: 116–24.

Gillespie, A. & Curzio, J. (1998) Blood pressure measurement: assessing staff knowledge. *Nursing Standard* 12 (23): 35–7.

Holyoake, D. (1998) Observing nurse–patient interaction. *Nursing Standard* 12 (29): 35–8.

Koivula, M. & Paunonen, M. (1998) Smoking habits among Finnish middle-aged men: experiences and attitudes. *Journal of Advanced Nursing* 27 (2): 327–34.

Li, M.K. (1997) Perceptions of effective clinical teaching behaviours in a hospital-based nurse training programme. *Journal of Advanced Nursing* 26 (6): 1252–61.

McLaughlin, C. (1997) The effect of classroom theory and contact with patients on the attitudes of student nurses towards mentally ill people. *Journal of Advanced Nursing* 26 (6): 1221–8.

Working Group on Living with Advanced Breast Cancer Hormone Treatment (1998) Living with advanced breast cancer hormone treatment: the nurse's perspective. *European Journal of Cancer Care* 7: 113–19.

CHAPTER 15

Experimental research

Peter T. Donnan

Experimental research is the gold standard method of demonstrating in a rigorously scientific manner that a new (or sometimes old) treatment or intervention is effective. In other words, it is the essential tool for a quantitative assessment of the efficacy of an intervention. It is a sobering thought to realize that a large proportion of current procedures have never been subjected to experimental research.

Experimental research, as the name suggests, involves conducting a study in which the experimenters do not know the outcome. There is little point in conducting an experiment if the outcome is well known. It also implies a great deal of control over the subjects and what happens during the study, in contrast to an observational study where the researcher has little or no control. This degree of control is essential in demonstrating the efficacy of an intervention, as it allows the preclusion of other explanations of the results. In addition, due to the high degree of control over what happens to the subjects, there is a strong ethical dimension to experimental research which is discussed later in the chapter.

As for all good research it is good practice to have a written document or protocol which details how the design was constructed, the aims of the study, the methods of analysis including any statistical techniques, and how the results will be reported.

Experimental research involves comparing one group, the intervention or treatment group, to a control or placebo group(s). The whole basis of an experiment is that the treatment or intervention group and the control group are similar in every respect other than the intervention. The reasoning then is that if the outcome differs between the groups, this difference must be *only* due to the intervention. I will mostly use the term intervention rather than treatment as the latter implies only drug therapy, while the term intervention has a much wider meaning and can include educational interventions, for example.

This description introduces the essentials of experimental research. First, a comparison group or groups known as controls are required to provide a standard by which we can gauge the effect of the intervention. Second, the subjects taking part in the experiment are randomly assigned to either the intervention group or the control group. Note that this does not necessarily guarantee that the groups are similar, but it is our best attempt! This leads to the most common design, the randomized-controlled trial (RCT), which will now be discussed in more detail.

Randomized-controlled trial

Examples

An example of a randomized-controlled trial was carried out by Rothert *et al.* (1997) to compare the effects of three educational interventions on menopausal women. Participants were randomly assigned to receive a brochure alone (the control group A) or to attend lectures/discussion groups (group B) or to receive a personalized decision intervention (group C). The outcomes were measures of knowledge, decisional conflict and satisfaction with the health provider pre-intervention, immediately post-intervention and at 6 months and 12 months. The results indicated that knowledge was significantly increased in groups B and C compared to group A and that this difference was maintained over time. Another example of the use of a RCT to test the efficacy of an intervention was in considering the introduction of screening for breast cancer in Britain. Previous trials of breast screening in New York (Shapiro *et al.*, 1982) and Sweden (Tabar *et al.*, 1985) had suggested that the introduction of this service would reduce mortality from breast cancer and a study was set up in Edinburgh in which women in general practices were randomly assigned to either be invited to breast screening or not be invited. The outcome would be the difference in mortality at a specified length of follow-up (Roberts *et al.*, 1990).

Lennox *et al.* (1998) is an example of a RCT in a General Practice setting with the aim of reducing cigarette smoking in patients following an educational intervention given by a set of health professionals. The educational intervention was randomly assigned to general practices and smoking status was measured at time intervals following the intervention. A recent example of a large international RCT was that designed to show that low-dose aspirin was effective in reducing hypertension (Hansson *et al.*, 1998).

These are all examples of how a RCT can provide valuable evidence of the efficacy of an intervention. The following paragraphs discuss some of the issues in a RCT.

The necessity of controls

When new treatments or interventions are proposed it is usually those who originate the idea – and are therefore most disposed to the new intervention – who implement it and often report on the results of the introduction. This has the potential for distortion (sometimes deliberate) of the outcomes from new interventions and their subsequent uncritical use. There is a great temptation to treat only the less ill in order to obtain good results, for example, or it is simply human nature to see only the positive side of an intervention. All of these points are very obvious, but it is only in the recent past that it has become accepted that a control group is essential in judging the efficacy of an intervention. The control group provides a standard set of results for the outcome by which the intervention group outcome can be judged. In other words, randomized-controlled trial outcomes are always relative to a control group. The selection of the control group is clearly critical in a RCT. In drug trials, the alternative to the drug under consideration can often be no treatment at all, that is, a placebo.

Eligibility of subjects

Depending on the purpose of the RCT, subjects who are likely to be representative of those in whom the intervention is to be applied are selected as potential entrants to the study. Usually, in a protocol there will be a list of inclusion and exclusion criteria for the study and each potential entrant is assessed against these criteria prior to entry. For example, there may be an age restriction so that those aged under 50 would not be admitted to a trial of a new arthritis drug.

Informed consent

It is necessary to obtain informed consent from patients to allow them to take part in the study. This requirement varies from country to country and in the United States this is a legal requirement. In order to do this the researcher must explain the study fully and carefully and point out that she does not know which intervention is most optimum for the benefit of the patients' health. As a consequence the mechanism by which the treatment is decided will be a random process, so that the treatment received will be a matter of chance. It should be explained that this is the only way in which an objective assessment of the treatments can be assessed. Sometimes a subject is too ill or too distressed to make such decisions and consent may be sought from a relative.

Random allocation

It goes against the grain for health professionals to take part in a study where they have to accept that they do not know which intervention is most optimum for the benefit of the patients' health. On the other hand, this is the whole point of mounting such a study. In addition, in a RCT through the use of randomization, control over which treatment patients receive is also relinquished. Nevertheless, it is only through the allocation of treatment by a chance mechanism that an objective assessment of the outcome can be obtained. The alternatives, such as a researcher selecting the less well patients for the control group, is likely to produce an assessment of the outcome which is biased. The mechanism of randomization is relatively simple, involving the production of a list which details which of the treatments the patients will receive on entry to the trial.

Blinding of treatment

A patient receiving a new treatment may feel that he is receiving something better than the standard treatment and so there may be a consequent psychological effect. Blinding the treatment to the patient is one way of trying to eliminate this effect in the comparison between treatments. It is also important to ensure that the researchers do not know the intervention to which the subject has been allocated. Of course, this is the ideal but in practice it is not always possible. In drug trials, it is often possible to blind the treatment by, for example, making the pills of the treatment under consideration the same colour and texture as the controls and with the same packaging.

It is also useful for those who measure or assess the outcome to be unaware of the intervention group to which the subjects belong. For example, personnel external to the study and blind to which group the subjects belong to could measure the outcome. If there is blinding of treatment and of assessment, then the trial is called a double-blind randomized-controlled trial. In practice, blinding is not always possible, simply because of the nature of the intervention. In a RCT of screening for breast cancer it would clearly not be possible to blind the subject as to whether they were invited to screening or not.

Analysis

Often the analysis in a RCT can be very simple. Through the use of randomization the groups in the trial should only differ according to which intervention group they belong and, hence, there should be no need to adjust the analysis for extraneous factors. Thus two group comparisons, such as t-tests (Chapter 31), are often used in the statistical analysis of RCTs in reporting the main analysis. This contrasts with more observational studies where allowance for confounders is necessary, requiring more sophisticated statistical modelling. Analysis is always by 'intention to treat' – that is, once randomized to a particular intervention, the subjects' outcome is included in that group whether they withdrew or did not comply with the therapy during the study period.

The hypothesis to be tested in the analysis is usually couched in neutral terms, and this is called the null hypothesis. The null hypothesis in a two-armed trial would be that there is no difference in outcome between the intervention subjects and the controls. If in the statistical test, for example, a t-test is significant then the null hypothesis is rejected and the intervention is said to be statistically different to the controls. For more details of hypothesis testing see Chapter 31.

Sample size

The appropriate sample size to show differences in outcome between the intervention group and the controls should be estimated at the planning stages of a RCT and details of the calculations included in the protocol. The difference in outcome used in these calculations should be a clinically worthwhile or scientifically meaningful difference. For example, selecting a large sample size in order to demonstrate, say, a reduction of 2% in mortality from breast cancer after the introduction of a breast screening service would be unlikely to be worth while. In contrast, a study designed to demonstrate a 20% reduction in mortality would be smaller in size and more meaningful to the researchers and policy makers.

The previous sections introduced some of the issues in mounting RCTs. For more details and a very readable description of the design and analysis of clinical trials, along with a historical perspective, see the text by Pocock (1996).

Difficulties with the randomized-controlled trial

Although the randomized-controlled trial is the gold standard for demonstrating efficacy, it is not always easy or even possible to organize such a study. Seeking the consent of a subject to enter a RCT does create difficulties. First, the patient will usually not be told which intervention he will receive. This has been discussed earlier under the heading of blinding. This goes against the grain for most health professionals but it is an essential part of the RCT. Second, the health professional must admit ignorance over which treatment is 'best' for the subject. If it is known which intervention has the optimal effect, then there would be no need to carry out a RCT in the first place.

Non-compliance

Once enrolled in a study, the subject may decide not to take the medication or not to take part in the intervention (for example, simply not take up an invitation to be screened) without the knowledge of the personnel running the trial. This non-compliance with the study protocol will dilute the effects of the intervention at the analysis stage, as they must still be included in the group to which they were allocated, whether they actually received the intervention or not. If non-compliance is extensive, the trial comparison may be so diluted as to be meaningless. Non-compliance is a serious problem in drug therapy such as lipid-lowering therapy where it is estimated that, in those surviving, only 50% were still compliant after 5 years (Avorn *et al.*, 1998).

Loss to follow-up

If the trial participants do not report back for the final outcome measurement for whatever reason, they will be lost to the study. As for non-compliance, if the loss to follow-up is extensive, the trial would collapse. The longer the study period, the greater will be the potential for loss to follow-up. It is good practice to inflate the estimate of sample size for the trial at the design stage, assuming a certain level of loss to follow-up.

The randomized consent design

In order to overcome the problem of removing patient choice inherent in a RCT, Zelen (1979) proposed a design which allowed the subject to refuse the intervention if he chose to do so. This is the randomized consent design, in which the subject is randomized to either seek consent or not seek consent. Those whose consent is not sought would simply be given the control intervention. Those randomly selected for the intervention would be asked whether they would accept the treatment or not (Fig. 15.1). This design will work as long as the number who refuse the intervention does not become excessively large. The analysis must be by 'intention to treat' so that although those who refused treatment did not receive the intervention they will be included in the analysis as if they did. In essence, the refusals will dilute the effect of the treatment.

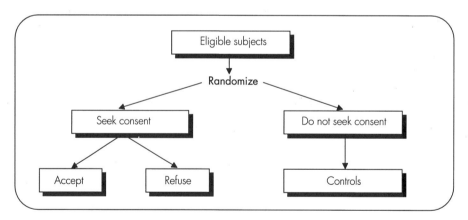

Fig. 15.1   Flow diagram of the randomized consent design (Zelen, 1979).

Cross-over trials

The main difference between the cross-over trial and the RCT is that each subject acts as his own control. This trial design is often utilized whenever it is difficult to obtain a balance in possible confounding factors between experimental groups. Each subject is exposed to each of the interventions at different time periods and only the order in which the subjects receive the interventions is randomized. If there are two interventions this is called a two-period cross-over trial (Fig. 15.2).

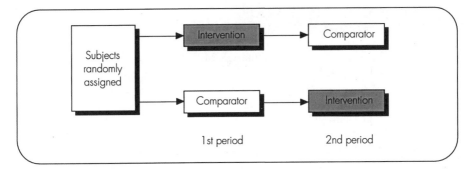

Fig. 15.2 The two-period cross-over trial.

This is a form of repeated measures design since each subject is assessed at different time periods. What makes this design also experimental is the fact that the order in which subjects receive different treatments is randomized. Of course for this design to be appropriate the effect of each intervention must wear off in time, and hence the need for a 'wash-out' period between interventions. This means that cross-over trials tend to be limited to chronic conditions which are stable such as asthma or hypertension in which the trial aims to consider short-term effects of therapy. One example of this design is in the assessment of bronchodilators in asthma sufferers. This design gives an unbiased measure of the difference between the intervention group and controls because of the random order in which the subject receives treatment.

Following cytotoxic chemotherapy for cancer, a common problem is the development of mouth sores and difficulty in swallowing. Anderson *et al.* (1998) carried out a randomized double-blind cross-over study to test the efficacy of oral glutamine. They found, statistically, that the duration of mouth pain was significantly less by 4.5 days in chemotherapy courses which had glutamine supplementation compared to placebo (glycine suspension).

Conclusions

This chapter has introduced some of the ideas involved in experimental research. The two main issues in randomized-controlled trials are concerned with having a comparator group or groups and reducing bias through the use of random assignment. Beware of studies that have only a 'before and after' design without an element of randomization or a comparison group. In many conditions subjects will improve with time, whatever the treatment. In addition to the RCT, cross-over trials were also discussed.

References

Anderson, P.M., Schroeder, G. & Skubitz, K.M. (1998) Oral glutamine reduces the duration and severity after cytotoxic cancer chemotherapy. *Cancer* 83: 1433–9.

Avorn, J., Monette, J., Lacour, A., Bohn, R.L., Monane, M., Mogun, H. & LeLorier, J. (1998) Persistence of use of lipid-lowering medications. *Journal American Medical Association* 279: 1458–62.

Hansson, L., Zanchetti, A., Carruthers, S.G., Dahlof, B., Elmfeldt, D., Julius, S., Menard, J., Rahn, K.H., Wedel, H. & Westerling, S. (1998) Effects of intensive blood-pressure lowering and low-dose aspirin in patients with hypertension: principal results of the Hypertension Optimal Treatment (HOT) randomised trial. *Lancet* 351: 1755–62.

Lennox, S.A., Bain, N., Taylor, R.J., McKie, L., Donnan, P.T. & Groves, J. (1998) Stage of change training for opportunistic smoking intervention by the primary health care team. Part I: Randomised controlled trial of the effect of training on patient smoking outcomes and health professional behaviour as recalled by patients. *Health Education Journal* 57: 140–9.

Pocock, S.J. (1996) *Clinical Trials. A Practical Approach*. Chichester: Wiley.

Roberts, M.M., Alexander, F.E., Anderson, T.J., Chetty, U., Donnan, P.T., Forrest, Prof. Sir P., Hepburn, W., Huggins, A., Kirkpatrick, A.E., Lamb, J., Muir, B.B. & Prescott, R.J. (1990) The Edinburgh Trial of Screening for Breast Cancer: mortality results at seven years. *Lancet* 335: 241–6.

Rothert, M.L., Holmes-Rovner, M., Rovner, D., Kroll, J., Breer, L., Talarczyk, G., Schmitt, N., Padonu, G. & Wills, C. (1997) An educational intervention as decision support for menopausal women. *Research in Nursing and Health* 20: 377–87.

Shapiro, S., Venet, W. & Strax, P. (1982) Ten to fourteen year effect of screening on breast cancer mortality. *Journal of the National Cancer Institute* 69: 349–55.

Tabar, L., Faberberg, C.J.G. & Gad, A. (1985) Reduction in mortality from breast cancer after mass screening with mammography: randomised trial from the Breast Cancer Screening Working Group of the Swedish National Board of Health and Welfare. *Lancet* I: 829–32.

Zelen, M. (1979) A new design for randomized clinical trials. *New England Journal of Medicine* 300: 1242–5.

CHAPTER 16

Action research

Jennifer E. Clark

Action research has been described as part of a new paradigm of nursing research and increasingly it is becoming the core research method for nurses and midwives, just as clinical trials are for medicine (Abbot & Sapsford, 1998). Action research is certainly becoming very popular among researchers as it is seen as a means of narrowing the theory practice gap and involving nurse practitioners, teachers and managers in the research process. The drive towards research-based practice and the need to change practice in the light of evidence rather than intuition has made research everybody's business. Action research is typically, but not exclusively, about professionals carrying out research into their own practice. It embraces the notion of doing research 'for' and 'with' people rather than 'on' people, which is the philosophical stance of the more traditional approaches to research. Action research, as its name implies, is about researching and bringing about improvements in practice. It may well be argued that all research aims to improve practice by producing and disseminating new theory and knowledge which is read and implemented by practitioners. However, the dissemination stage of the research process has traditionally been a difficult stage to fulfil, largely because it is an indirect process and totally dependent upon the will of practitioners to read, understand, and implement the research findings. Research has demonstrated (Hunt, 1987; Funk *et al.*, 1991) that nurses and midwives are indeed, for many reasons, reluctant to translate the findings of research into their practice. One reason postulated for this reluctance is that they fail to see the relevance of the research and its resultant theory to their own situation and that researchers are out of touch with the realities of current practice. The obvious solution to this widening theory–practice gap is for practitioners and others to become personally involved in research and to investigate issues that are relevant to their situation and to generate findings that are both feasible to implement and are ultimately self-owned. The dissemination of findings is integral to the research process in action research and not an adjunct to it, as is so often the case with more traditional methodologies.

Action research has tended to be classified as a qualitative research approach; however, this is not always the case. A wide spectrum of approaches may be used within action research ranging from the positivist to naturalistic. Bussey (1995) identifies three categories of research, namely:

- theoretical research
- evaluation research
- action research.

He distinguishes between them by emphasizing that theoretical research attempts to describe, interpret and explain events without making any judgements. Evaluation research attempts to describe, interpret and explain events so that others may make judgements, but action research attempts to describe, interpret and explain events while seeking to change them for the better.

Definitions of action research

While nursing is keen to embrace the concept of action research and views it as an important means not only of bridging the theory–practice gap, but of empowering nurses and midwives to exercise autonomy within their own sphere of work, there is still some confusion about what exactly is meant by action research as it appears to encompass a variety of approaches. Some action researchers (Hart & Bond, 1996; Holter & Schwartz-Barcott, 1993) have attempted to shed light on the confusion by suggesting typologies, and these will be discussed later in the chapter. However, at this point in the narrative it would be helpful to suggest some definitions that clarify to the reader at least some basic principles that underpin the action research process.

> 'Action research is a form of self reflective enquiry undertaken by participants in social situations in order to improve the rationality and justice of their own practices, their understanding of those practices and the situations in which those practices are carried out.' (Carr & Kemmis, 1986: 150)

> 'Action research aims to contribute both to the practical concerns of people in an immediate problematic situation and to the goals of social science by joint collaboration within a mutually acceptable ethical framework.' (Rapoport, 1970: 499)

> 'The systematic study of attempts to change and improve practice by groups of participants by means of their own practical actions and by means of their own reflections upon the effects of those actions.' (Ebbutt, 1985: 156)

These three definitions pinpoint four main principles or characteristics that underpin action research. Action research involves:

- collaboration between researchers and practitioners;
- the solution of practical problems;

- change in practice;
- the development of theory.

The context of action research

Historically, action research can be seen to have developed from two distinct perspectives. The first originated from the work of Lewin (1947), a social psychologist who developed a particular interest in the study of group dynamics. The second arose from psychoanalysis and work of the Tavistock Institute of Human Relations, whose agenda involved the study of organizational behaviour.

Lewin (1947) was a German psychologist of the Gestalt School who was forced to emigrate to America in the late 1930s to escape Nazi persecution. In America, Lewin and his colleagues were particularly interested in the social concept of learning. At that time the behaviourist learning themes were very popular. Behaviourist theory attempts to explain learning by the passive response of an individual to stimuli in the environment. The gestalt theorists, however, challenged that notion and suggested that learning is more insightful and that individuals learn through understanding the 'whole' and by determining how the various parts within a system work together to create the 'whole'.

Through their research into learning, Lewin (1947) and his colleagues became very interested in the concept of changing behaviour. As a gestalt psychologist, he hypothesized that to change a person's behaviour required helping that person to view things in a new way. This contradicted the thinking of the Behaviourist School which argued that change was primarily brought about by rewarding good behaviour and not rewarding bad.

Lewin was not only interested in changing behaviour but also in finding out that change actually had occurred and the processes that were responsible for bringing about that change. He developed the action research process as a consequence of this research. Lewin saw action research as a form of rational social management whereby social change was brought about through consensus democracy. He postulated that action research was a type of field experiment which was conducted under controlled conditions and where the researcher was an expert brought in from outside. Within his field experiment he identified three clear stages.

1. An analysis of the situation prior to the change experiment (fact finding).
2. The instigation of an event or happening designed to bring about a change (action).
3. Evaluation of the situation after the change experiment as compared to the 'before' situation (evaluation).

From this it is clear to see why Lewin described action research as proceeding in a series of steps or cycles that involve fact finding, action and evaluation at every stage. At each cycle, fact finding would lead to the development of an action plan that would be implemented and then evaluated. Following evaluation the action may be modified, re-implemented and re-evaluated to determine whether or not the action had led to improvement. This feedback mechanism was utilized by Lewin within the action research experiment to create a cyclical framework whereby the feedback from the previous stage would inform change in the next stage.

At the same time that Lewin was developing his action research ideas in America, a parallel, but independent development in action research was happening in England by a group of researchers who developed the Tavistock Institute for Human Relations (Rapoport, 1970). These researchers involved psychologists, social anthropologists and psychiatrists from a psychoanalytical background. They were involved with solving organizational problems during and immediately following World War II. They used a social technical system approach founded on systems management and systems theory as a framework for their action research programme.

Lewin and the Tavistock Institute have been the two major influences on the development of action research. In more recent years, however, action researchers from education, management, health and social sciences have utilized and interpreted action research from their own philosophical orientation, which has led to the development of a variety of epistemological stances. However, Holter & Schwartz-Barcott (1993: 299) emphasize that:

'Regardless of these differences, the four characteristics of collaboration between researcher and practitioner, solution of practical problems, change in practice and the development of theory remain central to all forms of action research.'

Since the early work of Lewin and the Tavistock Institute researchers, a variety of different action research methodologies have arisen. Rolfe (1996) suggests that these differing methodologies can be considered using a continuum. At one extreme lies the traditional approach advocated by Lewin (1947), where the researcher becomes involved in the project from the outside and is bought into the project by nature of her expertise to plan the project, collect the data and advise the action organisation as to the best way forward. At this end of the continuum also lies the sociological approach where the researcher tests out theories in real-life scenarios to determine their relevance and effectiveness. It is clear that, in both these methodologies, staff within the action organization are not directly involved in determining the action to be taken and are being 'researched' rather than participating in the research process. In more recent years the new paradigm of research thinking, particularly in the field of education, has led to the development of more participative or collaborative action research methodologies. These can be placed at the other end of the continuum to the more scientifically based positivist action research methodology described by Lewin. In participative action research the researcher collaborates actively with staff in the action organization to design, collect data and decide on an appropriate action and evaluate the effectiveness of the change. However, Rolfe (1996) emphasizes that in this approach it is important to ensure that the changes brought about through the research are indeed improvements and, to ensure this, a stage of reflection must be introduced into the cyclical framework. This type of action research, which Rolfe (1996) entitles reflexive action research, has obvious advantages over the more traditional approaches in that practitioners are actively involved in the research process. They are part of the creative thinking behind the determined changes and are therefore more likely to own the whole process and, in consequence, narrow the theory–practice gap.

The attributes of action research

Before looking at some of the specific attributes of action research it would be wise to consider briefly how action research differs from the traditional research methodologies. Waterman (1995) suggests that the differences can be demonstrated by considering the following criteria:

- The conceptual framework
- The research process
- The methods of data collection
- The role of the researcher
- Ethical considerations
- Reliability and validity.

The conceptual framework

Within traditional research there is an assumption that we can view society and human behaviour in much the same way as we understand biological and physiological phenomena (Carr & Kemmis, 1986). Within traditional research there is an assumption that outcomes can be proved and theory developed, and that theory, once proved, can be applied generally across other similar situations. Within the positivist traditional research approach, theory is determined scientifically and applied to practice (see Fig. 16.1).

In action research, theory and practice are intertwined and dynamic and interact with each other. Action researchers tend to view situations from a sociological or philosophical stance rather than the biological or physiological perspectives used in the more traditional methodologies. Here the conceptual framework reflects a spiral of theory–practice development, as illustrated in Fig. 16.2.

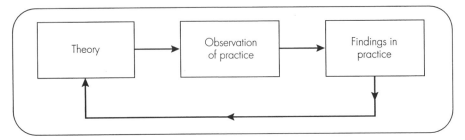

Fig. 16.1   Traditional positivist research framework.

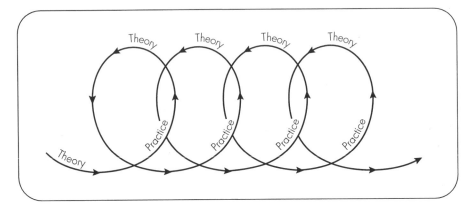

Fig. 16.2   Action research conceptual framework.

The research process

Differences exist within the research process used by action researchers and those used within other research approaches. Action research utilizes a cyclical approach where feedback from action taken in a previous stage determines the action in a subsequent stage. It is therefore a flexible and unpredictable process, unlike the more traditional methods which are planned, articulated and conducted to a predictable and relatively inflexible framework. Within action research it is possible to have an overall plan at the onset of the project; however, consideration must be given to the fact that this plan may change as the project progresses. This may be quite disconcerting for the researcher embarking on an action research project for the first time. There is comfort in being able to structure and plan a research project and to predetermine measurable objectives. This, however, is not the case within action research, therefore the task can seem more daunting at the outset.

The methods of data collection

Within traditional research there is a strong emphasis upon quantitative data that is statistically proved and generalizable. Traditional researchers from the positivist school tend to favour the experimental controlled trials and survey methodologies, which lend themselves to the generation of numerical statistically tested data. Within action research the field is spread much wider and although many action research projects, by their very nature, generate qualitative data some have also utilized quantitative data very effectively. Within action research the data tend to be analysed concurrent with their collection while in the more traditional approaches data collection and analysis occur sequentially. The wide range of data-collection methods open to action researchers requires them in many aspects to be multi-skilled. They need to be familiar with both quantitative and qualitative research methods, whereas in the more traditional approaches there is a tendency for researchers to 'specialize' and develop expertise in one approach. McNiff *et al.* (1998) also suggest that, on top of this, action researchers should also possess skills in interface management, collaborative skills, listening skills, intrapersonal and communication skills.

The role of the researcher

A fundamental difference between the two approaches lies in the role played by the researcher. In the traditional approach every care is taken to ensure that the researcher is neutral, without bias, objective and outside of the research situation. Indeed many researchers go to great lengths in justifying their approach to exclude bias and to ensure their objectivity. In action research, however, the researcher is part of the research process; she is inside the research situation:

> '...And the boundaries between the action researchers and the researched are blurred simply because they could be the same people. Action researchers tend to argue that detachment of oneself from a research setting in order "to see it as it really is" is impossible and cannot lead to understanding. Generally they propose that familiarity creates opportunity for insight. The objectives and the course of action research projects are negotiated between research participants; and with collaboration and co-operation between participants being the key themes.' (Waterman, 1995: 20)

Ethical considerations

As with traditional research, ethical issues are important albeit less straight-forward in action research. Meyer (1993), recounting her own experience of action research, identifies that action research is often written as case studies and this presents a potential problem in protecting the anonymity and confidentiality of participants. The collaborative nature of action research suggests that participants 'own' the findings and therefore it becomes more complicated in terms of protecting their anonymity. In traditional controlled trials or projects using surveys it is relatively straightforward to ensure confidentiality of participants. In action research the researcher may well ensure that no participant is named in the report, however the participant can be easily compromised by the fact that the researcher is known to be associated with a particular ward or department, thus making key players very vulnerable. Meyer (1993) also emphasizes that the issue of informed consent is also a potential problem in action research. She states:

'Consent really centres around the participants' willingness to take part in the project ideas and acceptance of the researcher as a facilitator of change. The proposals for change come from within the group of participants and as such is a step into the unknown for individual players. Informed consent is therefore not really possible and once the project is underway it is difficult for individuals to withdraw as they are part of a group committed to working together for change.' (Meyer, 1993: 1069)

In traditional research it is much easier for participants to opt out of the research situation by refusing to be interviewed or by simply discarding the questionnaire, but participants in action research are to some extent 'trapped' in the situation by the fact that they are committed and deeply involved in the change process.

Reliability and validity

Since its inception in the 1940s, action research has received much criticism regarding its scientific basis and in some instances has been considered not worthy of the label 'research'. Much of this criticism centres around debates as to its validity and reliability. Traditional researchers use statistical tests to prove reliability of their findings and validity is addressed using a variety of techniques, for example, a panel of experts to determine that the chosen research instrument measures what it is intended to measure. Action researchers, however, tend to adopt a different stance. Waterman (1998) argues that validity in action research can be determined by analysing its three major qualities: dialectual validity, critical validity and reflexive validity.

Dialectual validity

By its very nature action research addresses the tensions and difficulties that arise in practice. This, Waterman (1998) stresses, is a strength of action research that demonstrates its validity. Likewise the dialectual process of action research – which involves theory, research and practice as a dynamic, intertwined process involved in bringing about change in the real world – is a positive indicator of the validity of action research.

Critical validity

Action research is involved with 'improving the justice of people's situations' (Carr & Kemmis, 1986). Waterman (1998) suggests that there is an emancipating element in action research which tries to make things better, albeit the degree to which it achieves this differs between projects. It is this attempt to improve people's lives rather than the degree to which it actually affects change that is crucial to assessing validity. Waterman (1998: 104) stresses that: 'Reports of action research should contain analyses of intentions and abilities to act and emphasise the ethical implications and consequences of actions and theories.'

Reflexive validity

Within action research, researchers are encouraged to question, search for opposing perspectives and to evaluate their courses of action collaboratively. It is this exhaustive process that is a quality of action research and indeed goes some way to quell fears regarding bias and vested interests. Current practices in action research also demonstrate a reflexive stance in which researcher prejudices are positively examined to determine their degree of influence on the project and how to use that influence most appropriately. All action research projects should present an analysis as to how decisions were reached and why the study was conducted in a particular way. Waterman (1998: 104) states that: 'Action researchers view the problem of bias from a different angle and consider the exploration of biases as a vital means of demonstrating validity.'

In summary

McNiff *et al.* (1998) summarize very succinctly the similarities and differences between action research and traditional research. They state that:

'Action research shares the following characteristics with other research because:

- it leads to knowledge;
- it provides evidence to support this knowledge;
- it makes clear the process of enquiry which underpins that knowledge;
- it links new knowledge to existing knowledge.

'Action research differs from other research because:

- it requires action as integral to the research process itself;
- it is focused by the researchers' professional values rather than methodological considerations;
- it is insider research in the sense that practitioners research their own professional actions.'

(McNiff *et al.*, 1998: 14)

The action research process

As mentioned previously, the action research approach is by necessity a flexible and dynamic approach which tends to develop as the project progresses. In fact it would be true to say that the action research process is often better described retrospectively rather than prospectively. However, Meyer (1993), utilizing her experience of action research, identifies six potential stages:

- The negotiation stage
- The assessment stage
- The planning stage
- The action stage
- The evaluation stage
- The withdrawal stage

Meyer is keen to stress, however, that these stages are not as discreet as they may first appear. Action research is a dynamic process and, in reality, some stages may merge into each other. Gill & Johnson (1991) similarly identify six stages which they classify as:

- Entry
- Contracting
- Diagnosis
- Action
- Evaluation
- Withdrawal

For ease of presentation the six stages described by Meyer (1993) will be used as a framework for the remainder of this section.

The negotiation stage

This stage denotes entry into the project. The researcher may perform an 'insider' or 'outsider' role. The 'insider' role involves the combined roles of change agent, researcher and clinical leader. The researcher is usually part of the action organization and, as stated by Titchen & Binnie (1993), the combination of authority with a research role is obviously advantageous. However, the 'insider' role also has its downside in that participants can often feel threatened by the fact that the researcher is an insider, and this may influence their willingness to disclose information. The 'outsider' role is that played by a researcher who comes from outside the action organization and has no authority in the situation. In this role the researcher prescribes change for change agents in the organization to implement. This obviously has potential problems of ownership of the change as the participants may well feel that the changes are being forced upon them.

Titchen & Binnie (1993) advocate a dual partnership double act role, which seeks to combine the advantages of both the insider and outsider roles. In this approach the researcher from outside the situation mutually collaborates with an insider change agent facilitator. Both roles are of equal importance and they work together collaboratively, combining authority with impartiality. It is crucial at the negotiation stage to identify the type of role to be fulfilled. Teamwork and effective group dynamics are also essential characteristics of action research and considerable time may require to be spent at the negotiation stage to develop effective group functioning.

The assessment stage

It is essential in this stage to collect data regarding the current situation to act as a base line against which to measure any future change.

The planning stage

This stage invariably involves diagnosing problems and determining possible solutions. This is achieved using a variety of data-collection techniques – for example, focus groups, brainstorming, questionnaires, interviews and observation.

The action stage

This stage may involve several action/reflection cycles, where varying approaches to change are implemented, reflected upon, re-implemented with innovations determined from the previous cycle and reflected upon again, etc. This stage is often lengthy and can be stressful for all participants. It is during this stage that participants challenge the status quo and critically appraise their current practices. This may raise particular sensitivities, therefore it is essential for effective group dynamics to be evident during this stage and for group members to work democratically and practise self-reflection.

The evaluation stage

At this stage the data-collection measures utilized within the assessment stage are repeated to determine:

- that change has taken place
- the effectiveness of the change.

The withdrawal stage

In action research the researcher becomes involved in the research situation and withdrawal from the project is often more complex than in other forms of research. It is sometimes difficult for the researcher to know when to withdraw if she is performing an 'outsider' role and when to conclude the project if she is fulfilling an 'insider' role.

Modes of action research: the use of typologies

Holter & Schwartz-Barcott (1993) identify three modes of action research that emerge from the literature. These they entitle as follows:

- The technical collaborative approach
- The mutual collaborative approach
- The enhancement approach

The technical collaborative approach

This mode of action research is similar to that originally described by Lewin (1947). The intention of the researcher in this approach is to test a particular intervention to see how effective it is to solve a problem in a specific situation. The researcher is usually an expert and an outsider to the research situation. In this approach change is generally imposed after gaining the co-operation of practitioners. However, the lasting benefit of the change is doubtful, as it is likely to lack ownership. The kind of knowledge that emerges from this approach is largely deductive since it involves the testing and refining of existing theory.

The mutual collaborative approach

In this approach and, as the title suggests, the researcher and a member of the action organization collaborate together to identify problems, determine solutions, test solutions and evaluate outcomes. This working together approach leads to a better understanding of the underlying problems and their causes and hence to longer lasting changes. The knowledge generated from this approach is generally descriptive and can lead to the development of new theory.

The enhancement approach

In this approach the researcher has two principal goals. First, to enable practitioners to use theory to explain and resolve problems and, second, to raise corporate awareness in practitioners regarding their underlying values and beliefs, both personal and collective, that are manifest within the organizational culture and may impact on the problems identified. Local theory generates from meaningful discussions held between practitioners and researcher. Longer lasting change is an outcome of this approach as it allows negative values and unhelpful cultural norms to be dealt with and thus more meaningful change established. The knowledge generated is both predictive and descriptive.

Hart & Bond (1996), while acknowledging the many strengths of the Holter & Schwartz-Barcott typology, suggest that it has two fundamental limitations. First, they stress that it deals with action research projects as though they were static, but by nature they are dynamic and a project may well change its orientation during its life span. Second, their typology does not address the philosophical stance of the action researcher, which has tremendous influence over the goals and the approach taken. Hart & Bond suggest an alternative typology which is more dynamic in nature. Their typology groups concepts together into four categories – namely, experimental, organizational, professionalizing and empowering. It suggests that these four types can be placed strategically along a continuum relating to two alternative models of society: the consensus model to the left and the conflict model to the right. It also suggests that the four types are related to the three distinguishing criteria of action research – that is, the educative base, the particular forms and the differing ways of conceptualizing improvement and involvement. The result is a typology that resembles a grid against which action research projects can be assessed for the 'best fit', acknowledging that most projects adopt an eclectic approach that may not fit neatly into any single category. Readers wishing to study this typology in more detail are advised to read the original source of Hart & Bond's work indicated in the further reading section at the end of this chapter (Hart & Bond, 1995).

Conclusions

Action research, as a research methodology, offers many advantages to nurses and midwives not least of which must be the fact that the dissemination of findings is integral to the research process. Action research solves practical problems in tandem with the generation of theory; it empowers nurses and midwives to exercise more autonomy over their own specific sphere of professional practice; and it substantially reduces the theory–practice gap. It is, however, a time-consuming process necessitating collaboration between participants and researcher, an attribute that predisposes the process to specific ethical problems relating to informed consent and participant anonymity. Despite its increasing popularity in the field of nursing research, it still receives considerable criticism relating to its scientific robustness. Action researchers do not purport to have generalizable findings as an outcome of their research, however they do claim to bring about change in practice – an attribute which most traditional research finds hard to emulate.

References

Abbott, P. & Sapsford, R. (1998) *Research Methods for Nurses and the Caring Professions*, 2nd edn. Buckingham: Open University Press.

Bussey, M. (1995) *Creating Education Through Research*. Newark: Kirklington Press.

Carr, W. & Kemmis, S. (1986) *Becoming Critical, Education, Knowledge, and Action Research*. London: Falmer Press.

Ebbutt, D. (1985) Educational action research. Some concerns and specific quibbles. In R. Burgess (ed.) *Issues of Educational Research, Qualitative Methods*. Lewes: Falmer Press.

Funk, S., Champagne, M., Wiese, R. & Tornquist, E. (1991) Barriers to using research findings in practice: the clinician's perspective. *Applied Nursing Research* 4 (2): 90–5.

Gill, J. & Johnson, P. (1991) *Research Methods for Managers*. London: Paul Chapman.

Hart, E. & Bond, M. (1996) Making sense of action research through the use of a typology. *Journal of Advanced Nursing* 23: 152–9.

Holter, I. & Schwartz-Barcott, D. (1993) Action research: What is it? How has it been used and how can it be used in nursing? *Journal of Advanced Nursing* 18: 298–304.

Hunt, M. (1987) The process of translating research findings into nursing practice. *Journal of Advanced Nursing* 12: 101–10.

Lewin, K. (1947) Frontiers in group dynamics. Social planning and action research. *Human Relations* 1 (2): 143–53.

McNiff, J., Lomax, P. & Whitehead, J. (1998) *You and Your Action Research Project*. London: Routledge.

Meyer, J. (1993) New paradigm research in practice: the trials and tribulations of action research. *Journal of Advanced Nursing* 18: 1066–72.

Rapoport, R.N. (1970) Three dilemmas in action research. *Human Relations* 23 (6): 499–513.

Rolfe, G. (1996) Going to extremes. Action research, grounded practice and the theory–practice gap in nursing. *Journal of Advanced Nursing* 24: 1315–20.

Titchen, A. & Binnie, A. (1993) Research partnerships. Collaborative action research in nursing. *Journal of Advanced Nursing* 18: 858–65.

Waterman, H. (1995) Distinguishing between traditional and action research. *Nurse Researcher* 2 (3): 15–23.

Waterman, H. (1998) Embracing ambiguities and valuing ourselves: Issues of validity in action research. *Journal of Advanced Nursing* 28 (1): 101–5.

Further reading

Bellman, L. (1996) Changing nursing practice through reflection on the Roper Logan and Tierney Model. The enhancement approach to action research. *Journal of Advanced Nursing* 24: 129–38.

Hart, E. & Bond, M. (1995) *Action Research for Health and Social Care*. Buckingham: Open University Press.

Lauri, S. (1982) Development of the nursing process through action research. *Journal of Advanced Nursing* 7: 301–7.

Manley, K. (1997) A conceptual framework for advanced practice. An action research project operationalising an advanced practitioner/consultant nurse role. *Journal of Advanced Nursing* **6**: 179–90.

Smith, G. (1986) Resistance to change in geriatric care. *International Journal of Nursing Studies* **12** (1): 61–70. (A mutual collaboration approach to action research.)

Webb, C. (1989) Action research philosophy and personal experiences. *Journal of Advanced Nursing* **14**: 403–10.

CHAPTER 17

Historical research

Anne Marie Rafferty

Historical research, once the enthusiasm of a few eccentric scholars, is now the preserve of a small but growing intellectual community. Reflecting the rise of research and higher education provision for nurses and midwives more generally, a number of nursing and midwifery departments have added history to their research portfolio. The fortunes of historical research have fluctuated with fashions of curricular change and oscillations in the political temperature. The status attached to history by society appears to reflect the esteem in which liberal values in education are held at any given time. Insofar as nursing reflects in microcosm the wider changes in society, history can be regarded as a metaphor for gear changes in liberal educational values more generally.

Shifting sands

Compared to the history of medicine or science, little has been written about the purpose of history and the function of the historian in nursing. Yet nursing is not without its historiological commentators. Prominent among these have been Lynaugh & Reverby (1986) in the USA and Davies (1980) and Maggs (1978) in the UK. Such commentaries have marked a watershed in the writing of nursing history on both sides of the Atlantic. What they have advocated and practised was a move from the hero-centred view of history, to a more critical form of research which located nursing within a wider social and political context. The movement within American nursing history culminated in the early 1980s in the edited collection of Lagemann (1982), which brought together a series of essays that asked new kinds of questions about nursing politics and nursing work.

Pre-eminent among these questions are those pertaining to race, class and gender in nursing. Innovative work stretching from South Africa to Scotland, India to England considers ways in which these questions intersect with and react upon each other (Marks, 1994; Strachan, 1995; Rafferty et al., 1997). Such research complements that of earlier American nurse historians, who were among the first to include questions of race and ethnicity within their research repertoire (Carnegie, 1991).

Throughout the 1980s sporadic methodological commentaries emerged from nurse historians keen to reflect upon their craft. McPherson & Stuart's (1994) review essay provides a compact and wide-ranging commentary on the state of the historical art in nursing in the 1990s. Tracking the tension between the humanistic ethos of nursing and technology, Fairman & Lynaugh (1998) remind us that the gendered, love–hate relationship between nursing and technology reflects cultural ambivalence towards technology more generally. Together, these works have helped to create a new intellectual community within nursing and an audience for the consumption and appreciation of nursing history.

Why study history?

People study history for a variety of reasons: for pleasure, as a form of intellectual training, for the light it sheds on contemporary problems and as a contextual guide to decision-making. Marwick (1970) and Evans (1997) argue that the study of the past contributes greatly to our understanding of contemporary problems, human behaviour and the forces driving social change. In Britain, the use of historical evidence in justifying the case for change in the United Kingdom Central Council for Nursing, Midwifery and Health Visiting *Project 2000* document owed much to the inspiration of Celia Davies as project officer and her research experience in historical sociology (UKCC, 1986). As individuals we tend to be attracted to different subject areas, kinds of work and social environments for various reasons: some people love laboratory work, others libraries; some thrive on social and collaborative contact, others solving problems solo; some rejoice in computer graphics, ruminating over data sets and statistical tests; while others prefer the *in-situ* analytic art of participant observation. But the key ingredient that unites many researchers is passion – emotional and often political commitment to their chosen subject of study. This can apply as much to scientists as to historians and the history of science provides ample evidence of cases where faith and political beliefs can be as important an impetus to innovation as reason (Pickering, 1992).

Context and chronology

Research is concerned with asking questions, gathering evidence, describing and explaining the nature and strength of the relationship between variables. Historical research is also concerned with such questions and although it may be difficult to calculate the precise nature of the relationships between historical variables, it is also worth recalling how difficult it is to pin down causation in health care too. What differentiates the historical enterprise from the scientific, however, is the former's focus upon context and chronology as explanatory power. As the historian E.P. Thompson reminds us

'The discipline of history is, above all, the discipline of context; each fact can be given meaning only within an ensemble of other meanings.' (Thompson cited by Lynaugh & Reverby, 1986: 4)

Intricacies of interpretation

Unlike the scientist, the historian is not concerned with exercising control over variables in the same way that a scientist might – reducing the number of variables for analysis – nor with holding these constant over time. Rather the historian has to work with 'natural' experiments; those which posterity, the preservation policies of organizations, gatekeepers and legal regulators of access to records allow. That does not mean to say that every historian will use the same piece of evidence in the same way or arrive at the same conclusions using a similar set of sources. Interpretation lies at the heart of the historiographical endeavour. Historians will attach greater or lesser significance to the influence of particular variables upon events and outcomes. Under the influence of post-modernism history has been convulsed by culture wars. Such debates revolve around the proposition that a text is a text is a text. Thus, the border between fact and fiction, authorship and authority, breaks down. The historian is merely an author like any other, having no apparatus of authority to which to appeal in the case of competing interpretations of events except their own. Evans (1997) rejects this view and has mounted a stirring defence of the discipline from what he implies are its academic assailants. His defence of a more liberal approach to history is far more pragmatic; we can know something about the past although there are no hard and fast rules about its intepretation.

Carr (1970) has defined history as 'the continuous interaction between the historian and his facts, an unending dialogue between the present and the past'. Although it may seem on the surface that historians are at the mercy of their sources, all researchers are in fact dependent upon their evidence and subject to economic and ethical constraints. Historical research is particularly sensitive to the chronology of the question(s) being asked. In attempting to identify the 'causes' of wound healing, for example, a historical survey of past treatments may cast light on the mechanisms underlying changes in the theory and practice of wound care. The Hippocratic and Galenic medical theory of the fifth century BC to the second century AD, for example, maintained that suppuration and the production of so-called 'laudable pus' was an essential part of wound healing (Cartwright, 1977). This reasoning contrasts vividly with the current theory of wound care, the object of which is to prevent infection. What the historian attempts to understand is how such theory was shaped and the factors that brought about change at any given point in time. Studying the history of nursing research helps us to understand that knowledge is provisional and apt to alter with the generation of fresh findings. While more sophisticated analyses of the theory–practice gap and implementation process in nursing research are beginning to emerge, historical studies of specified nursing 'interventions' can enhance our understanding of the politics of innovation and research utilization.

Calculating change

Unlike research involving calculations and statistical inference and interpretation, history does not lend itself easily to estimating the precise effect of confounding variables, those which produce an interactive effect and therefore require correction to ascertain the effect of each individually. History is not, however, devoid of, nor divorced from, the world of statistics. Indeed there is a subdiscipline of history called *cliometrics* which deals precisely with this. History and computing are growing areas of interest for researchers skilled in the management of large data sets, working at the interface between demography and history. The advent of information technology had penetrated every sphere of life, including history. Quantitative methods in the history of medicine were the subject of a book by Porter & Wear (1988). Yet some historians have gone as far as talking about the strength of their evidence in terms of causation. Stone (1972), in his discussion of the causes of the English Civil War, divides the causal factors into three chronological groups: long-term preconditions, medium-term precipitants, and short-term triggers. 'Causes' here may be more readily conceived of in terms of necessary and sufficient conditions rather than ranked precisely into a hierarchy of contributory factors.

Let us take a recent example in this country: if studying the origins of *Project 2000* and the 'causes' of its success, one of the major questions the historian would ask is 'Why has *Project 2000* apparently succeeded as a reform strategy where others seem to have failed?' (UKCC, 1986). What factors have promoted its implementation? The merits of the case? Demographic pressures? The social, political, and economic environment? The fit with government policy? Administration of the health, educational and social services? Or all of these? And, if so, were all equal in importance? Immediately, we are confronted with the problems of historical evaluation. What in historical terms counts as success or failure? How can we measure historical change? Which outcome variables should we consider? Whose view(s) should we take into account – practising nurses, nurse leaders, the project team, government officials? Which sources should we use and how should we prioritize them? My own view is that successful state-sponsored change in nursing can often be explained as the product of three overlapping forces: context, convergence and contingency. These were all present in *Project 2000*. Thus the context and backdrop was the so-called demographic timebomb which threatened to explode in the employment market for nurses. Convergence consisted in the fit that the mobility and multi-purpose employment ethos of *Project 2000* had with Thatcher's policy on flexible workforces, casualization of the labour force and deregulation of the public sector. Finally, contingency resulted from the fortuitous timing that coincided with wider policy changes within higher education. A similar set of forces can be seen at work in the entry of nursing into higher education itself. Although as far back as 1948 it was recognized that 10–15% of the nursing workforce qualified for university entrance, the seismic shift in policy only occurred when the context of government objectives for higher education changed in the late 1980s. For once, the female dominance of the workforce converged with government's agenda as canny vice-chancellors and policy-makers cashed in on nursing's generous dowry of gender. Together, contingency ensured that nursing and health sciences made a significant contribution to the growth of higher education by broadening access, especially to women.

Value of and value in history

Perhaps the value of historical research in nursing can best be illustrated by an example which has provided a corrective to the historical record. This revisionist approach is admirably illustrated by Baly's (1986) study of Florence Nightingale and the politics of the Nightingale Fund. Much of Baly's research is devoted to the exposure of a number of myths concerning the Nightingale School and its training methods. Contrary to popular wisdom, St Thomas's was not originally considered by Miss Nightingale as an ideal institution for the Nightingale School on account of its insalubrious location and its matron, Mrs Wardroper, whose competence to supervise nurse training was doubted by Miss Nightingale. Furthermore, far from providing a codified scheme of instruction and a model of training ready for export, the training provided was haphazard, the wastage rate high, and only modest numbers of well-educated women came forward to be inculcated with the *new* spirit of reformed nursing. Diaries, for example, which were kept by the probationers for inspection by Miss Nightingale, indicated that most of the probationers' time on the wards was unsupervised and that the intellectual content of lectures was pitched deliberately low and required supplementary interpretation and coaching from the Home Sister (Baly, 1986: 174).

Continuity and change

History helps us to understand the process of change, be it in methods used to treat pressure sores or the introduction of new ways of organizing care. One of the first evaluation studies of team nursing, for example, was published in the late 1950s by a Canadian nurse (Jenkinson, 1953). Where did the idea and method originate? Was it significant that this innovation was promoted by a nurse from North America? What was it about the organizational climate at the hospital in question (St George's, London) that favoured the introduction of new ideas? Was the then matron, Muriel Powell, a crucial influence in supporting the change? In relation to nursing research, historical research can help us to understand more fully the factors which transform a 'good idea' into standard practice and help to explain why some research findings are implemented and not others.

Historical research provides one way of investigating the dynamics and direction of change. The historian's own views, opinions and preconceptions as well as research funding policy may be crucial determinants of the questions selected for study and the mode of investigation adopted. Individuals may be attracted to different disciplines, topics and techniques in research for a variety of reasons, some of which may be very personal. In qualitative research, the researcher's belief system may be taken for granted as intrinsic to the research process and even formally integrated into the fabric of the account and analysis (Walker, 1994). In scientific research, the accent is on eliminating the influence of the investigator, although studies in the history and sociology of science confirm that researchers' values, personal histories, belief systems and ambitions can be important motivators of research (Pickering, 1992).

Sources and sampling

It may at this point be worth-while considering the range of resources upon which the historian of nursing might draw in order to construct an account. First I shall discuss access and availability. While both historians and scientists may have to negotiate access to the research site through gatekeepers such as ethics committees, health service managers and keepers of manuscripts, the historian may have her work predetermined by virtue of the preservation or destruction of records. The potential to generate data anew rests with the scientist. The historian traversing unknown territory may have little idea of what, if anything, sources, once located, will reveal. Historical sources are subject to a particular set of regulations concerning access and closure which may be crucial in determining the research that can be undertaken. The '30 year rule' in the UK closes access to public records for 30 years after the date of the last item in the file. 'Public' may be defined as those records deriving from organizations which are accountable to public bodies such as Parliament, but all records of the National Health Service authorities also fall into this category. Medical records of patients in the UK are only open to the public after 100 years. In exceptional cases, organizations may decide to waive the rules normally governing access to material under their jurisdiction and open files earlier than the statutory period to *bona fide* researchers, provided precautions to safeguard anonymity and the conditions of the Data Protection Act in publications are adhered to.

Public records may be stored at the Public Record Office (PRO), the Scottish equivalent, Scottish Record Office (SRO), or a local repository such as the Metropolitan Record Office (GLRO) or regional records offices such as County

Records Offices or local repositories such as (in Scotland) the Lothian Health Trust Medical Archives Centre housed in Special Collections at Edinburgh University Library. Some hospitals store their own records, but the stage of preservation varies enormously. Private organizations such as the Royal National Pensions Fund for Nurses may also maintain their own records. The Royal College of Nursing (RCN) employs a full-time archivist for this purpose, who is based at the Scottish Headquarters in Edinburgh. The Wellcome Institute's Contemporary Medical Archive contains a number of different sources that are relevant to nursing, including the Queen's Institute of District Nursing and the records of the Community Practitioners and Health Visitors Association.

The scholarly and innovative merit of an historical work may hinge upon the extent to which it is based upon primary sources or reinterprets secondary sources in a novel way. Primary sources are the raw unedited data (the minutes, papers and correspondence of organizations such as the now defunct General Nursing Council for England and Wales), upon which historical interpretation is based. Secondary sources refer to the digested, interpreted or reported data of primary historical material. Generally, the secondary literature is mastered before the primary data are mined to provide the necessary contextual material for the account, but this order may not be strictly adhered to as new lines of inquiry emerge. Arguments will usually be suggested by the data, and are subject to change as different types of sources emerge and are explored and re-read at different stages in the research. Interpretation is a dynamic and interactive process. In keeping with developments in other areas of historical research, notably that in the history of medicine, the scope of nursing has broadened recently to encompass a wide range of sources. There is no standard method for the organization or compiling of sources or evidence. These might include not only official and semi-official printed or written documents and private papers, but also literary accounts, biography, autobiography and fiction. More recently, oral testimony has yielded useful data on the experiences of working nurses. Little account as yet has been taken of patients' views but film, television, video, architecture, art and photographic material have recently been incorporated within the inventory of sources and methods (Hudson-Jones, 1988). It remains to be seen what the impact of the telephone and on-line archives are likely to be in supplying the sources of the future. The Center for the Study of the History of Nursing within the School of Nursing at the University of Pennsylvania (established in 1985) has developed a strong track record in promoting research in the area and cultivating a community of scholars, actual and virtual in the discipline. Similarly, the Australian Nursing History Project, launched in November 1998 by the Postgraduate School of Nursing at the University of Melbourne, is one of the first to provide a register of nursing historical resources, profiles of significant nursing individuals, organizations, events and links to other sources through its website. One of the major advantages of using a range of tools and sources as data is the potential for verification of evidence and interpretation. Thus, official documents may be used in combination, if possible, with private diaries and oral testimony to check and confirm a line of enquiry. Different perceptions of the same situation or event are likely to emerge from different individuals with different agendas and interests. The uncovering of 'multiple realities' may be the very point of the investigative exercise and is especially important in tracking the pathways of decision-making in policy analysis. In many ways, historical research has much in common with qualitative research in its acknowledgement of multiple realities and triangulation of methods.

Voyage of discovery or journey without maps?

On a practical level, historical research can be both frustrating and rewarding. Hours spent searching for a particular source of evidence may yield little. Equally, it is possible to stumble on a goldmine of information: a personal diary, an album of photographs, a clutch of newspaper cuttings. The records of the past were not written with the needs of the historian in mind, although public bodies do have preservation policies implemented by officials trained to evaluate the historical importance of documents. These policies may be regulated by resources and other factors not necessarily within the control of historians themselves. As nurses and historians, we should take an active role in trying to influence preservation policies to maximize their utility for future generations of historians, nurses and researchers. Ideally, research projects should be based around a solid set of records, which assumes that the archives have been used by, or are known to, the researcher. Such effort presupposes that the researcher has already undertaken sufficient work to have refined the research question in order to identify specific sources. Few may be able to afford the luxury of such in-depth preparatory or pilot work before submitting proposals for funding to vetting agencies. Nonetheless, it is possibly inadvisable to depend upon only one source of data no matter how potentially rich.

The direction and outcome of the research will depend upon the use that can be made of the sources and, consequently, the question asked may change dramatically in the course of the investigation. The order of enquiry is negotiated and loose; there is no orderly progression of steps or stages to follow. Commuting between primary and secondary material in response to the data is common. Practicalities such as the employment of an archivist may be crucial in determining the use of sources. The listing of holdings and cataloguing of material greatly enhances the efficiency of information retrieval. Much may also depend upon the experience and efficiency of the researcher. While nurses who have a first degree in history will have an advantage in undertaking historical research, nurses who do not have to learn by other means much of what trained historians perhaps take for granted. Generally speaking, however, the problem of historical research is not one of finding sufficient material, but of containing the huge volumes of paper generated by organizations. Documents, journals and personal papers should be systematically screened for relevant material and this can mean hours of laborious scrutiny and scanning. All research has its routine tasks, but this is a labour that may be crucial to how the account will be organized and presented. In determining the division of labour, it may be advisable to tackle the records of one organization at a time. If events are particularly current, it is desirable to interview the participants themselves.

Oral history requires specific methodological and ethical considerations and has acquired the status of a subdiscipline within history itself (Thompson, 1978). It may serve a variety of purposes: to fill gaps in the documentation, to uncover details of decisions, to generate evidence missing from the records or to allow the clarification of factual points. In some cases it may be the only evidence available. There are many pitfalls, as well as great potential, in the use of oral testimony, some of which have to do with the power relations and social characteristics of the interviewer and interviewee. Oral history may be invaluable as an insight into an individual's thought processes, the discovery of new and important information and, more generally, in enriching the quality of data. As a testament to its commitment to nursing history and leadership, the Royal College of Nursing (RCN) sponsored a project concerned with collecting the career histories of a cohort of retired nurse leaders. This top-down history is being supplemented more recently by a bottom-up approach to the oral history of nurses who trained and practised in the 1930s. Training in oral history technique is available and a number of nurses involved in the RCN project have benefited from courses offered by the National Lifestory Collection (address is given at the end of this chapter).

Social and socializing history

What, therefore, have been the characteristic features of historical research in nursing? Much of nursing history has been used to serve a number of professional even 'professionalizing' ends (Rafferty, 1991). Early writing in nursing history was more concerned with synthesizing existing knowledge rather than producing new knowledge through fresh investigation. The use of previously unexploited primary evidence and the development of novel interpretations is the *raison d'être* of research. Both characteristics have been exemplified in studies of British nursing since the early 1960s. The innovative edited collection of social scientific aspects of historical nursing research referred to earlier (Davies, 1980) provided a focus for feminist and labour history interpretations of nursing history. Maggs (1978) was one of the first nurses to treat nursing history as a case study in social history.

Pilgrims of progress

It may be tempting to view the changes of the past as somehow inevitable and as the fulfilment of progress, and much history has been written from this point of view. This assumes that the past is governed by law-like mechanisms and ignores the conflict and complexities of rival forces competing for power. Much of the recent research in the history of nursing rejects this view as failing to account for the tensions between historical agencies and the intricacies of power differentials which favour one set of conditions rather than another. The past as representing progress, while psychologically gratifying, prejudges the past, and forces it into a mould which empirical research may contradict. For example, although increases in nurses' pay in the UK have occurred since the introduction of the National Health Service, the fluctuating pattern of relativities suggests that the story of nurses' pay has not been one of 'onward and upward' (Gray, 1989). Indeed ground gained politically in one decade may be lost in another as the 'crisis' in nurse leadership following the implementation of general management demonstrated.

The politics of history

Historical research may be driven by fashion as well as by the dual dynamic of the data and contemporary concerns of professional politics. Although the hospital, for example, has been criticized by historians as the root of economic evil and its harnessing of hierarchy and the power relations that it promotes, it still stands at the peak of the historiographical pyramid. For it was here that modern medicine and nursing were formed in scientific silhouette and formed the crucible for clinical careers. How then, given the serial assaults on its reputation, has the hospital retained its force as a cultural power? Part of the reason might be through its 'invention of traditions'. These are the trappings of prestige, the myths, rituals and ceremonial orders of the clinic that help to define the identity, cultural, political and ultimately economic power and status of institutions (Hobsbawn & Ranger, 1993). History has an important role to play in the moral and political economy of the hospital and its resilience over time.

Conservative and radical, the current incarnation of the hospital as a technological theme park merely reflects the latest stage in its evolution: from religious foundation, secularized philanthropy, organ of state bureaucracy to model of modernization. Hospitals have become beacons of modernity, re-engineered economic entities through which patients pass at lightning speed, struggling to fathom the symbolic trappings of the new regimes of care. In practical terms, history and the strength of the 'invented tradition' through which they operate may exert a strong but under-acknowledged influence upon the success and sustainability of any re-engineering schemes. Similarly, the success or failure of mergers may depend in part upon those self-same processes. Thus the past is very much present in contemporary change.

Mining metaphors

In many ways, historical research may be compared to mining: extensive exploratory work may be necessary to refine an area for further investigation, or diligent excavation may reveal a wealth of resources. For this reason, and the fact that only in exceptional cases will records be susceptible to computer analysis, the process of extracting and analysing the data and formulating interpretations is time consuming and labour intensive. One cannot readily feed the data into a computer and run a battery of tests or a statistical package to identify trends or characteristics. Much of the analysis has to be conducted without such aids to efficiency. Historical research can be expensive in time and resources, and there are no immediate practical spin-offs in terms of a product to justify research investment. It also tends to be an individualistic enterprise and less frequently undertaken as part of a multi-disciplinary project. Few projects are group efforts, although the history of the International Council of Nurses has been written as a team effort and collaborative project (Brush *et al.*, 1999). Historical research has helped to shed important light upon the multiple metaphorical meanings of nursing and therefore contributed towards a challenging political agenda for nurses.

Repertoire of resources

Access to historical research in nursing is mediated through normal academic channels, but enquiries are welcomed by the History of Nursing Society based at the Royal College of Nursing in London, which also holds conferences and meetings and publishes the *International History of Nursing Journal*. In theory, one can study nursing history wherever there are resources to do so; the Public Records Office in London and the Greater London Records Office both produce broadsheets outlining their holdings on nursing history, and the Wellcome Institute has a large collection of relevant archival material in their Contemporary Medical Archive.

The task of research, whether it involves registering for a higher degree or not, is eased considerably where there is intellectual and practical support. Help and advice can be offered by members of the RCN Society and also through the Wellcome Units for the History of Medicine based in Glasgow, Manchester, Oxford, Norwich, the Wellcome Institute in London and the Department of Nursing and Midwifery Studies at the University of Nottingham. In the USA, a Center for the Study of the History of Nursing and Archival Repository is affiliated to the University of Pennsylvania School of Nursing, and the *Nursing History*

Review is in its seventh volume. The Center has its own archivist. A second centre has been established at the University of Virginia. The Mary Adelaide Nutting Collection at Teachers College, Columbia University, New York, contains important educational and clinical material and texts. Historical options are offered in masters and doctoral programmes at the University of California at San Francisco jointly between the School of Nursing and the Department of History of Health Sciences. Fairman (1987) has produced a useful inventory of the repository holdings of nursing history archives in the USA and Sioban Nelson, together with Judith Parker have been prime movers in establishing the Australian Nursing History Project at the University of Melbourne referred to above.

Conclusions

The above discussion represents only the briefest outline of some signposts to historical research in nursing. Until the early 1960s, the writing of nursing history was dominated by nurses and nurse leaders who used history as a vehicle to justify professionalization. The arrival of researchers whose primary academic training was not in nursing – for example, sociologists, historians of medicine, feminist, labour and social historians – exerted an important impact upon the direction of the discipline. The pre-eminence of the professionalization agenda, which characterized the early writing in nursing history, was not necessarily broken by social scientists but was theorized and researched in a different way.

Interest in nursing by social and feminist historians and historians of medicine has led to a new set of questions being asked about nursing as women's work, the effect of race, class and gender, and other socio-political and economic factors upon the working experience of nurses, their place within the health care division of labour, the labour process and relationships with patients. McPherson's (1996) excellent monograph from Canada explores some of these themes in admirable detail. The latter has paradoxically proved to be the most intractable form of analysis. History has implications for nursing research. Above all it can provide a powerful tool for helping us to understand the theory–practice gap in nursing research. Historical research has much to contribute to reflective practice, the management of change and our understanding of the process and politics of innovation. It could facilitate the framing of a research policy for nursing and help us to unravel and celebrate the genius of nursing's inventiveness, past, present and, hopefully, to come.

References

Baly, M. (1986) *Florence Nightingale and the Nursing Legacy*. London: Croom Helm.
Brush, B., Lynaugh, J., Boschma, G., Rafferty, A.M., Stuart, M. & Tomes, N. (1999) *Nurses of All Nations: A History of the International Council of Nurses 1899–1999*. Philadelphia: Lippincott.

Carnegie, M.E. (1991) *The Path We Tread: Blacks in Nursing 1854–1990*, 2nd edn. New York: National League for Nursing.

Carr, E.H. (1970) *What is History?* London: Macmillan, p. 24.

Cartwright, F.F. (1977) *A Social History of Medicine*. London: Longman.

Davies, C. (1980) The contemporary challenge in nursing history. In C. Davies (ed.) *Rewriting Nursing History*. London: Croom Helm, pp. 1–17.

Dzuback, M.A. (1982) Nursing historiography, 1960–1980: an annotated bibliography. In E.C. Lagemann (ed.) *Nursing History: New Perspectives, New Possibilities*. New York: Teachers College Press, pp. 181–210.

Evans, R.J. (1997) *In Defence of History*. London: Granta.

Fairman, J. (1987) Sources and references for research in nursing history. *Nursing Research* **36** (1): 56–9.

Fairman, J. & Lynaugh, J. (1998) *Critical Care Nursing: A History*. Philadelphia: University of Pennsylvania Press.

Gray, A.M. (1989) The NHS and the history of nurses' pay. *Bulletin of the History of Nursing Group at the Royal College of Nursing* **2** (8): 15–29.

Hobsbawn, E. & Ranger, T. (eds) (1983) *The Invention of Tradition*. Cambridge: Cambridge University Press.

Hudson-Jones, A. (ed.) (1988) *Images of nurses: Perspectives from History, Art and Literature*. Philadelphia: University of Pennsylvania Press.

Jenkinson, V. (1953) Case assignment method of nursing. *Nursing Mirror* **116**: i–iv.

Lagemann, E.C. (ed.) (1982) *Nursing History: New Perspectives, New Possibilities*. New York: Teachers College Press.

Lynaugh, J. & Reverby, S. (1986) Thoughts on the nature of history. *Nursing Research*, **36** (1): 68–9.

McPherson, K. (1996) *Bedside Matters: The Transformation of Canadian Nursing, 1900–1990*. Toronto: Oxford University Press.

McPherson, K. & Stuart, M. (1994) Writing nursing history in Canada: issues and approaches. *Canadian Bulletin of Medical History* **11** (1): 3–22.

Maggs, C.J. (1978) Towards a social history of nursing, parts I and 2. *Nursing Times* **74** (occasional papers): 53–8.

Marks, S. (1994) *Divided Sisterhood; Race Class and Gender in the South African Nursing Profession*. London: Macmillan.

Marwick, A. (1970) *The Nature of History*. London: Macmillan, p. 17.

Pickering, A. (1992) *Science as Practice and Culture*. Chicago: University of Chicago Press.

Porter, R. & Wear, A. (eds) (1988) *Problems and Methods in the History of Medicine*. London: Croom Helm.

Rafferty, A.M. (1991) Historical knowledge. In J. Robinson & B. Vaughan (eds) *Knowledge for Practice*. London: Heinemann.

Rafferty, A.M., Robinson, J. & Elkan, R. (eds) (1997) *Nursing History and the Politics of Welfare*. London: Routledge.

Stone, L. (1972) *The Causes of the English Revolution*. London: Routledge & Kegan Paul. pp. 47–144.

Strachan, G. (1995) 'A good nurse cannot be bought with money': the development of the professional and industrial roles of the nursing organisation in Queensland, Australia, 1904–1950. *Nursing History Review* **3**: 235–56.

Thompson, P. (1978) *The Voice of the Past*. Oxford: Oxford University Press.

UKCC (1986) *Project 2000: A New Preparation for Practice*. London: United Kingdom Central Council for Nursing Midwifery and Health Visiting.

Walker, K. (1994) Confronting 'reality': nursing science and the micropolitics of representation. *Nursing Inquiry* **1** (1): 46–56.

Appendix 17.1: Useful addresses

UK

Royal College of Nursing
Scottish Board
42 South Oswald Road
Edinburgh, EH9 2HH

Wellcome Institute for the History of
Medicine
183, Euston Road
London NW1 2BE

Department of Nursing and Midwifery
Studies
Queen's Medical Centre
University of Nottingham
Nottingham, NG7 2UH

For further information regarding the
National Lifestory Collection, contact:

The Curator, Oral History
The British Library National Sound
Archive
96 Euston Road
London, NW1 2DB

USA

Center for the Study of the History of
Nursing
School of Nursing
University of Pennsylvania
420, Guardian Drive
Philadelphia, PA 19104–6096

Center for Nursing Historical Inquiry
School of Nursing
University of Virginia
Health Services Center
Mcleod Hall
Charlottsville
Virginia, 22903–3395

University of California at San Francisco
c/o The Library
School of Nursing Collection
Special Collection
San Francisco, CA 94143–0840

Mary Adelaide Nutting Collection
Columbia University
Teachers College
Milbank Memorial Library
Special Collections
New York, NY 10027

CHAPTER 18

Descriptive research

Diana E. Carter

If something is descriptive it is concerned with description or classification rather than explanation. Description can include description of types, classes, qualities, or characteristics of a focus of interest. Almost inevitably description is integral to any verbal or written communication we have with one another, and while personal experience suggests that such exchanges may not always be accurate, complete or unbiased, the process of describing is familiar to all of us.

The aim of descriptive research is to discover new facts about a situation, people, activities or events, or the frequency with which certain events occur. This is achieved through the systematic collection of information about the phenomenon of interest and forms an essential phase in the development of nursing knowledge in that it provides the basis for future research, generating questions and hypotheses for experimental study. As with other types of research, descriptive research begins with the identification of a problem or problematic situation. The description and analysis of that situation may reveal relevant factors or relationships hitherto undetected which, in turn, could form the basis of further research.

Many areas of nursing, midwifery and health visiting have been investigated in descriptive studies, such as the pain experienced by patients post-operatively (Ferguson *et al.*, 1997), coping strategies and quality of life of patients with chronic conditions such as end-stage renal disease (Lindqvist & Sjoden, 1998), the environment in which nursing care is given, and nursing practices and their actual or potential effect on patient well-being, as in Callaghan's (1998) study of bacterial contamination of nurses' uniforms. The characteristics of patients and nurses (for example, nurses' attitudes) have also been studied and described (McLaughlin, 1997), as have numerous other areas.

The nature of descriptive research

The focus of descriptive studies is on the situation as it is, the researcher making no attempt to manipulate variables. This focus might include conditions that exist, practices that prevail, beliefs and attitudes that are held, ongoing processes, and developing trends. The data which are obtained can then be used to assess and justify current conditions and practice, or to make plans for improving them.

Descriptive studies vary enormously in their scope and complexity. For example, a large sample of subjects drawn from a defined population may be studied. This is referred to as *survey research* (see Chapter 22). At the other extreme, a case study design involves the extensive study of a single unit (an individual, family, or group). In this instance, while the number of subjects is small, the number of variables examined tends to be large because there is a need to investigate all the variables that may have an effect on the situation being studied, as explained in Chapter 20. Similarly, the information obtained in descriptive studies may be quite diverse, ranging from data on easily defined objective facts such as age, gender, income, and education level, to subtle and personal realms of human experience such as feelings or attitudes. The methodology of descriptive studies can also show wide variation – the methods of data collection, including the use of questionnaires and interviews which sometimes incorporate rating scales (for example, Likert scales), visual analogue scales, and observation techniques.

Descriptive research frequently precedes experimental studies as it often serves to generate predictions (hypotheses) about the relationship among the various phenomena studied which can then be tested in an experimental study which may confirm or reject the prediction.

Descriptive studies are generally guided by research questions and/or research objectives rather than a research hypothesis as such. As mentioned above, in descriptive research there is no attempt to introduce anything new or to modify or control the situation being studied, and because there is no manipulation of the variables under study, and no attempt made to establish causality, descriptive researchers do not use the terms 'dependent' and 'independent' when referring to variables. While relationships between variables are identified in order to obtain an overall picture of the phenomena being examined, examination of the types and degrees of relationship is not the primary purpose of a descriptive study.

However, in common with all types of research, the descriptive researcher is trying to achieve a clear picture of the situation, and protection against bias is an important consideration. Measures taken to achieve this protection include the definition of variables, sample selection, the use of valid and reliable instruments, and methods of data collection.

Defining the variables

Conceptual and operational definitions are the two types of definition to which researchers refer. As with a dictionary definition, a *conceptual* definition conveys a general meaning, but does not help in relation to the measurement of a particular variable. The researcher has to go further than this and describe what is to be measured and how this will be carried out. This is known as an *operational* definition (or operationalization), and involves specifying the tools or instruments required to make the observations or measurements (see Chapter 7). Having operationalized a variable the findings of the study will be more reliable and it will also be possible for others to replicate the study.

Sample selection

Samples vary considerably in the extent to which they represent the population, but the researcher who pays particular attention to the representativeness of the sample increases the possibility of generalizing the findings to a larger group. Many descriptive studies include a large number of subjects obtained through random sampling which, it is hoped, will increase the generalizability of the findings to a wider population. However, some studies use non-random sampling techniques, and while they may produce important relevant findings, such findings cannot automatically be extrapolated to similar situations. More details of sampling techniques can be found in Chapter 22.

Valid and reliable instruments

Instruments to be used for the collection of data must first of all be tested for reliability and validity. Reliability refers to the degree of constancy or accuracy with which the instrument measures an attribute, while validity is the degree to which it measures what it is supposed to be measuring. There are many methods of assessing aspects of an instrument's reliability, and also a variety of approaches in relation to validity which are referred to elsewhere in this text. Perhaps an important point to note here is that even though an instrument has been previously tested in another study, it is advisable to re-test it as it has been shown that neither reliability nor validity is constant and both can change over time.

Data-collection methods

As mentioned above, data collection in descriptive studies may involve the use of interviews, questionnaires, and observation techniques.

Interviews and questionnaires

Interviews and questionnaires both involve direct questioning of subjects. Qualitative descriptive research frequently employs unstructured interviews, while quantitative descriptive studies, which call for instruments that will facilitate the collection of numerical (quantifiable) data, often use questionnaires and structured interviews. Interviews and questionnaires are both useful for obtaining data about the subjects of a study. The data may pertain to:

(1) *personal background information*: which includes demographic information such as age, marital status, educational level, and professional qualifications;

(2) *behavioural information*: which may describe (a) what the subjects did in the past, as in the study by Foxall *et al.* (1998) which investigated the frequency of breast self-examination of nurses over the 12 months prior to the study, (b) what people currently do, as for example the coping strategies used by the patients in Linqvist and Sjoden's (1998) study; or (c) subjects' intended/expected future behaviour, as in the study of occupational stress by Quine (1998) which included asking respondents whether they were likely to look actively for a new job in the next year;

(3) *level of knowledge or information on a particular topic*: as in the studies by Gillespie & Curzio (1998) which investigated and described the nurses' knowledge of blood pressure measurement, and Neilson & Jones (1998) of women's knowledge of cervical cancer and cervical screening;

(4) *opinions, attitudes and values, or how the subjects feel, or what they believe*: as exemplified in the study of the beliefs of people with non-insulin-dependent diabetes about diabetes and diabetic complications by Dunning & Martin (1998) and that by McLaughlin (1997) of student nurses' attitudes towards people with mental illnesses.

Questionnaires may also incorporate the use of Likert-type rating scales where, in relation to each item, subjects are asked to indicate the point on the scale which most effectively represents their opinion. In their study of student nurses' approaches to studying, French *et al.* (1998) asked their respondents to score a number of items according to whether they definitely disagreed, disagreed with reservations, whether the item did not apply or it was impossible to give an answer to whether they agreed with reservations or definitely agreed. Likert scales are discussed in more detail in Chapter 23.

Visual analogue scales can also be employed and have been found particularly useful in obtaining descriptions of the severity of pain experienced by patients. Figure 18.1 shows an example of a scale on which respondents could be asked to indicate their pain severity, with 0 representing no pain and 10 the most severe unbearable pain.

The use of visual analogue scales is not confined to the assessment of pain.

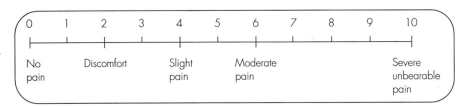

Fig. 18.1   Visual analogue for pain.

Similar scales have also been used in the assessment of dyspnoea, as described in a study of the application of measurement instruments for the assessment of dyspnoea in patients with advanced cancer (van der Molen, 1995), while patients' perceived overall efficiency of coping with end-stage renal disease was measured by Linqvist & Sjoden (1998) using a 10-point visual analogue scale in relation to physical, psychological, social and existential aspects of the disease.

Observation

Observation techniques are frequently used in descriptive research studies. The focus of observation may be the behaviours and characteristics of individuals, and may include physical appearance, verbal and non-verbal communication behaviours, and actions as in the observation of tutorials which formed part of a study by French *et al.* (1998) of students' learning approaches. Environmental characteristics may also be observed as an individual's surroundings can have a considerable effect on behaviour. Where a particular situation is being observed, the researcher's participation in that situation can range from one of non-participation (French *et al.*, 1998), where the emphasis is solely on the observation and recording of events, to one of participation, where the researcher is actually a part of the situation as well as an observer and recorder of events.

Irrespective of whether interviews, questionnaires or observation are selected some consideration needs to be given to the validity of each of these methods. For example, subjects' verbal or written responses to interview questions or questionnaire items about how they actually carry out a particular task, may bear little or no resemblance to how they actually perform it. Similarly, there is no guarantee that the behaviour observed is a true reflection of how subjects behave when there is no observer present. Interviews, questionnaires, and observation are dealt with in more detail in Chapters 24, 25 and 26. The remainder of this chapter will look at the different types of designs that can be used when conducting descriptive research.

Descriptive designs

Exploratory descriptive design

As the name suggests, this type of design is appropriate for areas about which nursing, midwifery and health visiting have little theoretical or factual knowledge. The researcher is exploring a particular area to discover what is there, the meanings attached to the discoveries, and how these can be organized. Opinions differ as to whether exploratory research should be classed as 'descriptive', and some research texts do not include exploratory designs in this category. A reason for this is that in descriptive studies the research question presupposes a prior knowledge of the problem and the researcher must be able to define what and who are to be measured and the techniques of doing so. However, description is integral to the process of exploration.

This type of study calls for intuition and insight on the part of the researcher. It also calls for a degree of flexibility so that any new leads can be followed up, moving the study into new areas as the researcher proceeds and as her knowledge of what is being studied increases.

The approach in such studies is frequently, but not exclusively, qualitative (see Chapter 12), integrating a variety of data-collecting methods such as participant observation and unstructured interviews. This type of approach does not rely on precoded instruments, and the possibilities of discovery and understanding unknown phenomena is enhanced.

Because of the exploratory nature of the study, the variables are not under the researcher's control and are simply discovered and observed as the researcher encounters them. On occasions, studies consist of an early exploratory phase which provides the basis for the development of data-collecting instruments such as questionnaires which are used in a later phase of the study, as in the survey of nurses' and physicians' perceptions of the impact that hormonal therapy has on patients' quality of life (Working Group on Living with Advanced Breast Cancer Hormone Treatment, 1998).

Simple descriptive design

In simple descriptive designs, the variables of interest have been previously studied, either independently (as in an exploratory study) or with other variables. The variables are partly controlled by the situation (as in exploratory designs) but they are also partly controlled by the researcher, who chooses the sample for the study. This design is used when the researcher wishes to examine the characteristics of a single sample, as shown in Fig. 18.2.

After determining the phenomenon of interest, the researcher identifies and defines the variables within this and then proceeds to use the appropriate data-collecting techniques in order to obtain data which describe the variables. The number of variables to be examined and described will be determined in part by

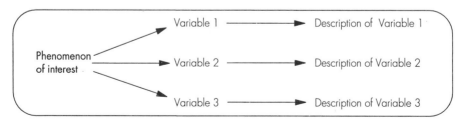

Fig. 18.2 Simple descriptive design.

the study. For example, in studying staff stress, Quine (1998) identified job satisfaction, occupational demands, staff support mechanisms and job control as important variables for description.

Comparative descriptive design

The comparative descriptive design is appropriate if the researcher wishes to examine and describe the variables in two or more groups, as illustrated in Fig. 18.3.

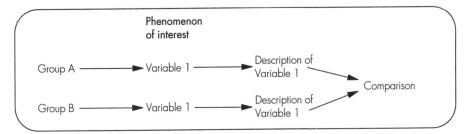

Fig. 18.3 A comparative descriptive design.

This type of design can be seen in the study carried out by Li (1997), which aimed to identify similarities and differences in nurse educators' and student nurses' perceptions of effective clinical teaching behaviours. Using a 7-point Likert scale all the respondents were asked to rate 48 identified effective clinical teaching behaviours according to their perceived degree of importance. The researcher was then able to identify the ten most important and the ten least important behaviours as perceived by each group, compare these and test the identified differences for statistical significance.

Case-control study designs

A case-control study is one in which a group of *cases* (for example, patients with a post-operative wound infection) is identified. A second group of *controls* is then selected. This latter group will comprise post-operative patients who are similar in many respects (for example, in terms of the surgical operation they have had) except that their wounds are not infected. The two groups can then be compared with respect to the particular variable (for example, skin preparation) which is thought to have precipitated the development of the wound infection post-operatively. From the data presented in Fig. 18.4 it can be seen that, in the majority of cases (that is, those patients who had developed post-operative wound infections), the pre-operative skin preparation had involved shaving the skin, whereas relatively few controls (patients whose wounds had not become infected) had had their skin prepared this way.

	Nature of skin preparation		
Group of patients	Pre-operative shower only (%)	Depilatory cream and shower (%)	Skin shave and shower (%)
Cases (patients with post-operative wound infection)	7	8	85
Controls (patients with no post-operative wound infection)	89	5	6

Fig. 18.4   Case control study of pre-operative skin preparation.

The majority of case-control studies are retrospective in that they look back into the history of the subjects and investigate and describe what happened to them in the past before they were selected for study.

Retrospective study designs

Retrospective studies are sometimes referred to as 'ex post facto' because they attempt to link the present situation with what happened in the past. In other words, both the proposed cause and the proposed effect have already happened, and the researcher is attempting to identify the factor(s) that have resulted in the effect. However, it has to be acknowledged that the researcher's knowledge of the proposed cause and proposed effect can sometimes bias the investigation. Additionally, there is the problem that if the researcher is interested in something that happened a long time ago and has resulted in the effect, then the subjects' ability to recall the information accurately may be somewhat suspect.

Longitudinal designs

Longitudinal designs facilitate the collection of data over a period of time, and are useful if, for example, the researcher wanted to examine changes in a group of subjects over time (Fig. 18.5).

If, for example, the researcher wished to study the development of a particular clinical skill in student midwives, she could select a cohort of students at the commencement of their pre-registration course and describe this group's performance of that skill at different stages of the course. As can be readily appreciated, the use of a longitudinal design can prove expensive if the time scale is extensive. Such studies also call for long-term researcher and subject commitment in many instances. On the other hand, it is generally recognized that research problems which involve trends, changes, or development over time, are best addressed through longitudinal designs.

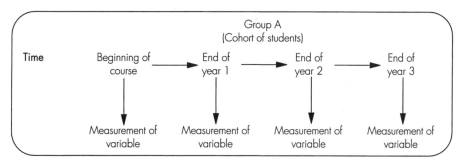

Fig. 18.5 Longitudinal design.

Cross-sectional designs

This type of design involves the collection of data at one point in time. It is a design that would be appropriate for examining simultaneously groups of subjects in various stages of development (Fig. 18.6). Taking the above example of the development of manual dexterity in student midwives, the researcher could employ a cross-sectional design to collect data to describe, at one time, groups of subjects at different stages of their pre-registration programme. Hence the collection of data could be 'telescoped' into one period, the duration of which is determined only by the length of time it takes to collect the data.

Group	Stage of course		At the same point in time
A	End of year 3	⟶	Measurement of variable
B	End of year 2	⟶	Measurement of variable
C	End of year 1	⟶	Measurement of variable
D	Start of year 1	⟶	Measurement of variable

Fig. 18.6 Cross-sectional design.

While this type of design may be more economical in terms of time and money than the longitudinal design, it does make the assumption that the stages of development are part of a process which will progress across time. A comparison of longitudinal and cross-sectional designs is shown in Fig. 18.7.

Prospective study designs

Prospective studies are very like longitudinal studies in that they start in the present and end in the future. Looking to the future, the researcher is interested in describing the effect(s) of a cause (or causes) which may already have occurred. Following her study of staff stress in an NHS trust, Quine (1998) suggested that a

Longitudinal	Cross-sectional
• Costly in terms of effort and money	• Less time-consuming; less expensive; more manageable
• Confounding variables could affect the interpretation of the results	• Confounding variables of maturation resulting from elapsing time not present
• Early trends in the data can be investigated	
• Subjects may respond in a socially desirable way that they believe is congruent with the researcher's expectations	

Fig. 18.7   Comparison of longitudinal and cross-sectional designs.

prospective study would be useful in helping draw firmer conclusions about cause (occupational stress) and effects such as levels of job satisfaction, health and movement to new jobs. However, such studies are less common than retrospective studies in that it can take a long time for the phenomenon of interest to become evident. It is acknowledged that prospective studies are stronger than retrospective ones because of the degree of control that can be imposed on extraneous variables that may confound the data.

Conclusions

Many variables in nursing are not amenable to experimental manipulation, and this is one reason why descriptive studies can be of great value. The descriptive researcher, in search of meaning, is concerned with observing, describing, and documenting aspect of events, phenomena, or situations as they occur naturally, and the information obtained can often form the foundation for the development of nursing, midwifery and health visiting theories.

This chapter has introduced some of the aspects related to descriptive research and has briefly considered a number of types of descriptive designs which are frequently employed by researchers conducting this type of research.

References

Callaghan, I. (1998) Bacterial contamination of nurses' uniforms: a study. *Nursing Standard* 13 (1): 37–42.

Dunning, P. & Martin, M. (1998) Beliefs about diabetes and diabetic complications. *Professional Nurse* 13 (7): 429–34.

Ferguson, J., Gilroy, D. & Puntillo, K. (1997) Dimensions of pain and analgesia administration associated with coronary artery bypass grafting in an Australian intensive care unit. *Journal of Advanced Nursing* 26 (6): 1065–72.

Foxall, M.J., Barron, C.R. & Houfek, J. (1998) Ethnic differences in breast self-examination practice and health beliefs. *Journal of Advanced Nursing* **27** (2): 419–28.

French, P., Callaghan, P., Dudley-Brown, S., Holroyd, E. & Sellick, K. (1998) The effectiveness of tutorials in behavioural sciences for nurses: an action learning project. *Nurse Education Today* **18**: 116–24.

Gillespie, A. & Curzio, J. (1998) Blood pressure measurement: assessing staff knowledge. *Nursing Standard* **12** (23): 35–7.

Li, M.K. (1997) Perceptions of effective clinical teaching behaviours in a hospital-based nurse training programme. *Journal of Advanced Nursing* **26** (6): 1252–61.

Lindqvist, R. & Sjoden, P.-O. (1998) Coping strategies and quality of life among patients on continuous ambulatory peritoneal dialysis (CAPD). *Journal of Advanced Nursing* **27** (2): 312–19.

McLaughlin, C. (1997) The effect of classroom theory and contact with patients on the attitudes of student nurses towards mentally ill people. *Journal of Advanced Nursing* **26** (6): 1221–8.

Neilson, A. & Jones, R.K. (1998) Women's lay knowledge of cervical cancer/cervical screening: accounting for non-attendance at cervical screening clinics. *Journal of Advanced Nursing* **28** (3): 571–5.

Quine, L. (1998) Effects of stress in an NHS trust: a study. *Nursing Standard* **13** (3): 36–41.

van der Molen, B. (1995) Dyspnoea: a study of measurement instruments for the assessment of dyspnoea and their application for patients with advanced cancer. *Journal of Advanced Nursing* **22** (5): 948–56.

Working Group on Living with Advanced Breast Cancer Hormone Treatment (1998) Living with advanced breast cancer hormone treatment: the nurse's perspective. *European Journal of Cancer Care* **7**: 113–19.

CHAPTER 19

Evaluation research

Senga Bond

What sets evaluation research apart from other forms of research is its prime intention of contributing to policy-making – be it at the level of an individual work unit like a school of health studies or a hospital ward or, at the other end of the continuum, the highest level of government. That the Secretary of State for Health has repeatedly spurned the collective proposals of the Royal Colleges that there should be evaluations of the proposed changes to the structure of the Health Service before they are introduced wholesale, points to the political context in which evaluations inevitably take place. All research is political, and evaluation research more so.

Well-conceived, well-designed and conducted and thoughtfully analysed evaluations have the potential to provide insights into how services or projects are operating, the extent to which they are meeting intended goals or the needs of recipients, their strengths and weaknesses, their cost effectiveness, and so potentially provide fruitful directions for the future. Evaluations should provide relevant information for decision-makers and so contribute to setting priorities, guiding the allocation of resources and the modification and refinement of project structures and processes. With such a broad range of possible functions it is not surprising that evaluations conform to a number of different models, differentially appropriate to a range of circumstances and interests and having particular strengths and weaknesses in different contexts.

The purpose of evaluation

Table 19.1 points to some different evaluation models and the particular characteristics they emphasize. This list immediately reveals the wide range of activities and meanings involved in the idea of 'an evaluation' and the range of investigative activities that could be involved. Usually, however, there are three main categories of purpose which guide the request for, or the decision to undertake, an evaluation. These are needs assessment, formative evaluation and summative evaluation.

Table 19.1   Some models of evaluation (based on Herman *et al.*, 1987)

Model	Emphasis
Goal-oriented evaluation	Evaluation should assess the extent to which the specified goals of an innovation are achieved, i.e. the effectiveness of an innovation.
Decision-oriented evaluation	Evaluation should facilitate intelligent judgements by decision-makers.
Responsive evaluation	Evaluation should describe the processes involved in a scheme or innovation and relate this to the value perspectives of key people.
Evaluation research	Evaluations should focus on explaining the effects of innovations and generating generalizations about with whom and in what circumstances they are effective.
Goal-free evaluation	Evaluation should assess the effects of innovations over and above their own specified goals and focus on the extent to which client needs are met as well as unintended consequences.
Advocacy–adversary evaluation	Evaluation should derive from the argumentation of contrasting points of view.
Utilization-oriented evaluation	Evaluation should be structured to maximize the utilization of its findings by specific stakeholders and users.

Needs assessment

The first is not evaluation of an existing project at all but a means of seeking an assessment of needs, problems or conditions which should be taken into account and addressed in future planning or in reviewing current services. In this kind of situation there is generally a need for information, or a feeling that things are not as they should be, and there is a need to clarify goals, assess the extent to which they are shared, identify whether clients perceive problems, and decide whether there needs to be new forms of action. Examples of this kind of enquiry would be:

- What is the size of the population requiring a service?
- What is the nature or range of services or facilities likely to be required?
- How will a new service be monitored?
- What do consumers feel about services being offered?

A needs assessment of palliative care services offers a useful example for planning purposes (Higginson, 1993).

Formative evaluation

This kind of evaluation has as its main thrust providing information which will improve the running or development of an ongoing service or a new project in relation to its value. It will involve monitoring the implementation process or the functioning of an existing service and whether it is on track. The thrust is to understand how well a service or project is moving towards its objectives so that remedial action may be taken when things seem to be going amiss and modifications are required, or to recognize when things are going well. Parlett & Hamilton's (1972) classic paper deals with conducting formative evaluations.

This time-consuming activity involves detailed assessments of the many processes involved in an innovation and feedback activities to the participants so that they can act on the insights gained. In some respects formative evaluation embodies components of action research (see Chapter 16) since its thrust is to make changes for improvements. These changes may involve personnel, their activities, organization, or technologies in use. An example of formative evaluation is work undertaken by Hart (1998) about community stroke services. The study builds on theories about the nature of chronic disease from patient and professional perspectives (Kaufman, 1988; Pinder, 1990) and finds a mismatch between patients' goals of recovery and professionals' goals of rehabilitation within a framework of uncertainty created by a chronic illness – in this case a stroke. For rehabilitation efforts to become more effective there needs to be ways of professionals recognizing patient and family goals and explaining the nature of stroke and consequences for rehabilitation. Clearly the study has theoretical relevance for other types of chronic illness.

Summative evaluation

The main goal of summative evaluation is to present information about the effectiveness and value of a service or innovation. It may inform whether to expand, reduce, continue or discontinue an innovation based on findings. Whether this is the case will depend on whether there is an improvement in outcomes, the cost–benefit equation is acceptable or the activity serves political ends.

Carrying out this kind of evaluation may involve only one example or case, or comparison, either between different types or levels of innovations within a programme or with a control group which is not receiving any intervention. Some evaluations are very large scale, involving thousands of people in many different cities (COMMIT Research Group, 1995a, 1995b) or several sites within a single country, for example a study of nurse practitioners in a range of hospital and primary care sites (Coopers & Lybrand, 1996). Most evaluations are carried out on a much smaller scale, however, for local purposes and involve only a single site or even a single health professional with consequent limitations for their generalizability.

Comparing evaluation and research

It should now be clear that there are many reasons for doing evaluations and many different ways of going about it. In some eyes, evaluating a service or project involves no more than participants sitting around a table, sharing their opinions and arriving at a conclusion. At the other extreme are large-scale, well-designed and resourced research studies which consider not only the *effects* of health interventions or social programmes but also attempt to reveal *the circumstances in which* they are effective and *explain why* this is the case. This is called getting inside the 'black box', rather than leaving it as unknown territory. Most evaluation falls somewhere in between.

Evaluation applies the methods of social research to provide information to answering questions about worth or value and hence inform decisions. The principles and methods which apply to the other kinds of research – how to design experiments or quasi-experiments, how to collect and analyse different kinds of data – that are described throughout this text apply here too. What distinguishes evaluation research is not method or even subject matter, but intent – the purpose for which it is done.

Table 19.2 compares some characteristics as they apply more to evaluation or to research. The focus in evaluations relates to the underlying purposes and, while evaluations are intended to inform decisions, and hence action, there is nothing inherently action-oriented about research *per se*. While nursing research tends to have an applied focus, it need not have, since the prime purpose of research is to seek new understandings and add to our store of knowledge. Thus evaluation research straddles the twin ideals of generating knowledge and also informing decisions, and has to adapt to fulfil both purposes. How it should do so inevitably raises tensions about the best way to achieve this.

Most evaluations are local, although they may have more general implications. Research has as a main characteristic the generalizability of its findings. Thus evaluation research must be set at this wider level and make clear the parameters which limit the extent of its generalizability. If we take as an example an evaluation of nursing homes in the NHS (Bond *et al.*, 1990a, 1990b) and compare differences between homes, there are some findings which have relevance for the private and voluntary nursing home sectors. However, because the study was wholly based in the NHS, and we know that clients in NHS nursing homes were more cognitively impaired than are those in private establishments (Bond *et al.*, 1990b) caution would be urged in deciding which findings can be extrapolated to homes with a different case mix. Some could be generalized since they do not depend on a particular case mix to retain their applicability (i.e. external validity).

Those who ask for evaluations should be interested in the worth of findings in terms of their value for decision-making. This tends to be their major criterion in considering whether the evaluator has done a good job. For research the essence

Table 19.2   Characteristics of research and evaluation

Characteristic	Evaluation	Research
1. Focus	Decisions – evaluation seeks understanding to facilitate decisions	Conclusions – research seeks understanding as its primary goal
2. Generalizability	Low – results are often applicable only to the setting studied i.e. poor external validity	High – results should be applicable to comparable situation; high external validity
3. Valuing in inquiry	Worthwhileness, utility	Truth
4. Measurement principles	Important	Important
5. Scientific principles	Important	Essential
6. Sampling techniques	Desirable	Crucial
7. Random selection of subjects	May be feasible	Important if possible
8. Descriptive and inferential statistics	Utilized	Utilized
9. Audience	Specific, identified and important	General scientific community
10. Politics	Recognized and accommodated	Usually considered improper
11. Replicability	Usually not possible or constrained	Very important
12. Setting	Very significant	Minimally important
13. Reporting	Internal, external and political	External, public and open
14. Theory building	Not usually	Central and important
15. Theory testing	Not usually	Central and important

lies more in the 'truth' of the findings than in their immediate utility. This position, of course, varies according to whether one takes the position that in social affairs there are many truths depending on perspective (Everitt, 1996). While there will always be differences in opinion about what makes interventions involving people and social circumstances work, the position taken here is that it is up to the evaluator to provide criteria against which claims can be judged and to furnish grounds for why a particular account is to be preferred – in other words, to provide evidence to decide what confidence can be placed in the findings, irrespective of any other value they may hold. Evaluation research then has to conform to the canons of science and measurement principles if it is to arrive at information that is valid, but because evaluations take place in the real and messy world they are the art of the possible. It takes ingenuity and creative flair to find ways of carrying out evaluations that provide answers about effects of interventions but also about the mechanisms that create them. For instance, it is not always possible to sample adequately those who are exposed to a service, for practical or political reasons, so that the evaluation exercise is carried out in such a way that the findings are restricted. For example, if we stick with ways of evaluating palliative care services, it is often not easy to obtain the views of patients who are or are not receiving the services because their doctors, nurses and family believe that people near the end of their lives should not be 'troubled' by being asked for their views. Those included in the study may well be atypical in some respects – more articulate or independent, further from death – hence offering a biased sample from which to draw conclusions.

Evaluations tend to be sought, or are carried out, in-house while a consultant may be employed. The customer and audience for the evaluation therefore is well identified in advance and should have had a major say in how the evaluation proceeds. The relevance of the findings, however, may prove to be of value to a wider audience, but this is not necessarily the case. In basic research, the audience is not targeted in advance, since the findings tend to be acted upon in some way before they are relevant to and become incorporated into the technologies of commerce, industry or public service. Indeed, fundamental research should in many respects be impartial to particular applications, and focus exclusively on a search for truth. Marie Curie had no application in mind in her life work to isolate a new chemical element. The search was to increase our knowledge. In research *per se*, then, the political context of research is played down while in evaluations and evaluation in research, the political context is both recognized and taken into account while the researcher, rather than the focus of the study, attempts to remain impartial. Thus, in doing evaluation research there has to be a balance between disinterest and the political context in which the results are to be produced and used.

In the NHS nursing home study, where care was nurse rather than consultant managed, there were obvious vested interests and the evaluation research had to take these on board while designing a study which had scientific rigour with samples large enough to offer sufficient power to draw conclusions based on statistical principles. This scientific approach to evaluation research meant that the study was long and time-consuming, and in this case when political views changed to a view that long-term care should be provided by the private sector rather than the NHS, the customer, the Department of Health, refused permission for the study to be extended to include private nursing homes. In this sense, while there were certainly findings of general interest in the provision of long-term care, the political implications of the NHS base for the work were important in how the study was conducted and the findings were viewed by the Thatcher administration.

In this case findings were published in lengthy in-house reports to the Department of Health and then, after agreement with the customers, in academic and professional journals. Evaluation findings are generally of more local interest with publication limited to local reports. What evaluation adds to the general body of knowledge depends not only on where it is published but how valid are its findings and how theoretically sensitive and searching are its design and methods. At this time there is a great movement to accept the randomized-controlled trial (RCT) as the only acceptable method for evaluating the effectiveness of treatment interventions with carefully controlled inputs and samples. While this general method is useful up to a point in studies where the effects depend on chemical/biological events (for example, the effects of pharmacological agents on the body) rather than social events (for example, whether to turn up for preconception care and act on the advice given), it has the disadvantage of averaging out effects by grouping together cases in which the intervention is effective and those in which it is less so. This is because typically RCTs do not get inside the 'black box' to understand why some women and some clinics do not respond to, in this case, preconception programmes and care. The contribution of RCTs is that while they may permit accumulation of knowledge of what works, they often fall short of revealing anything about within-group variation in the success of different groups of subjects, and often there is little to add to a general body of knowledge or to theory-building. Contributions to theory are of central importance to research. Thus evaluation research should inform theory as well as provide information which has relevance in its own right. On the other hand, evaluations which only approximate the requirements of research are unlikely to contribute to theory and are empirically driven.

The above discussion indicates why there is a distinction between many evaluations and research and, even within research, this is often atheoretical. It should now be clear that it is possible to do evaluations which are acceptable as research, as long as the study can accommodate theory testing, methodological rigour and the political and practical requirements of evaluation. Evaluation research is an endeavour which is partly social, partly political, partly technical and should always be theoretical.

Determining the evaluation approach

While a clear specification of the reasons for undertaking an evaluation should be established at the outset, it is equally important to ascertain what evaluation customers will accept as credible information. This is where the professional standards of researchers are challenged to find ways of carrying out credible work within the constraints laid down both by customers and the situation in which the researchers are being asked to work. Nevertheless, evaluation research has itself developed the range of methods it uses since the 1960s.

Like most of social science, early evaluation looked to logical positivism to justify its method choices. Congruent with this approach was the preference for using goals articulated in advance as a basis for formulating causal hypotheses which could then be tested experimentally. This kind of thinking relies on assumptions that the implementation of a programme or policy is homogeneous across sites and unvarying over time, that goals are explicit and shared and that there are effects which are amenable to valid measurement using experimental designs. This approach to evaluation was epitomized in the classic texts of Suchman (1967) and Campbell (1969), which advocated methods approximating experiments. However, field experiments are only feasible where, according to Booth (1988):

(1)   the programme under trial is a simple one with clearly defined aims;
(2)   there is a need to establish its effectiveness;
(3)   inputs are specific and measurable;
(4)   people can agree on how outcomes can be measured;
(5)   randomization is both politically feasible and administratively possible;
(6)   diverse clinical objectives do not intrude;
(7)   non-co-operation or attention can be kept within acceptable limits;
(8)   results are likely to be useful and timely.

Few innovatory programmes and evaluation studies meet such guidelines.

The assumptions of the value of experiments have come under attack not only in evaluation research but also in science as a whole. A basic difficulty lies in the nature of experiments themselves which, while probing connections between 'independent' and 'dependent' variables, cannot assign causality or explain why a treatment is or is not effective. Full explanation of why and in what circumstances an innovation achieves its effects is extremely useful in specifying the factors that have to be present if an innovation is to be successful when transferred elsewhere (Cronbach, 1982). Together with a recognition of the need for explanatory knowledge, i.e. the development of middle range theories, came the recognition that it is important to let evaluation issues emerge from intensive on-site knowledge rather than formulate them prior to data collection at the outset. Innovations based on social interchanges and in different social contexts change in unanticipated ways; they are not stationary targets, and are conceptualized by actors – with different viewpoints, realities and meanings – who make choices.

Thus evaluators who came to recognize the social nature of innovations and change, introduced qualitative and constructivist paradigms and shifted their gaze from outputs to processes (Guba & Lincoln, 1989). In so doing, they are prepared to use methods which take on board different perspectives. This approach involves constructing and testing explanations of what is observed from the data, and seeking data to enable explanations to be constructed rather than setting out hypotheses in advance and predetermining the data to be collected. The evaluators involve the participants more closely at all stages in the evaluation process by finding from the range of relevant stakeholders whether and how the proposed interventions have affected them. The trouble with this approach is that while recognizing that there are different views, interpretations and perspectives among different stakeholders, influence will eventually be determined by those holding the power, and the contexts and institutional structures in which the interventions are operating will be major determining influences. Those who adopt a constructivist/naturalistic/phenomenological approach to evaluation thus only include part of the story.

More recently, case study research (Yin, 1993) has gained prominence as an evaluation strategy. Multiple case studies include the collection of a range of theory relevant information to assess whether a pattern of cause–effect relationships can be discerned in existing cases.

These developments in different philosophical and methodological approaches to evaluation underscore the values of a pluralistic approach to evaluative research (Rossi & Freeman, 1993). There are merits in the different approaches, and each adds in different ways to carrying out successful evaluations for different purposes to encompass the interrelated activities that comprise the interventions. In the field of educational research Cronbach (1963: 672) wrote:

'The program may be a set of instructional materials distributed nationally, the instructional activities of a single school, or the educational experience of a single pupil. Many types of decisions are to be made, and many variations of information are useful. It becomes immediately apparent that no one set of principles will suffice for all situations.'

It is clear that there are choices to be made and that breadth and depth have to be considered. There is also a need to understand whether an intervention has had an effect, as well as why this is so and in what circumstances. If the latter is the case then there is no option but to move beyond the pragmatic RCT (Schwartz & Lellouch, 1967) which tell us nothing of why something works to uncover the sequences of intention, action, interaction and reaction which constitute the day-to-day implementation of a service or policy. Here, Chen's (1990) emphasis on theory-driven evaluation comes into play.

'The domination of the experimental paradigm in the program evaluation literature unfortunately draws attention away from a more important task in gaining understanding of social programs, namely developing theoretical models of social interventions.' (Chen & Rossi, 1983: 283)

What makes an intervention work? If diabetic women are to plan their pregnancies, take folic acid and strictly control their blood glucose level before they become pregnant then we need to understand why some women do this and others do not, what it is about the behaviour of some clinicians that causes some women to feel they are being criticized or disempowered and about the organization of some services that mean they are not accessed. In developing new interventions to be evaluated Pawson & Tilley (1997) call for theory-led evaluations. New interventions should be considering and testing theoretical insights drawn from previous work – that is, setting up hypotheses or explanatory propositions that can be tested while taking into account the social context in which interventions are taking place, the macro and micro processes that constitute the intervention and the outcomes that follow from stakeholders' choices and the resources they bring to the situation. So if women are ill informed about the relationship between blood glucose and the likelihood of having a baby with a congenital abnormality, would informing them make them think and/or behave any differently and what would be the mechanisms at work in doing so? How does the association between knowledge about the effects of controlling/not controlling blood glucose and acting in such a way as to control it actually come about? Does the manner in which the information is presented – whether once only, or reinforced, or who provides it – make any difference? How is it influenced by the social and other contingencies of the situation in which the woman finds herself? Do they enable or disable the mechanisms between knowledge and behaviour? If a woman's social context is such that she has problems in, or is not interested in, or has no motivation to regularly test and manage her blood glucose level, will providing her with information make any difference?

If we take this approach, then irrespective of the particular methods adopted to gather the data, empirical evaluation research will only be as good as the theory that guides it. There is a needed respect for a diversity of approaches. Because of the desirability of not only knowing what works, but why and in what circumstances, it seems entirely appropriate to include different approaches within a single study. This kind of research is expensive and time-consuming, but its comprehensiveness not only enables decisions to be taken about the most appropriate policy to adopt, but also contributes to understanding the means whereby the policy may successfully be disseminated to some settings but not others, effective with some patients but not others, and useful in the hands of some kind of health professionals but not others.

Undertaking evaluations in an environment with an accelerating rate of change creates yet other methodological dilemmas. However, strategies which cannot be adaptive are 'doomed to reflect only that which stood still long enough to be measured' (Rist, 1984).

Conclusions

New services, clinical interventions and educational initiatives are difficult to evaluate. They are multi-dimensional, complicated, elusive and always 'on the move'. The evaluation methods employed must also be subtle, sophisticated and valid; they must be sufficiently dynamic to adapt to or account for both the changing characteristics of clients or students, setting and context and changing perceptions of needs. They must also be responsive to changing social, political and economic climates – as anyone doing research in the NHS will be only too aware. All too often exciting new schemes are introduced without thought to their evaluation, with consequent loss of opportunity and increased difficulty of obtaining baseline data or data about how the scheme was introduced. Nevertheless, attempting to provide as rigorous and as theoretically relevant information as possible for service or educational development is an infinitely interesting and challenging occupation. When policy-makers are willing to take account of the findings produced through evaluation research, and actually use it in policy-making; the rewards are rich indeed. It is worth stressing again the importance of the political process that involves relevant policy-makers in understanding the evaluation process and gaining their commitment to the implications of the findings.

Evaluation researchers need to acknowledge that they operate in a changing social world that is quite unlike the physics laboratory when empirical systems can be devised to mirror theoretical models fairly well. The open system in which they operate means that inevitably there will be new forces at work that create new contexts and challenge existing mechanisms. In carrying out their craft they need to bring together realism with intellectual and methodological rigour.

References

Bond, J., Bond, S., Donaldson, C., Gregson, B. & Atkinson, A. (1990a) Evaluation of an innovation in the continuing care of very frail elderly people. *Ageing and Society* 9: 347–81.

Bond, J., Atkinson, A., Gregson, B., Hughes, P. & Jeffries, L. (1990b) *The 1984 and 1987 Surveys of Continuing Care Institutions in Six Health Authorities*. Vol. 4: *Evaluation of Continuing-Care Accommodation for Elderly People*. Health Care Research Unit, University of Newcastle upon Tyne.

Booth, T. (1988) *Developing Policy Research*. Aldershot: Gower.

Campbell, D.T. (1969) Reforms as experiments. *American Psychologist* 24: 409–28.

Chen, H. (1990) *Theory-Driven Evaluation*. Beverly Hills, CA: Sage.

Chen, H. & Rossi, P. (1983) Evaluating with sense: the theory-driven approach. *Evaluation Review* 7: 283–302.

COMMIT Research Group (1995a) Community Intervention Trial for Smoking Cessation (COMMIT). I: Cohort results from a four-year trial. *American Journal of Public Health* 85: 183–92.

COMMIT Research Group (1995b) Community Intervention Trial for Smoking Cessation (COMMIT). II: Changes in adult cigarette smoking prevalence. *American Journal of Public Health* 85: 193–200

Coopers & Lybrand (1996) *Nurse Practitioner Evaluation Project. Final Report*. London: Coopers & Lybrand.

Cronbach, L. (1963) Course improvement through evaluation. *Teachers College Record* 64: 672–83.

Cronbach, L.J. (1982) *Designing Evaluations of Educational and Social Programs*. San Francisco: Jossey Bass.

Everitt, A. (1996) Developing critical evaluation. *Evaluation* 2: 173–88.

Guba, E.G. and Lincoln, Y.S. (1989) *Fourth Generation Evaluation*. New York and London: Sage Publications.

Hart, E. (1998) Evaluating a pilot community stroke service using insights from medical anthropology. *Journal of Advanced Nursing* 27: 1177–83.

Herman, J.L., Morris, L.L., & Fitz-Gibbon, C.T. (1987) *Evaluation Handbook*. New York and London: Sage Publications.

Higginson, I. (1993) Quality, cost and contracts of care. In D. Clark (ed.) *The Future for Palliative Care*. Buckingham: Open University Press.

Kaufman, S.R. (1988) Stroke rehabilitation and the negotiation of identity. In S. Reinharz & G.D. Rowles (eds) *Qualitative Gerontology*. New York: Springer, pp. 82–103.

Parlett, M. & Hamilton, D. (1972) *Evaluation as Illumination: A New Approach to the Study of Innovatory Programs*. Occasional Paper, Centre for Research in the Educational Sciences, University of Edinburgh.

Pawson, R. & Tilley, N. (1997) *Realistic Evaluation*. London: Sage.

Pinder, R. (1990) *The Management of Chronic Illness: Patient and Doctor Perspectives on Parkinson's Disease*. London: Macmillan.

Rist, R. (1984) On the application of qualitative research to the policy process: and emergent linkage. In L. Barton & S. Walker (eds) *Social Crises and Educational Research*. London: Croom Helm.

Rossi, P.H. & Freeman, H.E. (1993) *Evaluation: A Systematic Approach*, 5th edn. Thousand Oaks, California: Sage Publications.

Schwartz, D. and Lellouch, J. (1967) Explanatory and pragmatic attitudes in therapeutic trials. *Journal of Chronic Diseases* 20: 637–48.

Suchman, E. (1967) *Evaluative Research*. New York and London: Sage Publications.

Yin, R.K. (1993) *Case Study Research: Design and Methods*, New York and London: Sage Publications.

CHAPTER 20

Single case study

David Pontin

There seems to be a growing consensus within the nursing, midwifery and health-visiting research community that the time for a re-evaluation of case study research is upon us. There is an acknowledgement that case study research is a form of research that has been with us for some time but whose praises have generally been unsung (Gray, 1998; Newell, 1998; Rolfe, 1998; Sharp, 1998; Fridlund, 1997; Sandelowski, 1996). This chapter sets out to provide an overview of the main characteristics of case study research and to illustrate the links between questions, research design and the data collected in case study research.

Robson (1993) provides a useful definition of case study research. He describes it as:

'. . . a strategy for doing research which involves an empirical investigation of a particular contemporary phenomenon within its real life context using multiple sources of evidence.'

From this description a number of things are evident regarding case study research. First, from a design perspective, case study research is not necessarily a form of qualitative research, because it does not rely solely on people's accounts of their perspectives and feelings regarding their life worlds. Although these sort of data may be included in the design, the aim of case study research is to develop as full a picture as possible of a setting, situation or an event by working with a variety of data sources and causal processes. This usually means using a variety of methods to generate different forms of data. These may be quantitative and/or qualitative depending on the questions being asked of the particular phenomenon being studied (Sandelowski, 1996; Patton, 1990; Hakim, 1987). Second, as its name suggests, the subject of case study research is likely to be one example of an entity which is investigated in depth and in detail (although, as we shall see later, more than one example may be investigated). The example chosen for investigation by researchers may be one of a number of quite different and varying things – a role or a relationship, a life-history, an organization, an event, a social group or a set of particular circumstances (Yin, 1994). Third, because case study research is carried out in 'real life' situations where it is difficult to conduct experiments, claims may be made by researchers for greater ecological validity of their results (Hammersley & Atkinson, 1995). Ecological validity refers to the way that experimental conditions for controlling variables may have a distorting effect on the phenomenon being studied. This possible distortion then affects the validity of the data generated by the research. By studying the phenomenon in the 'real world' it is argued that there is less likely to be distorting effects from experimental conditions, which makes the findings more valid for the particular phenomen in question – that is, they have greater ecological validity. Finally, the boundaries of case study research overlap with other research designs and strategies. Hakim (1987) points out that research strategies such as action research is a particular form of case study research, albeit with an additional requirement for change and emancipatory working practices.(see Chapter 16).

Flexibility and versatility

Perhaps one of the reasons why the place of case study research within nursing, midwifery and health-visiting research is being re-evaluated has something to do with the flexibility and versatility of the research design (Meier & Pugh, 1986). The 'problem' for many is that the phenomena they wish to investigate cannot be replicated in laboratories and/or do not lend themselves easily to experimental research designs such as randomized controlled trials. The subject matter for many researchers exists in 'real life' settings far away from controlled, experimental conditions. In many ways, case study research is one of the most flexible of research designs available to clinicians wishing to enquire into their practice, its effects on clients and the settings in which it takes place. Hakim (1987) makes a very powerful analogy between the use of case study research and the use of a spotlight to illuminate a particular aspect of a setting, or a microscope to examine a phenomenon in detail. This idea of focusing on a particular phenomenon, setting or aspect of a situation is a hallmark of case study research. Because focusing is such a hallmark of the design, it stands to reason that the trustworthiness of any findings from case study research depends on how well the study is focused by researchers to provide appropriate findings so that the questions which they pose may be answered. This idea of making sure that the methods of a study are appropriate to generate the necessary findings to answer the research question is called methodological appropriateness (Patton, 1990).

The flexibility of case study research may be seen from the range of possible designs open to researchers. You will see, from the examples given below, that it is common practice to use more than one method to generate or collect data (Stake, 1994; Yin, 1994; Hakim, 1987). This triangulation of methods (Denzin, 1978) is essential in order to build up the richly detailed picture of the context within which the case is set. What will also become apparent is the place of time within the design. Some designs are cross-sectional (one point in time) others are longitudinal (either continuous or a number of discrete time periods). The use of time in the research design is dependent on the case being studied and the questions being asked. At one end of the continuum presented in Fig. 20.1 are simple descriptive accounts of one or more cases.

Descriptive - - - - - - - - - - - - - -	- - - - - - - - - Exploratory - - - - - - - - -	- - - - - - - - - - - - - - Explanatory
Simple, illustrative accounts of 1 or more cases	Identification and definition of ideas and assumptions present in illustrative accounts	Rigorous testing of well-defined ideas and assumptions about the phenomena in question

Fig. 20.1   A continuum of the range of focus possible for case study research designs.

Descriptive case studies

These are illustrative examples of a particular phenomenon in question. For example, Eden & Foreman's (1996) work describes the problems associated with an under-recognition by nurses of delirium in patients in critical care settings. In order to do this they present a detailed case history of one client admitted to a critical care unit. They relate information regarding his home medication, laboratory blood values during admission, daily haemodynamic values, blood gas values and a chronology edited from his care plan. This tracks the precursors and manifestation of delirium and is then used as a baseline against which interviews with nursing staff from the unit can be combined and analysed. From this examination of the events leading to under-recognition of delirium, Eden & Foreman (1996) discuss the implications for nursing practice within critical care units. Moving on from descriptive case study research we come to exploratory case studies.

Exploratory case studies

The aim of this design is to move beyond description and identify the ideas and assumptions behind the phenomena which have been previously described. Luker et al. (1998) provide an example of this form when they explore the context within which district nurses and health visitors make decisions about prescribing from a nurse's formulary having successfully completed a nurse prescribing course. Over a one-year period the original group of nurse prescribers became less in number due to job mobility and maternity leave. Nurses were interviewed every three months. The interviews were initially semi-structured, and the findings from each round were used to structure subsequent interviews along with data from the Prescription Pricing Authority on nurses' prescribing activity in the eight sites involved. As a result of their work, Luker et al. (1998) identify a number of difficult decision-making areas faced by these community nurses when prescribing for their patients. In the main these difficulties centre around managing uncertainty in decision-making in clinical practice when incorporating new roles into practice.

Explanatory case studies

As we move along the continuum through exploratory work, we come to case study research which sets out to provide explanations of phenomena which are present within the case or cases that have been selected for investigation. Researchers using these explanatory designs set out in an intellectually rigorous manner to test well-defined ideas and assumptions about the phenomena in question (Yin, 1994; Hakim, 1987). We are able to see this process taking place in the work of Watkins & Redfern (1997) in the evaluation of a night nursing service for elderly people with dementia. In this particular case, Watkins & Redfern wished to link outcomes of the project to specific forms of nursing intervention, and to do this they established clearly differentiated standards for structure, process and outcome factors. This allowed Watkins & Redfern to collect data on the relationship between the structure of a night nursing service for elderly people, nursing interventions and actions, and patient and care outcomes. They used patient activity observation rating scales completed by nurses and carers, and self-rating scales completed by carers at six-monthly intervals over an 18-month period. These data were analysed in conjunction with non-participant observation data of patient activities, patient attendance data and interviews with carers.

Watkins & Redfern's (1997) findings show that over a six-month period patients did not become more dependent, which indicates a possible slowing down of their deterioration; attending the night nursing service facilitated independence in the client group; and carers with an emotional attachment to the client valued the service as it allowed them to continue providing care and support.

Experimental isolation

The way in which explanatory case study research is able to test rigorously the ideas and assumptions about specific phenomena is by means of experimental isolation. A precise account of the processes that take place within specific cases is developed by researchers. This is rich in detail and allows the researchers to tease out the causal processes and factors which are thought to have a bearing on the phenomena being studied. Researchers then identify which of these factors and/or processes are present in the case(s) to be studied and they decide which of these factors and/or processes will be included or excluded in the case study research. The decision about which factors should be isolated for inclusion or exclusion within the explanatory case study research design depends on their relevance to the explanation being tested. If they are relevant they are included, if not they are excluded (Yin, 1994; Hakim, 1987). This isolation of factors and/or processes is a powerful alternative to the randomized allocation of subjects to treatments characteristic of experimental research design. In experimental research design, researchers claim to control for an infinite number of variables and rival explanations but fail to specify what they are (Campbell, 1988). In contrast to this, explanatory case study research is very specific about the factors and/or processes that are included or excluded.

Variations on the explanatory case study design

Critical/strategic

The use of experimental isolation within case study research means that there are a number of variations of the explanatory design. Critical case studies or strategic case studies examine the evidence from situations which provide positive illustrations of the phenomena in question. Turner Shaw & Bosanquet (1993) provide an example of this in the evaluation of four nursing development units which were supported by the King's Fund Centre for Nursing Developments programme for a $2\frac{1}{2}$-year period. Their aim was to identify 'best practice' from the programme. In order to achieve this they developed a two-phase design: phase one collected baseline data and explored the methods/tools used to measure the key elements of the nursing development unit framework; phase 2 explored the ongoing development of the nursing development units. They used a variety of methods to gather data: participant observation; semi-structured interviews with nursing development unit staff, key decision-makers and other health care professionals; surveys of nursing development staff; analysis of King's Fund documents and District Health Authority data regarding costings and patient activity. The result of this evaluation was the production of 'recommendations' for other areas who might be considering developing nursing in a similar fashion.

Deviant

Another variation of the explanatory design is the deviant case study where the findings from the case study research are used to show an exception to the general rule. An example of this can be seen in the works by Pontin (1997), Pontin & Webb (1995, 1996), and Webb & Pontin (1996, 1997) in their examination of the effects of introducing primary nursing onto four demonstration wards. Again a variety of methods were used to collect data: participant observation of clinical areas; non-participant observation of business meetings; documentary analysis; and interviews with clinical staff, nurse managers and patients. During the two-year period of the project, one of the clinical areas failed to move forward in its development of nursing practice and staff considered the end result to be worse than when they started (Pontin, 1997; Webb & Pontin, 1996, 1997; Pontin & Webb, 1995, 1996). This provided evidence of the effects of key factors within the case study design and, as with Turner Shaw & Bosanquet's (1993) work, identified 'recommendations' for other areas considering developing nursing practice in this way.

Classification by case

We have seen from the preceding section that we may classify case study research by its focus – descriptive, exploratory and explanatory – but in addition to this we may classify case study research according to the type of case used in the study. The most widely used classification is shown in Fig. 20.2.

Individual case histories	(e.g. Turton, 1995)
Community studies	(e.g. Brown, 1996)
Social groups	(e.g. Woods, 1997)
Organizational and institutional studies	(e.g. James et al., 1993)
Specific events, roles and relationships	(e.g. Symes, 1997)

Fig. 20.2   Classification of case study research by case (Rolfe, 1998; Sandelowski, 1996; Hakim, 1987).

Individual case histories

Individual case histories, as the term implies, are detailed accounts of specific personal experiences or events which people have lived through. The accounts which are provided by researchers explore the possible causes, processes and experiences that directly or indirectly contribute to the outcome of the study. They are particularly useful in studying less well represented groups or groups of people where access is difficult. The work of Turton (1995) is a good example of the use of this form of enquiry. She reports on her experiences of setting up a district nursing service for people with human immunodeficiency virus and uses field diaries and interviews to trace the chronology of events and causative factors which shaped the development and delivery of the service. While personal accounts are the main focus in this type of work, they are by no means the only sorts of evidence used. Documentary evidence, administrative records, non-participant observation and interviews with key informants are also necessary to build up rich, detailed pictures of settings and situations (Rolfe, 1998; Yin, 1994).

Community studies

Brown's work (Brown, 1996) is an example of case study research with a single local community: in this case, the development of a home play project in a locality of Sheffield. He describes and analyses the pattern of relationships between parents' feelings about their children's behaviour, the level of resources in the area for children and the outcomes of a community development programme with a home-visiting component. Typically, community studies describe a particular community and also address specific questions relating to policy and theory – in this case the use of outcome measures in community development.

Social groups

Social group case study research is typically either of small groups of people in direct contact with one another, such as work teams, or larger groups of people who share a common identity, activities or interests. Occupational groupings are a good example of the latter. Woods (1997) reports on case study research carried out with a group of nurses who were undergoing higher degree preparation for advanced nursing practice. By examining the progress of a strategically different group of nurses – i.e. those preparing for advanced practice – Woods hopes to describe and evaluate the impact of advanced nursing practice on usual nursing and medical activity. Research into work practices often involves some form of observation, either participatory or non-participatory, with all of the attendant advantages and disadvantages each method brings to case study research (see Chapter 26).

Organizational and institutional studies

The variety of methods that may be used in organizational and institutional case study research can be seen to good effect in James et al.'s (1993) work on neo-natal services in one city between 1990 and 1992. Four main methods were used – unstructured interviews with ancillary, nursing and medical staff from the neo-natal services and nurse managers in related paediatric and maternity services within the town; participant observation; visits to peripheral special care baby units and interviews with staff there; and analysis of internal policy documents relating to the provision of neo-natal services within the city and adjoining areas. Organizational or institutional case study research is a useful design to highlight 'best practice' initiatives in terms of implementing policy, or addressing managerial/organizational issues. In particular, it may be used when organizations or institutions are facing change or going through a refocusing of their usual activity.

Specific events, roles and relationships

The final type of case study research mentioned here is concerned with events, roles and relationships. Hakim (1987) suggests that this is a more diffuse form of research and that the overlap between this form of research and organisational/

institutional and social groups research is quite large. Indeed, if we examine the examples given to illustrate the two previous forms of case study research it is possible to see how they could be seen as examining either social groups or organisational change. However, the characteristic of this particular form of case study research is that the investigation is concerned with specific events, roles and relationships. This concern with roles and relationships may be seen in the work of Symes (1997). She uses a series of focus groups and follow-up depth interviews with midwives who have worked in community-based midwifery teams. By allowing the midwives to talk about the changes in their work patterns and the changes in their relationships with their clients, Symes is able to tease out the implications for the changes in the role of community midwives. What becomes apparent from her work is that there is ambivalence from midwives about this change in role – the opportunity to practise 'true' midwifery is welcomed but there is great concern about the effects of such practice on the lives of midwives away from work and the impact on family and home life.

Generalizability

I mentioned earlier that the praises of case study research have been unsung for some time and it is fair to say that there has been a great deal of criticism of case study research regarding its 'scientific' nature and, in particular, the generalizability of case study research findings (Frankfort-Nachmias & Nachmias, 1996; Black, 1993; Smith, 1975). The rehabilitation of case study research is in some part due to a rethinking of what is actually meant by 'generalizability' of findings (Campbell, 1988). A strong argument has been put forward to distinguish between two forms of generalization. Unfortunately the debate is at a stage where a number of different terms are being used to refer to broadly similar phenomena, so I shall endeavour to group them together here to provide an overview. However, it is important to remember that there are differences within each broad grouping (as well as between them) and readers should be wary of assuming that the debate is closed. Far from it! Purely for ease of expression I shall adopt the terms used by Sharp (1998) when describing the broad groupings – that is, empirical generalization and theoretical generalization (see Fig. 20.3).

Empirical generalization

When researchers use empirical generalization they select a random sample from a population and calculate the probability that the sample is representative. Any statistical inferences which are made by the researchers from their work can only be made from a known and finite population. This is difficult to do in most nursing research because we have great problems in identifying known and finite populations. It is further complicated by the fact that findings from this sort of

Sharp (1998)	Empirical generalization	Theoretical generalization
Sandelowski (1996) Fraenkel (1995) Eisner (1991) Silverstein (1988) Lincoln & Guba (1985) Stake & Trumbull (1982)	Nomothetic (law like) generalization	Idiographic (naturalistic) generalization
Rolfe (1998) Yin (1994) Hakim (1987)	Statistical generalization	Analytical generalization

Fig. 20.3   Different forms of generalization within research.

research may only be generalized to the sample population. It may not be legitimately generalized to future events, situations or settings to make predictions (the very things with which nurses, midwives and health visitors are concerned!). Also empirical generalizations do not allow researchers to work out the relationships that might exist between variables, they only show whether a correlation exists or if a causal relationship is likely to exist. The nature of these relationships can only be worked out and explained by researchers by using theories to describe the world. Sharp (1998) illustrates this well when he talks about the relationship between social class and health. He argues that an explanation for the relationship cannot be induced from the data alone; researchers have to use models, theories and concepts to produce explanations.

Theoretical generalization

Theoretical generalization, on the other hand, is a way in which researchers can generate a theory about phenomena which explains the relationships between them. The generation of the theory is achieved by in-depth study of one case, or a larger limited number of cases, and the aim is to make a generalization based on the plausibility of the link between the characteristics of the phenomena being studied (Rolfe, 1998; Mitchell, 1983).

Case study research allows researchers to make in-depth studies of one or more cases and to generate and test theories about particular phenomena. However, as well as making theoretical generalization from case study research, researchers are also able to make empirical generalization by using multiple cases. Hakim (1987) argues that as the number of sites in which a case study is conducted increases, the 'general significance and robustness' of the findings also increase. The biggest increase in robustness occurs when a case study moves from one site to two (Sudman, 1976). This not only provides a strong justification for using multiple cases in case study research, but also provides a rationale for replication studies.

Conclusions

Perhaps the most compelling advantage of case study research for nurses, midwives and health visitors is the wide diversity of research designs open to them. They may range from simple, descriptive, cross-sectional, one case, single researcher projects to large, explanatory, multiple case, longitudinal, multi-researcher programmes. This means that complex health care phenomena may be studied in 'real life' settings and, to a greater or lesser degree, empirical generalizations and theoretical generalizations may be generated.

However, the value of case study research findings is dependent on the strength of the design which, in turn, rests on the fit between the questions asked, the methods used and the cases selected. Therefore, before beginning this type of work, clear statements have to be formulated by researchers about the research question, the case study research focus and classification type, the factors for inclusion/exclusion (if it is explanatory), the number of cases to be studied, the methods to be used and forms of data to be analysed as well as the analytical processes involved. Because of its flexibility, case study research has great potential for nurses, midwives and health visitors in practice to investigate clinical phenomena (Rolfe, 1998). However, care must be taken to maintain the intellectual rigour of the approach.

The disadvantage of case study research is paradoxically the very flexibility of design, and in particular the methods, used to generate data. It is highly unusual for researchers to be proficient, let alone expert, in every single form of research method possible. Researchers develop skills and expertise in certain forms of enquiry in much the same way that practitioners develop clinical skills, and as we don't expect every practitioner to be 'expert' in every field of clinical practice we cannot expect researchers to be 'expert' in every form of research. When 'the researcher' is also 'the practitioner' this problem becomes magnified by the pressure of everyday workload management. Therefore, to do justice to the enquiry practitioners will need to either negotiate reductions in workload when they carry out the research or work in partnership with researchers who do not have clinical caseload responsibilities. Ideally, this situation will be resolved by applying for research grants to fund research time (see Chapters 4 and 10).

References

Black, T. (1993) *Evaluating Social Science Research*. London: Sage.

Brown, I. (1996) Outcome measures, health visiting and community development. In *Evidence Based Community Development*. London: Community Development Interest Group, Health Visitors Assoc.

Campbell, D. (1988) *Methodology and Epistemology for Social Science: Selected Papers*. London: University of Chicago Press.

Denzin, N. (1978) *The Research Act: A Theoretical Introduction to Sociological Methods*, 2nd edn. New York: McGraw-Hill.

Eden, B. & Foreman, M. (1996) Problems associated with under recognition of delirium in critical care: a case study. *Heart and Lung* **25** (5): 388–400.

Eisner, E. (1991) *The Enlightened Age: Qualitative Inquiry and the Enhancement of Educational Practice*. London: Macmillan.

Fraenkel, P. (1995) The nomothetic-idiographic debate in family therapy. *Family Process* **34**: 113–21.

Frankfort-Nachmias, C. & Nachmias, D. (1996) *Research Methods in Social Science*, 5th edn. London: Arnold.

Fridlund, B. (1997) The case study as a research strategy. *Scandinavian Journal of Caring Science* **11** (1): 3–4.

Gray, M. (1998) Introducing single case study research design: an overview. *Nurse Researcher* **5** (4): 15–24.

Hakim, C. (1987) *Research Design: Strategies and Choices in the Design of Social Research*. London: Allen & Unwin.

Hammersley, M. & Atkinson, P. (1995) *Ethnography: Principles in Practice*, 2nd edn. London: Tavistock.

James, N., Arthur, T. & Pittman, A. (1993) *Nursing Quality Counts: A Case Study of Neonatal Services 1990–1992. Nursing Policy Studies 9*. Nottingham: Dept of Nursing & Midwifery Studies, University of Nottingham.

Lincoln, Y. & Guba, E. (1985) *Naturalistic Inquiry*. London: Sage.

Luker, K., Hogg, C., Austin, L., Ferguson, B. & Smith, K. (1998) Decision making: the context of nurse prescribing. *Journal of Advanced Nursing* **27**: 657–65.

Meier, P. & Pugh, E. (1986) The case study: a variable approach to clinical research. *Research in Nursing and Health* **9**: 195–202.

Mitchell, J. (1983) Case study and situational analysis. *Sociological Review* **31** (2). 187–211.

Newell, R. (1998) Single case experimental design: controlling the study. *Nurse Researcher* **5**, (4): 25–39.

Patton, M. (1990) *Qualitative Evaluation and Research Methods*, 2nd edn. London: Sage.

Pontin, D. (1997) *The effect of primary nursing on the quality of nursing care: an action research study of nursing development work*. Unpublished PhD thesis, University of Manchester.

Pontin, D. & Webb, C. (1995) Assessing patient satisfaction. Part 1 – The research process. *Journal of Clinical Nursing* **4**: 383–9.

Pontin, D & Webb, C. (1996) Assessing patient satisfaction. Part 2 – Findings: nursing, the hospital and patients' concerns. *Journal of Clinical Nursing* **5**: 33–40.

Robson, C. (1993) *Real World Research*. Oxford: Blackwell Science.

Rolfe, G. (1998) *Expanding Nursing Knowledge: Understanding and Researching your Own Practice*. London: Butterworth Heinemann.

Sandelowski, M. (1996) One is the liveliest number: the case orientation of qualitative research. *Research in Nursing and Health* **19**: 525–9.

Sharp, K. (1998) The case for case studies in nursing research: the problems of generalisation. *Journal of Advanced Nursing* **27**: 785–9.

Silverstein, A. (1988) An Aristotelian resolution of the idiographic versus nomothetic tension. *American Psychologist* **43**: 425–30.

Smith, H. (1975) *Strategies of Social Research: The Methodological Imagination*. London: Prentice Hall.

Stake, R. (1994) Case studies. In N. Denzin & Y. Lincoln (eds) *Handbook of Qualitative Research*. London: Sage, pp. 236–47.

Stake, R. & Trumbull, D. (1982) Naturalistic generalisation. *Review Journal of Philosophy and Social Science* 7: 1–12.

Sudman, S. (1976) *Applied Sampling*. London: Academic Press.

Symes, N. (1997) *Great expectations: midwives' views and experiences of continuity of care*. Unpublished MSc thesis, University of Bristol.

Turner Shaw, J. & Bosanquet, N. (1993) *A Way to Develop Nurses and Nursing*. London: King's Fund Centre.

Turton, P. (1995) *Developing a community nursing service for people with HIV disease: an action research project incorporating ethnographic methods*. Unpublished PhD thesis, University of Manchester.

Watkins, M. & Redfern, S. (1997) Evaluation of a new night nursing service for elderly people suffering from dementia. *Journal of Clinical Nursing* 6: 485–94.

Webb, C. & Pontin, D. (1996) Introducing primary nursing: nurses' opinions. *Journal of Clinical Nursing* 5: 351–8.

Webb, C. & Pontin, D. (1997) Evaluating the introduction of primary nursing: the use of a care plan audit. *Journal of Clinical Nursing* 6: 395–401.

Woods, L. (1997) Designing and conducting case study research in nursing. *Nursing Times Research* 2 (1): 48–56.

Yin, R. (1994) *Case Study Research: Design and Methods. Applied Social Research Methods*, Vol. 5. London: Sage.

CHAPTER 21

Longitudinal research

Tricia Murphy-Black

Overview of longitudinal research

Longitudinal research uses data collected over time. This is a flexible research design that can have data collected by quantitative or qualitative methods. In these days of evidence-based health care, one very attractive aspect is that it is possible to make stronger causal interpretations from the data than is possible from other forms of non-experimental design. While the randomized-controlled trial (RCT) may be the gold standard for measuring the cause and effect of an intervention, there is much in health care that cannot be manipulated. One such example is the effect of smoking. Even when the ill effects of smoking were not appreciated, a RCT in which the control group was not allowed to smoke and the experimental group was forced to smoke would have considerable difficulties with both compliance and ethical approval.

Some longitudinal studies are both small scale and serendipitous, such as the 1998 event when, aged 77, John Glenn returned to space, 36 years after his first space flight in 1962. The possibility of comparing physical data from the first flight with data to be obtained 36 years later was probably not even a gleam in the most avid longitudinal researcher's eye. The second flight will provide information about the same person as well as the effects on a senior citizen.

Definition

Longitudinal research is a nice example of the differences between research design and research methods. The design (longitudinal) is a description of the research strategy or the overall map of how the problem will be examined, while the methods give the detail of how to carry out the practicalities of the study. Both quantitative and qualitative methods may be used to collect data for longitudinal research. Menard (1991: 4) has defined longitudinal research as

'. . . research in which (a) data are collected for each item or variable for two or more distinct time periods; (b) the subjects or cases analysed are the same or at least comparable from one period to the next; and (c) the analysis involves some comparison of data between or among period.'

The elderly patients with dementia in the study by Watson & Deary (1997) had data collected about their feeding difficulties at 18-month intervals. Midwives' professional development was followed for three different phases and compared two groups: those who qualified in 1979 and in 1983 (Robinson, 1994). Both these studies fulfilled the criteria of the definition above.

Types of longitudinal research

Essentially longitudinal research is aiming to measure differences or changes in a variable between one time period and another. The intervals may be short or long and the data are used to analyse cause and effect relationships (Bowling, 1997). Menard (1991) describes a number of different types.

Prospective panel design

In this type, data are collected at least twice, at different time periods, during those time periods. These time differences may be short (a month apart) or long (10 years apart). The panel, that is, the sample (sometimes also called a cohort, see below) comprises the same cases (individual nurses, patients, hospitals,) and the same variables (attitudes, symptoms, outcomes of care) which are measured at each time point.

An example is the examination of the outcomes of nurse education and subsequent patterns of employment which are being studied by Robinson *et al.* (1998). This is an ongoing study (1997–2001) of a nationally drawn cohort of approximately 3000 newly qualified nurse diplomates from the P2000 courses of all four nursing branches. The nurses were recruited just before qualification and postal questionnaires were distributed at 6 months (1998) and 18 months (1999). Further questionnaires are planned for three years after qualification and possibly longer. This survey is prospective – that is, the data are collected from a fixed starting point and continue forward. This is the most common type.

Retrospective panel design

In this design data are collected at a single time period but the questions ask about several time periods in the past (recent episodes of ill health; experiences of different jobs). It is similar to prospective panel design but the data-collection activities by the researcher only cover one time period. This design shares the same disadvantages as other retrospective designs (the data may have been originally recorded for reasons other than research; or the individual may have difficulty in remembering accurately over a long period of time). A study of the mortality rates in nine neo-natal intensive care units used data from the clinical notes over the previous seven years. This included the abstraction of the gestation, birth weight, congenital malformation and routine physiological data from the first 12 hours after birth of babies less than 31 weeks' gestation or birth weight less than 1500 g. These data were then re-analysed to allow for a more detailed comparison of the performance of each of the hospitals during the years 1988–1994. This study demonstrated the value of longitudinal design – annual league tables were unreliable indicators of performance, did not demonstrate best practice and did not show consistent differences between hospitals. As the apparent performance of individual hospitals fluctuated substantially from year to year, the annual differences were random rather than significant (Parry *et al.*, 1998). The common factor in both these designs is that the research subjects or cases and the variables to be measured remain the same at the different time periods.

Repeated cross-sectional design

In this design the data are collected on the same set of variables for two or more time periods. The essential difference is that the cases will be comparable (all first-year students or patients with the same disease) but are not identical. As with the panel design, this may be prospective (measurements at different times) or retrospective (all measurements at the same time). The commonest form of study using this design is the political opinion poll. In the weeks leading up to a general election, the same variables (attitudes to the political parties) are measured again and again. The time intervals may be short (monthly, weekly, or daily) but the cases or the sample will be different. The polling organizations take considerable trouble to ensure that each sample is representative of the population of the country as a whole. The measures used include age, gender, socio-economic grouping and race. A new sample will be picked for each of the data-collection intervals. These political opinion polls plot the change of attitude to the different political parties. Polls from the same organizations, or even different organizations, are compared one with another in daily news reports. The polls are considered by the political parties to be highly significant.

Summary

Although Menard (1991) reported that there is not a consensus on the definition of longitudinal research, some researchers narrow it to prospective panel designs only, which is especially true in developmental studies in psychology. Other disciplines, however, consider this to be too restrictive. There are a number of different features of the full range of methods, which are useful in answering a range of different research questions in human sciences.

Advantages and disadvantages

Advantages

Longitudinal research offers a number of advantages (see Barley, 1995; LoBiondo-Wood & Haber, 1998; McNeill, 1990; Menard, 1991; Robinson *et al.*, 1998; Seed, 1995):

1. It is possible to record the progress of the developmental process, including normal development and the progress of disease.
2. There is reduction in the risk of bias in sample selection, especially in cohort samples – that is, those chosen because they share a particular life event at the same time, such as date of birth or starting school or university.
3. It allows measurement and analysis of change in the individuals and in the whole aggregated sample.
4. The measurement of change also allows the exploration of cause and effect in events, or other variables.
5. It is possible to explore the effect of time on events or other variables, such as change in political views with increasing age.
6. It reduces the problems associated with remembering events accurately, especially in studies that revisit the sample regularly.
7. As all the subjects in the study have repeated measurements of the same variables, all subjects serve as their own controls.
8. The regular follow-up, especially when collecting qualitative data, gives an increased depth of responses.
9. Early trends in data can be followed, especially in qualitative data, but questionnaires or other instruments can also be tailored to the individual's experiences.
10. There can be exploration of both relationships between and differences in variables.
11. It is possible for the researcher to record the development of an individual's reality or experience and to be verified.

Disadvantages

The disadvantages of longitudinal research (see Goldstein, 1979; LoBiondo-Wood & Haber, 1998; McNeill, 1990; Menard, 1991; Robinson *et al.*, 1998) are:

1. Difficulties in recruiting subjects, especially if they know the study will continue for a long time.
2. Difficulties in maintaining the subjects in the study; keeping in touch over many years – they may drop out, move, emigrate or die (this is known as attrition).

3. Changing the research subjects – inclusion in the study may make them less like the population from which they were chosen, that is, they become atypical.

4. Subjects included as children may decide against continuing in the study when they become adults.

5. As the sample gets smaller, whatever the cause, it becomes less representative of the population from which it was drawn.

6. It can be difficult to keep a research team in place through many years of the study.

7. Any study that continues over many years is costly. Few are funded as an ongoing project and it may be difficult to attract funding for later parts of the study.

8. The feature that is the main advantage – the length – becomes a disadvantage with the length itself contributing to problems of data quality. These include validity; reliability, interaction between the researchers and the subjects; the relevance of the research (what was an important feature at the start of a study 10 years ago may no longer apply).

The purpose of longitudinal research

The purpose of longitudinal research is to examine change over time (Menard, 1991) – a change may be of natural growth and development (Goldstein, 1979) such as the British National Child Development Study. The purpose may also be to measure the effects of events (e.g. childbirth, bereavement), policies (changes to the social benefit system, introduction of new form of education) or natural disasters (radiation fallout from Chernobyl; the greenhouse effect on climate). Longitudinal studies can identify service needs – for example, the need for provision of psychological support was recognized in a study which identified a deterioration of emotional status after unsuccessful IVF treatments (Slade *et al.*, 1997). The change measured may be of the patterns of change; to establish the direction (better or worse; positive or negative) and the extent of the change (Menard, 1991).

Conducting longitudinal research

Defining the research questions

The progress from the research problem to the research question is always the most important part of developing a research proposal. While this is true for all research, it is vital in longitudinal research. An ill-defined, poorly focused or wrongly directed question could lead to years of data collection that will have very limited value. The nature of longitudinal research must always be kept in mind, the extent of change and the direction of change. What is this study measuring? How can it be measured? The study by Robinson *et al.* (1997) not only had specific research questions (what are the career plans and the careers followed by a cohort of nurses?; what aspects of their health care experience is relevant to retention in nursing?) but also, was sufficiently sophisticated that the plans reported in one questionnaire could be reiterated in a later one so that each respondent could reflect on her own plans and actual experience.

Choosing methods in longitudinal research design

There are a number of different methods that can be used in longitudinal research. If the method chosen is a survey, it may be referred to as an analytic survey (rather than a descriptive survey).

Quantitative

Physical measurements, of children and adults, are obvious methods of data collection in longitudinal studies of development such as the 1958 birth cohort (Davie *et al.*, 1972). The follow-up to this cohort included a range of other methods such as an investigation of the relationship between psychological health and occupational class, undertaken at 23 years and linked to data from the subjects when they were 16 years old (Power & Manor, 1992). As another possibility with such a study, the interest from different disciplines can be combined – for example, an investigation of the relationship between birthweight and socio-economic disadvantage during childhood and adolescence (Bartley *et al.*, 1994). This study collected data from males of the 1958 cohort at birth and at 7, 11, 16 and 23 years of age.

Qualitative

Longitudinal designs are also amenable for use with qualitative methods. For instance, the examination of work and family decision-making processes of 61 couples by Zvonkovic *et al.* (1996) or the in-depth study of 20 families caring for a severely disabled child (Beresford, 1996). The major difference between qualitative and quantitative data collection lies with the researcher. In qualitative research, data collection can be a more or less continuous process (Seed, 1994) while the quantitative researcher will collect data at intervals over a number of months or years.

Long and short

Some longitudinal studies continue for many years and involve a large number of subjects. The national census occurs every ten years and involves the whole population. In Scotland, the first census was conducted in 1801 and since then has only missed 1941, during World War II (GROS, 1997). Other studies are much shorter, but still fulfil the definition of longitudinal research as there are repeated measurements over time. Examples include a three-month study of postnatal care (Murphy-Black, 1989a) or the study to measure any association between HIV infection and neurological and psychological impairments 12 months after testing (Burgess *et al.*, 1994).

Planning

The planning of a longitudinal study should be detailed in order to protect against as many of the disadvantages as feasible. Sometimes it has to be accepted that this is only 'as detailed as possible'. Some studies, for instance, the Midwives Careers' Project, started off with an educational purpose to compare those who had two different forms of training (Robinson, 1994). As the latter stages were only planned after the first round of data collection, it was too late to include questions, which may have contributed to the total picture after additional data collection at different times.

Sometimes a design that has a theoretical or clinical basis may in itself cause problems. For example, a series of interviews were planned with all the mothers who had babies during a specific month, at ten days (when daily visits by midwives stopped), at one month (when postnatal care by midwives ended formally) and at three months after the birth of their babies. There was a short period when the interviews at ten days overlapped with the interviews at a month. Foreseeing such a problem might have resulted in employing additional interviewers, or staggering the data-collection period (two weeks at the beginning of one month; two weeks at the end of the following month). These possible solutions have implications for the planning, costing and organizing of the project.

Pilot study

Although all projects benefit from a pilot study, with a longitudinal study this can sometimes seem daunting. In a study that has a number of complex issues to deal with, planned over a number of years, it would rarely be feasible to have a pilot study for ten years preceding an actual ten-year project. One way of dealing with this difficulty is to have a pilot sample. This sample 'runs ahead' of the main study by a few months, to allow the researchers to test instruments and procedures in advance of each phase of the project. Robinson *et al.* (1998) used this technique to examine the issues surrounding the selection, recruitment and maintenance of the sample and the design and development of questionnaires. In a study where the main sample was in the region of 3000, the pilot group was 600. This sub-group will never form part of the main sample but will remain the pilot group for the whole life of the study, allowing for piloting of questionnaires at each stage, i.e. 6 months, 18 months and 3 years after qualification.

Methodological issues

Sampling

The descriptions of longitudinal research described at the beginning of this chapter (prospective panel, retrospective panel; repeated cross-sectional) refer not only to the pattern of data collection but also to the sampling.

Prospective panel

The panel – that is, the sample – such as groups of graduates from specific pro-grammes – is chosen by certain criteria and then followed up for a specified period. There may be considerable efforts made by the research team to ensure that this panel is representative of the population from which it is chosen. For instance, Robinson *et al.* (1998) – studying nurses qualifying in 1997–98 – needed to have a sample that would be representative of each branch and dip-lomates as a whole. So the adult branch, with the greatest number, had a sample size between one-eighth and one-sixth of all the nurses due to qualify, and between one-third and one-half of nurses in the mental health and children branches. The learning disability branch, the smallest, included all those about to qualify.

Cohort

A sample with a shared characteristic, such as age or date of birth, is known as a cohort. The children in the British National Child Development were all the babies born in Britain in the second week of March 1958 (Davie *et al.*, 1972), sometimes known as the 1958 birth cohort.

Retrospective panel

In this instance the sample is chosen after an event. There will be just as much care given to the selection but an element of the selection will be out of the control of the researchers. Having identified an event or condition, the researcher then looks back to collect the data. If the focus of the research is the beginning of pregnancy, a very large sample would be required if all the women of fertile years were included until the correct sample size was reached. In practical terms, it is better to pick women who are already pregnant. One of the problems is that certain groups (those having spontaneous or therapeutic abortions) will have been excluded.

Repeated cross-sectional

A cross-section of the population is chosen (perhaps from each year of students at university, or each ward in a hospital) and later the same data collection is repeated but with a different sample. An audit that questions a certain number of patients each month, or year, from a ward or department is using this method of sampling. A slightly different version was the sample of midwives qualifying in 1979 who were questioned about their educational experience. This was repeated with midwives qualifying in 1983. As these two samples had different educational experiences (12 months versus 18 months) it was possible to compare the outcomes of the courses. As both of these panels were followed up subsequently, this study combined the prospective panel with the repeated cross-sectional (Robinson, 1994).

Population

The population is the total number of a group, all the residents in the UK, all students or all nurses, for example. The most familiar population study is the census which provides a picture of the country as it is each decade but also allows follow-up from one time period to the next. Usually this is at the aggregate level where all the data from 1981 is compared with that of 1991 (size of the population, number of households with children; proportion of people who speak Gaelic or Welsh). Sometimes there is a follow-up of samples following the census, as shown in the work of Sloggett & Joshi (1994) who used a random sample of nearly 300 000 people aged between 16 and 65 at the 1981 census. The follow-up for the next nine years demonstrated a significant positive relationship between the degree of deprivation of the ward of residence and premature death.

Attrition

The major challenge in the longitudinal study is to maintain the representativeness of the sample. Even a sample which is assumed or demonstrated to be representative of a particular population may have deteriorated by the time of data collection. This deterioration is due to attrition, that is, non-responders or drop-outs. The viability of studies can be compromised by loss of respondents. This may include a decision to withdraw, loss of contact with the research team through mobility, change of status or, the ultimate loss, death. For studies planned over a number of years, attrition at each stage can result in the increasing loss of representativeness (Goldstein, 1979).

In some studies, the nature and design of the study can aid the completion of all phases of the study and, at the same time, result in some subjects being excluded mid project. One hundred and forty-four couples who entered for a programme of *in vitro* fertilization treatment also agreed to take part in a prospective study of their emotions and relationships until six months after the identification of pregnancy or discontinuation of treatment following three unsuccessful cycles (Slade *et al.*, 1997). There was, however, an irregularity in the longitudinal design (those pregnant after the first cycle of treatment, $n = 28$, had their final data collected between six and seven months after the first set while those who had three treatment cycles, each with a three-month interval between treatments, had their final measurements between 12 and 14 months after the first). Even a study such as this, which may expect high compliance with the treatment if not the research, experienced nearly 10% of the subjects failing to complete all the data sets. In this particular study, admittedly, half ($n = 7$) had to be excluded because they no longer fulfilled the unit's criteria for treatments (such as divorce proceedings or hysterectomy) while an additional seven did not complete the data collection.

Studies with small samples are not immune to problems of attrition. Lathlean (1996) planned a year's in-depth study of five lecturer practitioners followed by a larger more superficial study. Because the job changed so much, she needed to follow them up for longer and carried on for another year, during which two of the lecturer practitioners left their posts.

Strategies for reducing attrition

One way of dealing with this problem is to address it at the planning stage of the project. Drawing on experiences of a number of longitudinal studies, the team undertaking the nurses and midwives careers' projects used the following strategies: developing and testing questionnaires for validity, reliability and length with a pilot group; checking addresses; asking responders for help to contact the non-responders; meeting students to invite them to participate, maintaining regular contact; following up non-responders three times, each time enclosing another copy of the questionnaire and using stamps rather than freepost return envelopes (Robinson, 1994; Robinson & Marsland, 1994; Robinson *et al.*, 1998). All of these strategies have time and cost implications for the study. A small study ($n = 645$) with three rounds of questionnaires employed a cross-over technique to see if the response improved if stamps were used rather than reply-paid envelopes. At each distribution of questionnaires half the sample was sent stamped and half reply-paid envelopes. The positions were reversed at the next round. The response rate was good overall (83% at the first round, 76% at the third). Of the 1935 questionnaires distributed almost equal numbers of each were returned, with only three more of the stamped than the reply-paid envelopes (Murphy-Black, 1989b).

Data analysis

Analysis of longitudinal data is complex. Such studies frequently involve large data sets and may be dependent on the return, data processing and analysis before the next round can be undertaken. It is vital that the quality control of the procedures to keep track of all the data is maintained throughout the life of the study. The analysis of the data is frequently both cross-sectional (the picture of the most recent data collection) and longitudinal (the most recent plus data from the previous times). As will have been appreciated from some of the studies referred to, data from the most recent phase of the study may be reported followed by a second report of the comparison with the previous data-collection period or periods. Establishing a correlation between an event and outcome may be straightforward. The 1958 birth cohort showed a highly significant increase in the incidence of congenital heart disease of babies born to smokers compared with those born to non-smokers (Fedrick *et al.*, 1971). Some measurements, however, may require closer examination. If the mean score of a sample for depression is compared with the mean score a year later, and is the same at both times, it would appear that there was no improvement in the incidence of depression. This, however, may hide the fact that some individuals have higher or lower scores and the group effect has cancelled out the differences (Bowling, 1997). In this example, it will be necessary to measure the difference in individuals as well as the group.

It cannot be emphasized too strongly that consideration of the analysis should be included in the planning stage. Where possible a statistician should be a member of the team; if this is not possible, it will be essential to have statistical advice.

Conclusions

Choosing a longitudinal design for a research project might seem too daunting for a novice researcher. It is possible to undertake such a project in a relatively short time period but it is important that both the advantages and the disadvantages are considered in making the choice. The golden rule of research should be paramount; that is, the design and methods should be chosen to answer the question and a longitudinal research design should be chosen only if no other method can meet these needs.

References

Barley, S.R. (1995) Images of imaging: notes on doing longitudinal fieldwork. In G.P. Huber & A. van de Ven (eds) *Longitudinal Field Research Methods: Studying Processes of Organizational Change.* Thousand Oaks: Sage.

Bartley, M., Power, C., Blane, D., Smith, G.D. & Shipley, M. (1994) Birth-weight and later socioeconomic disadvantage – evidence from the 1958 British cohort study. *British Medical Journal* **309**: 1475–8.

Beresford, B. (1996) Coping with the care of a severely disabled child. *Health and Social Care in the Community* **4** (1): 30–40.

Bowling, A. (1997) *Research Methods in Health: Investigating Health and Health Services*. Buckingham: Open University Press.

Burgess, A.P., Riccio, M., Jadresic, D., Pugh, K., Catalan, J., Hawkins, D.A., Baldeweg, T., Lovett, E., Gruzelier, J. & Thompson, C. (1994) A longitudinal-study of the neuro-psychiatric consequences of HIV-1 infection in gay men. 1: Neuropsychological performance and neurological status at base-line and at 12-month follow-up. *Psychological Medicine* **24** (4): 885–95.

Davie, R., Butler, N.R. & Goldstein, H. (1972) *From Birth to Seven*. London: Longman.

Fedrick, J., Alberman, E.D. & Goldstein, H. (1971) Possible teratogenic effect of cigarette smoking. *Nature* **231**: 529–30.

Goldstein, H. (1979) *The Design and Analysis of Longitudinal Studies*. London: Academic Press.

GROS (1997) *The Census in Scotland*. General Registrar Office, Scotland http://www.open.gov.uk/gros/histcens.htm

Lathlean, J. (1996) The challenges of longitudinal ethnographic research in nursing. *Nursing Times Research* **1** (1): 38–43.

LoBiondo-Wood, G. & Haber, J. (1998) *Nursing Research: Methods, Critical Appraisal, and Utilization*, 4th edn. St. Louis: Mosby.

McNeill, P. (1990) *Research Methods*, 2nd edn. London: Routledge.

Menard, S. (1991) *Longitudinal Research*, Series No. 76: Quantitative Applications in the Social Sciences. Newbury Park: Sage.

Murphy-Black, T. (1989a) *Postnatal Care at Home: A Descriptive Study of Mothers' Needs and the Maternity Services*. Nursing Research Unit, University of Edinburgh.

Murphy-Black, T. (1989b) *Appendix to Postnatal Care at Home: A Descriptive Study of Mothers' Needs and the Maternity Services*. Nursing Research Unit, University of Edinburgh.

Parry, G.J., Gould, C.R., McCabe, C.J. & Tarnow-Mordi, W.O. (1998) Annual league tables of mortality in neonatal intensive care units: longitudinal study. *British Medical Journal* **316**: 1931–5.

Power, C. & Manor, O. (1992) Explaining social-class differences in psychological health among young adults – a longitudinal perspective. *Social Psychiatry and Psychiatric Epidemiology* **27**: 284–91.

Robinson, S. (1994) Professional development in midwifery: findings from a longitudinal study of midwives' careers. *Nurse Education Today* **14**: 161–76.

Robinson, S. & Marsland, L. (1994) Approaches to the problem of respondent attrition in a longitudinal panel study of nurses' careers. *Journal of Advanced Nursing* **20**: 729–41.

Robinson, S., Murrells, T. & Marsland, L. (1997) Constructing career pathways in nursing: some issues for research and policy. *Journal of Advanced Nursing* **25**: 602–14.

Robinson, S., Marsland, L., Murrells, T., Hickey, G., Hardyman, R. & Tingle, A. (1998) Designing questionnaires in a longitudinal study of nurse diplomates' careers. *Nursing Times Research* **3** (3): 195–8.

Seed, A. (1994) Patients to people. *Journal of Advanced Nursing* **19** (4): 738–48.

Seed, A. (1995) Conducting a longitudinal study an unsanitized account. *Journal of Advanced Nursing* **21** (5): 845–52.

Slade, P., Emery, J. & Lieberman, B.A. (1997) A prospective longitudinal study of emotions and relationships in in-vitro fertilization treatment. *Human Reproduction* **12** (1): 183–90.

Sloggett, A. & Joshi, H. (1994) Higher mortality in deprived area – community or personal disadvantage. *British Medical Journal* 309: 1470–4.

Watson, R. & Deary, I.J. (1997) A longitudinal study of feeding difficulty and nursing intervention in elderly patients with dementia. *Journal of Advanced Nursing* 26 (1): 25–32.

Zvonkovic, A.M., Greaves, K.M., Schmiege, C.J. & Hall, L.D. (1996) The marital construction of gender through work and family decisions: a qualitative analysis. *Journal of Marriage and the Family* 58 (1): 91–100.

CHAPTER 22

Survey design and sampling

F. Ian Atkinson

The intention of this chapter is to introduce the general principles of survey research design and methods of random sampling. Broadly, survey research can be seen as either descriptive or analytical in purpose. Descriptive surveys aim to make descriptive statements about a study population. The intention of analytical surveys is to explore associations between the different variables under study. While it is useful to distinguish these two main purposes, in practice, much survey work is carried out for both descriptive and analytical reasons.

A major feature of a survey is that information is obtained from a sample of subjects who are selected from a study population and then, on the basis of this information, the whole study population can be described. In other words, population parameters can be estimated on the basis of sample statistics. Already this has introduced terms which need to be defined.

The term *population* refers to all those people about which a researcher wishes to make statements. In research, the investigator defines the population of interest; for example, if you wanted to make statements about the prevalence of smoking among registered nurses in a single Health Board area, then the population would be all registered nurses employed in that Health Board. Populations for surveys are not always people, they may be items. If hospital managers wanted to make a statement about the quality of a consignment of disposable syringes delivered to a hospital then every syringe in that consignment would constitute the population of interest. A *sample* refers to the group of people that a researcher selects from a defined population and these are the individuals about whom information will be collected. This information can be summarized as 'sample statistics' (for example, the mean age of a sample). A population parameter refers to a measurable characteristic of a study population which is not known but which is estimated on the basis of a sample statistic in descriptive surveys.

By their very nature, descriptive survey findings do not allow statements of 'fact' to be made about a population parameter. Indeed, any statement about a population based on sample findings can only be a *probability* statement, meaning that there is a chance that it could be wrong. The challenge is to reduce the chance of this final statement being wrong to an acceptable and calculable level. This can only be achieved by giving attention to the design of surveys and the principles which need to be applied are outlined below.

At this point it might be reasonable to ask: If there is a chance that the final statements about a population will be wrong then why bother doing surveys at all? Why not get information from everyone, for example all the registered nurses, then statements of fact could be made about how many smoked and no one could question the findings?

If information is collected from all individuals in a defined population, this is referred to as a *population census*. Although the idea of carrying out a census may hold some attractions, a brief consideration of the nature of censuses as compared to sample surveys shows the latter to have definite advantages. First, it is very difficult to get information from everybody in a defined population, there are always some who either cannot be contacted or decline to help with an investigation. Even in the national census where people are compelled by law to complete and return a form there are still those who refuse. As a consequence the researcher may still be unable to make factual statements about the population. Second, a census can be very expensive to carry out and it can be shown that after a point any increase in the number of people from whom information is sought will not increase the accuracy of population estimates in proportion to the extra costs involved. In other words, the law of diminishing returns begins to take effect. Third, in some instances it might be entirely impractical to get complete information from a population. In the example of a consignment of disposable syringes, if each was tested for contamination then none would be left for the hospital to use. Also some populations change so that they cannot be counted in any event, or they may be so large or inaccessible that counting them becomes impossible.

For practical reasons survey designs and methods may have to be used in order to study populations. In Britain, much of what is known about the nation's health, social conditions, standards of living, work, education, social attitudes and behaviour is based upon survey findings (see, for example, Thomas *et al.*, 1998, and Government Statistical Service, 1998).

One of the major objectives of any survey research is to achieve the highest possible degree of accuracy in the findings. Generally there are seen to be three main sources of inaccuracy, or error, in survey work. These are known as sampling error, non-response error and response error. Each of these concepts is discussed later in this chapter. The avoidance of errors is central to the design of surveys and by giving attention to the procedures employed they can be controlled.

Sample selection

The first problem for the researcher is how to select a sample which will represent the population under study. A system of selection is needed to ensure that the researcher, and factors extraneous to the research, have no influence whatsoever on the selection procedure. If there is a possibility that individuals with particular characteristics might stand a higher chance of being included in a sample than do others in the population, then the final sample could represent a population different from the one intended for study. Consequently, the research findings could be inappropriately applied to what is essentially a different study population.

For example, imagine you needed to assess the number of midwives with a positive or negative view towards proposed changes in salaries and conditions of service. In order to estimate the feeling of the profession in a particular hospital it is decided to sample midwives and ask them how they will vote on the proposed changes. The population here would be all midwives both qualified and in training at the hospital. A sample might be taken by a convenient procedure involving the researcher sitting in a hospital corridor and asking the views of all who came by. Unfortunately and unbeknown to the researcher this corridor leads to an area stocked with journals and daily newspapers which were publishing detailed comment on the issue. The outcome of this might be that a high proportion of midwives who answered the questions were aware of the full implications of the proposed agreement and would not support it. Had the sample been obtained by other means or in another part of the hospital then an entirely different picture could have emerged in the findings because a less-well-informed group of midwives would have been selected. As it was, the sample selected was biased and did not represent the whole population of midwives in the hospital.

How then can a sample that might represent a defined population be selected? In order to obtain such a sample a method is needed that will remove all biases in selection. The only way this can be achieved is by incorporating a system of randomness into the selection procedure. The term *random* does not mean haphazard or careless but refers to a precise method of selection where all individuals in a defined population stand an equal chance of being selected for inclusion in the study sample.

Simple random sample

There are many types of sample design which incorporate the principles of random selection. Here the methods of selecting a 'simple random sample' are outlined to introduce the basic principles of random sampling. An easily understood and full exposition of variations in the design of random samples is provided by Moser & Kalton (1985). The procedures involved in selecting a simple random sample are illustrated here with a practical example of sampling to estimate the mean age of 100 patients who attended an outpatient clinic. The procedures involved in this exercise are identical to those that would have to be followed in real sample selection.

Sampling frame

After having defined a study population the first stage of sample selection is to obtain a list of all individuals in that population. This list is known as the *sampling frame* and from it the sample is chosen. It is essential that the sampling frame gives a complete coverage of the population otherwise it will not be adequate for its purpose. Clearly if some members of the population are not included in the list they stand no chance of being selected and the resulting sample could be biased. Obtaining an adequate sampling frame often poses problems for research which involves human populations.

Once the sampling frame is obtained individuals are numbered consecutively starting at zero. For purposes of the practical exercise the population is represented by all the people included in Fig. 22.1. The members of this population have already been given consecutive numbers starting at 00 and finishing at 99. The two-digit number underneath each person represents his or her number in the sampling frame. The number above each person represents his or her age.

Sample selection

Imagine that a sample of 15 people is required; all that is needed is a list of 15 two-digit random numbers and the people on the list with corresponding numbers are taken for the sample. Random numbers can be obtained in several different ways but the example of the tombola drum method gives the clearest understanding of the nature of randomness. To generate random numbers using a tombola involves marking ten discs with a single digit from 0 to 9. The discs are placed in the drum which is spun and a single disc selected. The number is written down, the disc is put back in the drum and the process is repeated until sufficient numbers have been obtained to select the sample. This process ensures that all numbers have an equal chance of being selected which, itself, is the property of randomness. If a tombola drum was used to select a sample of 15 people from a population of 100 then the procedure would have to be repeated a total of 30 times. This would provide 15 two-digit numbers between 00 and '99', therefore covering every numbered individual in the population. Such a procedure could become rather tedious if a large sample was required so random numbers are published in sets of statistical tables (Lindley & Scott, 1984) or can be easily generated by a computer. Figure 22.2 is a table of random numbers which were generated by a computer.

For our sample, 15 two-digit numbers between 00 and 99 have to be found and they are chosen in the following way. First, select a point in any row and any column of Fig. 22.2. Imagine that the third column along and the fifth row down is chosen, that is number 8. A two-digit number is required, so two columns have to be used. The first number then is 87 and the person who has number 87 in the sampling frame (Fig. 22.1) is selected for the sample. The second number is then selected by going down the column, so the next person to be included in the

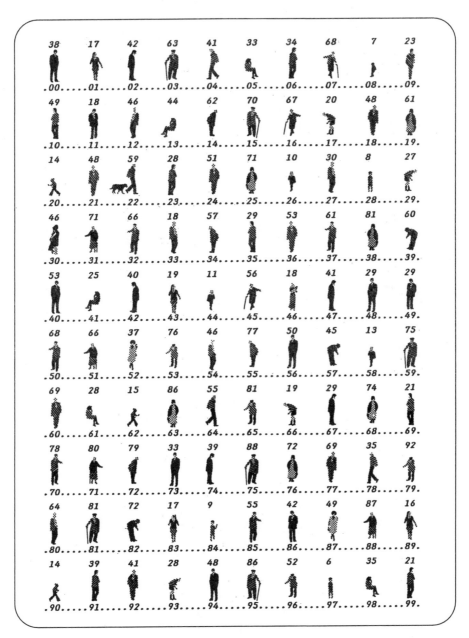

Fig. 22.1 The population: one hundred patients who attended an outpatient clinic.

sample is number 81. This process is repeated until a list of 15 random numbers have been obtained. If by chance the same number is encountered twice, then that person is not included in the sample twice. Rather, selection continues until a set of unique numbers (15 for this sample) have been obtained. The sample selected in this example is shown in Fig. 22.3.

28	98	16	42	02	52	11	94	58	65
07	48	17	11	90	06	44	16	83	92
44	96	27	13	38	71	70	45	61	13
96	18	84	58	25	95	37	10	12	77
75	**87**	41	62	61	84	62	35	84	02
69	**81**	00	90	65	10	96	03	27	94
40	**96**	08	06	39	39	51	43	13	59
35	**21**	62	59	92	62	57	03	02	74
44	**74**	29	57	32	57	52	12	39	41
82	**25**	38	03	30	96	74	70	86	33
59	**80**	06	78	09	29	10	43	09.	68
76	**34**	71	58	48	34	86	09	31	34
37	**04**	36	11	74	28	03	79	12	52
68	**89**	13	93	80	58	75	32	40	47
74	**45**	59	62	02	15	87	95	63	44
31	**20**	12	19	74	32	71	10	51	35
53	**51**	86	80	74	48	56	06	15	30
52	**28**	75	45	61	22	01	03	47	89
57	**41**	82	32	86	09	02	01	98	12
47	43	77	34	65	32	83	34	20	36

Note: The 15 highlighted numbers are those selected for the example given in the text.

Fig. 22.2   Random numbers.

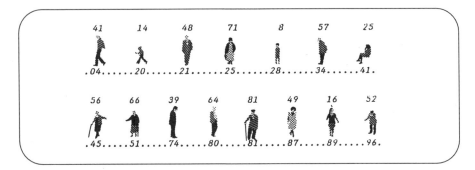

Fig. 22.3   The sample selected.

In some sample designs, a particular subject might be included in the sample more than once, and this is called sampling with replacement. In social surveys this is not generally done and is termed sampling without replacement.

Having completed this procedure a simple random sample consisting of 15 individuals has been selected. A sample has no particular property that could be tested to see if it is representative of our population. All that is known about it is that it was just as likely to be chosen as any other sample. Any 'test' of randomness can only be applied to the process by which the sample was selected.

Generalization

In order to introduce the idea of how survey findings can be generalized to a whole population – in other words, how population parameters can be estimated on the basis of sample statistics – a sample mean is used to illustrate the general principles. Estimation from other types of sample statistics (for example, proportions, variance and differences) are in principle similar to procedures applied to the mean and are considered by Armitage & Berry (1987).

Sampling error

The reason for selecting this sample was to calculate the mean sample age in order to estimate the mean age of the population. As already noted, the number above each person in Fig. 22.1 represents that person's age, in years, so the mean age of the sample can be calculated as 45.8 years. In real research the value of a population parameter is not known but in this case the true population mean can be calculated as 46.09 years. Notably these two numbers are not the same and if more samples were taken it is likely that they too would have mean values which were different from the true population mean. The difference between a sample statistic and the true population parameter is referred to as sampling error. This raises the question: 'If sample means can vary, then how can the true population mean be estimated with any confidence on the basis of one sample?'

The answer to this lies in the fact that although the mean values obtained are determined randomly, the mean values obtained begin to vary in an astonishingly predictable way if a large number of different samples are selected. If a very large number of samples were taken from the population and the mean age of each was plotted on graph paper, eventually a symmetrical bell shaped curve, approximating the profile of a 'normal' distribution, would be produced. (Readers not familiar with the normal distribution should consult Chapters 30 and 31.) The curve produced by this graph is known as the sampling distribution of the mean and is very important in establishing levels of confidence in survey findings. If an infinite number of samples were taken and the mean of all the sample means calculated, the result would be exactly equal to the true population mean. In terms of the sampling distribution curve this implies that the value at its centre equals the true population mean. Further, the larger the sample size used to make these calculations, the more compact this curve would become. These phenomena can only be guaranteed to occur when the samples are selected using random methods.

Levels of confidence

The actual calculations required to estimate the levels of confidence in the estimated population parameter are outwith the scope of this chapter. However, an understanding of the use of the normal distribution indicates that it is many times more likely that a sample is picked with a mean near to the centre of the sampling distribution than one with a mean at the tails of the curve. Areas enclosed by the standard normal distribution represent the probability of observing a value, in this case a sample mean, from a normally distributed variable such as the sampling distribution of the mean. Using this knowledge the chances of a sample mean falling different distances from the true population mean can be calculated. It is by using these tools for analysis that levels of confidence in survey finding are estimated. Readers who wish to follow up the subject of making population estimates and calculating confidence limits are referred to Chapter 31 of this book and to Armitage & Berry (1987).

In practice, obtaining truly random samples of human subjects is extremely difficult and often impossible. Even surveys of highly visible populations frequently depend upon convenience samples; for example, patient surveys generally recruit respondents sequentially when they are admitted to hospital (Mitchell, 1997). Faugier & Sargeant (1997) discuss some populations – e.g. prostitutes and drug users – that are hidden and pose particularly difficult sampling problems, and although researchers cannot expect to obtain sampling frames for these populations, each has been the subject of survey type research (e.g. Rhodes *et al.*, 1994). Unfortunately, if samples are not randomly selected then the statistical model upon which descriptive surveys are based ceases to apply. This is not to say that survey research becomes invalid because of this difficulty, rather it just becomes difficult to extrapolate the findings to wider populations. Often it is the insights attained through the analysis of associations between different variables affecting a sample which prove to be the most valuable part of survey findings.

Sample size

There are no simple answers to the question: How big a sample should be recruited for survey work? There are formulae in the literature (Armitage & Berry, 1987; Moser & Kalton, 1985) which can be applied to the problem but still they alone cannot provide definitive answers. These formulae take into account factors including the levels of confidence which need to be attained in the findings, the size of the population, and the variability of our measures when they are applied to the study population.

Accuracy in survey work is determined by careful design and execution of the research and large samples alone do not in any way guarantee the accuracy of findings. To illustrate this point, many research textbooks describe an American survey which aimed to predict the results of a presidential election and used a sample size of ten million people. Because of the ways in which the sample was selected, incorrect conclusions were drawn about the forthcoming election result.

In practice, sample size is to a large extent determined by the ways in which the data are to be analysed. If it is intended that the information should be tabulated, this means that respondents will have to be divided into different categories – for example, male and female; young, middle aged and old; those who are ill or not ill (see Fig. 22.4). Figure 22.4 illustrates the rapid reduction in the sizes of subgroups for analysis after dividing a sample of 100 people by only three variables (sex, age band and illness). In this example it would be impractical, because of the small numbers after the third division, to control for the influence of both age and sex when examining the effects of another factor on the health of the sample. In Fig. 22.4 the splitting into subgroups is made equally at each division. In research practice this equality rarely occurs and after three divisions it may be found that some subgroups contain no respondents at all.

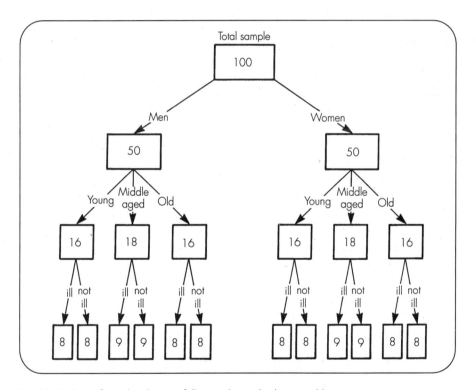

Fig. 22.4 Sizes of sample subgroups following division by three variables.

The process of dividing and subdividing can only be continued as long as there remain workable numbers of respondents in the subgroups and, even with a large initial sample, only a few divisions can leave such small numbers that conclusions could not be drawn from them. It is important, therefore, to clarify which sub-division of the sample will be the final one, and what would be the smallest desirable number of respondents to have within it for the purposes of analysis.

This procedure can, of course, lead an investigator to estimate that enormous samples are required but unavoidable constraints can thwart these intentions: the limitations of time and resources. The process of collecting data from respondents can be costly and time consuming so, inevitably, considerations arising from the organization and funding of research impinge upon the nature and size of research endeavours.

Sources of error

As already noted, there are three major causes of error which affect survey findings. The nature of sampling error has been described and the methods for dealing with this type of inaccuracy were outlined. The problems of non-response and response error are now considered.

Non-response error

An essential part of sampling is to determine precisely who is to be included in the study. This has to be followed by ensuring that information is obtained from all those included. If some of the sample either refuse to help with the survey or, for some reason, cannot be contacted then there is a risk of introducing error into the findings through non-response.

To illustrate the mechanics of this type of error, imagine that for the survey of the numbers of registered nurses who smoked a simple random sample was taken, but only one-half of the nurses agreed to help with the research. Their decisions to help or not might have been influenced by their own smoking behaviour. Imagine that those who did smoke felt threatened by the thought of having to answer questions on the subject while the non-smokers felt no inhibitions. As a result a high proportion of non-smokers and a low proportion of smokers would provide data for the research. The consequences for the survey findings would therefore be to underestimate the prevalence of smoking.

In dealing with respondents every effort must be made to encourage them to provide the information required. A careful choice of research topic, clear explanations as to the purpose and importance of the study, well-constructed questionnaires and interview schedules all contribute towards motivating respondents to co-operate.

When faced with a non-response problem the question which has to be addressed by the researcher is: Do those people who have responded differ from those who have not responded, in ways relevant to the aims of the research? Finding an answer to this question may not be easy but could be crucial for the validity of research findings.

Response error

The next source of inaccuracy is termed 'response error' and this takes two forms, random error and systematic error.

Random error

Random error broadly refers to making mistakes in measurement and/or in the recording of data. This type of error always occurs in any endeavour which involves measurement of any kind and there is a well-developed 'law of errors'. Because mistakes in this type of error behave in a random way, in the long run they even each other out and will not unduly affect the findings of research involving groups of respondents. This can be illustrated using the example of estimating the mean age of a sample. An interviewer might inaccurately record a respondent's age because of fatigue or a lapse of concentration but the recording made is just as likely to be above as below the respondent's true age. If it is truly random error, then an equal number of overestimates and underestimates will be made in the course of collecting data from the whole sample. When the mean age is calculated the numbers will balance each other out and a correct mean age will be produced. In other words, random error tends to control itself statistically.

Systematic error

Systematic error is rather different in its mode of operation and arises from problems in the way in which phenomena are measured. Using the example of age, imagine the phrasing of the question predisposed respondents to say that they were younger than they really were. The outcome of this would be to systematically underestimate the age of the whole sample. Because the researcher may be unaware of the bias in the question these errors would not be accounted for in the presentation of research findings. Even if the biased question was eventually recognized, it would be impossible to make corrections to the data obtained. Consequently systematic error has to be guarded against from the outset of the research. This will involve the careful testing of questions used in interviews or questionnaires and precise calibration of all measuring instruments being used for the research.

Conclusions

This chapter has attempted to acquaint the reader with the basic principles upon which survey research is based. The main sources of error in survey findings, how they operate and how they might be controlled have been discussed. This short consideration can only offer an intending researcher an introduction to survey design and sampling but it is hoped that it will provide an initial grounding for further study in the area. Survey research can be applied in many fields of enquiry and its principles will continue to provide an indispensable tool for planners, policy-makers and all those who, for whatever reason, need to describe and analyse the characteristics of populations.

References

Armitage, P. & Berry, G. (1987) *Statistical Methods In Medical Research*, 2nd edn. Oxford: Blackwell Scientific Publications.

Faugier, J. & Sargeant, M. (1997) Sampling hard to reach populations. *Journal of Advanced Nursing* **26**: 790–7.

Government Statistical Service (1998) *Social Trends*, No. 28. London: The Stationery Office.

Lindley, D.V. & Scott, W.F. (1984) *New Cambridge Elementary Statistical Tables*, Vol. 78. Cambridge University Press.

Mitchell, M. (1997) Patients' perceptions of pre-operative preparation for day surgery. *Journal of Advanced Nursing* **26**: 356–63.

Moser, C.A. & Kalton, G. (1985) *Survey Methods in Social Investigation*. London: Gower.

Rhodes, T., Donoghoe, M., Hunter, G. & Stimson, G.V. (1994) HIV prevalence no higher among female drug injectors also involved in prostitution. *AIDS Care* **6** (3): 269–76.

Thomas, M., Walker, A., Wilmot, A. & Bennett, N. (1998) *Living in Britain. Results from the 1996 GHS*. Office of National Statistics Social Survey Division. London: The Stationery Office.

Further reading

Marsh, C. (1982) *The Survey Method: The Contribution of Surveys to Sociological Explanation*, Contemporary Social Research Series No. 6. London: Allen & Unwin.

C: Data collection

The selection of a data-collection instrument offers considerable scope and choice. This section is not intended to present a comprehensive range of data-collection methods, but to introduce a small variety of techniques.

Each of the data-collection methods selected for inclusion has been well tested, and has been more or less widely used in health care research.

The material presented in relation to attitude measurement, interview, questionnaire, observation, the critical incident technique and physiological measurement provides a *basis* for understanding each of these methods and, for potential researchers, an overview of a number of data-collection methods for consideration and further study using the references in each chapter.

CHAPTER 23

Attitude measurement

Robert J. Edelmann

What are attitudes?

Attitudes are one way of describing differences between people; that is, with regard to their differing likes and dislikes. Attitudes are not, however, transient feelings or moods but consistent and enduring thoughts, beliefs and feelings that people have about particular attitude objects – that is, about issues, people or events (Aranson *et al.*, 1994). An attitude is thus a disposition to evaluate something in a particular way. This evaluative component of attitudes is generally studied in relation to the *beliefs* people hold about a particular issue and the *actions* they take towards it.

Attitudes thus consist of three aspects: an *emotional* or *evaluative* component; a *belief* or *cognitive* component; and an *action* or *behavioural* component. For example, a person might hold a belief that blood donors are altruistic (the belief/ cognitive component), feel very positively about the idea of donating blood for health care (the emotional/evaluative component), and may donate blood whenever they can (the action/behavioural component). The emphasis placed on these three components varies greatly in both attitude theory and research. Social psychologists for several decades have investigated the links between beliefs and evaluations on the one hand and evaluations and behaviours on the other.

Beliefs – the thoughts or cognitions that we hold – show a general correspondence to whether something is positively or negatively evaluated. It is perhaps not surprising that if someone holds positive attitudes towards, say, nursing staff they will also have predominantly favourable thoughts about them – perhaps that they are caring, understanding people. Conversely, if someone holds negative attitudes towards nursing staff they will have predominantly unfavourable thoughts – perhaps that they are distant and unapproachable.

The relationship between evaluations and behaviours is, however, less clear. For many years social scientists regarded attitudes as the causal element in relation to behaviour. People with positive attitudes towards a particular object or event were assumed to engage in positive behaviour towards it, while the converse applied for people with negative attitudes. However, a review in the

1960s of work investigating the link between attitudes and behaviour (Wicker, 1969) reported that there was little more than a modest link between attitudes and behaviour. Subsequent research, exploring the reasons for this poor relationship, suggested that attitudes did indeed relate to behaviour but only in certain circumstances (Fishbein & Ajzen, 1975). For example, attitudes do seem to be better able to predict behaviour if both are defined with an equivalent level of specificity or generality. Just as an attitude object can be defined very generally – for example, nursing staff, or, more specifically, nursing staff on ward X – behaviours too can be defined very generally – for example, all behaviours of nursing staff, or, more specifically, behaviours of those particular nursing staff on ward X.

It is also important to bear in mind, however, that attitudes are not the only factor predictive of behaviour. Indeed, factors such as expectations of significant others – that is, normative beliefs, in addition to issues such as perceived control over the behaviour in question – are often found to be better predictors of behaviour than attitudes themselves (Fishbein & Ajzen, 1975). One might, for example, be very favourably disposed towards the idea of donating blood but still not actually donate any. Factors such as general anxiety about the procedure involved, concern about the time commitment required, or lack of blood-donating behaviour from family or friends may prevent a favourable attitude being turned into direct action.

Thus, while people's beliefs or thoughts may relate quite closely to whether an attitude object is evaluated positively or negatively, such evaluations do not necessarily relate to subsequent behaviour. It is clearly important to bear this in mind when measuring attitudes. The cognitive, evaluative and behavioural components of attitude systems can each be assessed and may provide results which differ from each other. While behaviours can be readily observed and quantified – for example, voting habits, or private versus state health care utilization – behaviours can only be assumed to reflect the person's tendency to evaluate the attitude object positively or negatively. Assessment of beliefs provides a clearer link with evaluative judgements. However, it is only within the last two decades that researchers have attempted, systematically, to assess the cognitive component of attitudes (Petty & Cacioppo, 1981). The most frequently used method of assessing attitudes is by questionnaire aimed at examining the evaluative component of attitudes and it is this manner of assessment which forms the major focus of the present chapter.

Attitude scales

Several different questionnaire methods have been developed to measure the evaluative component of attitudes. These generally consist of a series of statements reflecting beliefs about the attitude object, to which the respondent indicates whether he agrees or disagrees. The belief statements selected are chosen to reflect certain criteria, which ensure that the statements do indeed assess favourable or unfavourable views towards an attitude object.

The four main scaling methods used to assess the evaluative component of attitudes are the Thurstone, the Likert, the Guttman and the semantic differential. Although the techniques differ they have basic assumptions in common. First, they assume that a person's attitude can be represented by some numerical score. Second, they assume that each item means the same to each respondent.

The Thurstone method

The first major method of attitude measurement was developed by Thurstone (1928). He assumed that it was possible to elicit statements about a particular issue which could then be ordered according to a dimension of favourableness/ unfavourableness towards that issue. He also felt that it was possible to order a series of statements so that the distance, in numerical terms, between any two statements was equal.

In order to provide a reasonable spread of views about a particular issue, a Thurstone scale is generally made up of about 20–40 statements which have been derived from a larger pool of statements. The first step in constructing a Thurstone scale involves collecting a large number of statements about the particular issue. These can be obtained from the relevant literature, from discussion with experts in the field or from direct questioning of people for whom the issue is of relevance. Any statements which are ambiguous, confusing, contain both positive and negative information or could be approved by people who hold negative attitudes are discarded.

As an example, let us consider a recent issue about which there has been some controversy: the suggested use of donated ovarian tissue (from mature women, from girls or women who have died or from aborted foetuses) in embryo research and assisted conception. In assessing people's attitudes towards this issue, a preliminary set of statements might include:

- The use of donated ovarian tissue in research and treatment is morally wrong in all circumstances.
- The use of donated ovarian tissue in research and treatment should only be permitted if the tissue is obtained from mature women.
- The use of donated ovarian tissue should be for treatment purposes only.
- The use of donated ovarian tissue in research and treatment is perfectly acceptable.

The next step is to ask a number of people to judge the extent to which each statement expresses a positive or negative attitude towards the particular issue, regardless of their own particular attitude. This is generally conducted in the form of a sorting task. Each statement is written on a card and the person making the judgements is asked to sort the cards into 11 piles placed along a continuum from positive to negative. The two ends and the middle pile are labelled. The middle pile is used for neutral opinions and the five piles on either side are used to represent varying degrees of positive or negative views towards the particular issue.

The ratings – that is, the number of the pile into which each statement is placed – from all the judges are then tabulated. From these data it is possible to calculate both the numerical scale position of each statement – that is, its average scale value – and the extent to which judges agreed on its placement – that is, its spread of ratings. Statements which have poor interjudge agreement are discarded. Finally, from the remaining statements, 20 to 40 are selected to constitute the attitude questionnaire. Statements should cover the full range of median scores assigned by the judges and every statement on the scale should be almost equidistant numerically from its neighbour. The questionnaire can then be given to any group of people who are asked to indicate agreement, disagreement or neutrality towards each statement. Given that each statement has a predetermined value as described above, each person's score – that is, the mean value on all the items with which they agree – can then be calculated.

The hallmark of a Thurstone scale is that the intervals between the statements are approximately equal, this being achieved by the method in which it is constructed. One obvious drawback, however, is that it is rather laborious and time consuming to construct. Indeed, one study suggested that it took a third as much time again to construct a Thurstone scale as it did a Likert scale (Barclay & Weaver, 1962), which no doubt explains why there are few references to the Thurstone method in recently published nursing research. Because measures made with the Thurstone and Likert techniques are highly correlated, many studies have relied upon some version of the more efficient Likert scaling procedure for attitude measurement.

The Likert method

The Likert scale (Likert, 1932) consists of a series of opinion statements about a particular issue, event or person. The person's attitude is the extent to which he agrees or disagrees with each statement, which is generally rated on a 5-point scale where 1 is strongly disagree, 2 is disagree, 3 is undecided, 4 is agree and 5 is strongly agree. A person's attitude score is the total of his ratings, with a higher score indicating a more favourable attitude. If strong disagreement with any item indicates a favourable attitude, scoring is reversed so that 5 always represents a positive view. Although the 1 to 5 format is widely used, a wide range of other formats have also been employed. For example, respondents have been asked to place a mark along a line labelled 'strongly agree' at one end and 'strongly disagree' at the other. In other instances they have been asked to circle a number between −10 and +10, or between some other numerical end-points, to indicate agreement or disagreement with various attitude statements. Whatever the format, the basic task remains the same, that is to indicate the extent to which the respondent accepts or rejects various statements relating to an attitude object.

The method of Likert scale construction is similar to that used for the Thurstone scale. Thus, an initial pool of statements is collected from relevant sources and edited accordingly. However, unlike the Thurstone scale there is no assumption that intervals on the rating scale are equal. Thus, the difference between 'agree' and 'strongly agree' may be much larger in the respondent's perception than the difference between 'agree' and 'undecided'. A Likert scale can thus indicate the relative ordering of different people's attitudes but does not indicate precisely how close or far apart these attitudes are. A further implication of a Likert scale is that all the items are highly correlated with each other and with the total scale score, as opposed to Thurstone's distinct and independent items.

Likert scales are widely used in research and there are numerous examples in the nursing literature. For example, Bowman *et al.* (1983) developed a 20-item Likert scale to collect information on nurses' attitudes towards the nursing process. That scale was adapted in a more recent study to assess nursing students' attitudes towards nursing models (McKenna, 1994). Ten of the items were negatively worded and ten positively. Each item was rated on a scale of 1 to 5 with 5 reflecting a positive attitude towards nursing models. Examples of questions are given in Fig. 23.1.

1. Nursing models improve care	SA	A	U	D	SD
2. Nursing models involve too much paperwork	SA	A	U	D	SD
3. Nursing models work well in practice	SA	A	U	D	SD
4. Nursing models are a waste of time	SA	A	U	D	SD
5. Nursing models can be used in any areas	SA	A	U	D	SD
6. There is not enough time to use nursing models	SA	A	U	D	SD

(SA – strongly agree; A – agree; U – undecided; D – disagree; SD – strongly disagree.)

Fig. 23.1   Likert scale items assessing attitudes towards nursing models.

Although widely used, Likert scales are not without their difficulties. One particular problem is that while a particular set of responses will always add up to the same score, the same total may arise from many different combinations of responses. For example, a score of 30 could be obtained from 15 items scoring 2, or 10 items scoring 1 together with 5 items scoring 4. Such different combinations might actually be quite rare but it would clearly be preferable if the same total score always meant the same thing.

The Guttman method

A further, though less widely used, method of assessing attitudes involves the Guttman method (1944, 1950), which was derived from early attempts to measure attitudes reported by Bogardus (1928). Bogardus was concerned with developing a social-distance measure which was really a measure of attitude towards ethnic groups. People were asked to indicate, with regard to a specific group, which of seven relationships ranging from intimate (for example, 'marriage') to most distant (for example, 'exclude members of the group from the country') they would be willing to accept. Guttman extended this method of scaling by assuming that an attitude towards any object, situation or event can be assessed by ordering a set of statements along a continuum of 'difficulty of acceptance'. Thus, statements range from those that are easy for most people to accept to those which few people would endorse. Acceptance of one item implies that people would also accept those which are less difficult to accept. An example of such a scale is given in Fig. 23.2.

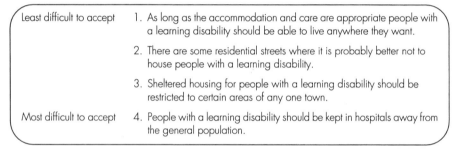

Fig. 23.2 Guttman scale items assessing attitude towards community care for people with a learning disability.

In order to construct a scale which represents a single dimension, subjects are presented with an initial set of statements and the extent to which they respond with specified answer patterns is recorded. These patterns, referred to as scale types, follow a certain step-like order. The subject may accept: none of the statements in the set (score 0), the first statement only (score 1), the first and second statements only (score 2), the first, second and third statements only (score 3) and so on. If the subject gives a non-scale response – for example, accepts the third statement but not the first and second – it is assumed that he has made a response error. By analysing the number of response errors it is possible to determine the extent to which the initial set of statements represents a unidimensional scale. Eliminating poor statements and retesting enables a scalable set of statements to be developed.

One problem with such a method is that it is almost impossible to develop a perfect unidimensional scale. People may actually be responding to their own perceived dimension or to multiple dimensions rather than to the one assumed to underlie the scale. This may well be because both attitudes and behaviour are rather too complex to be encompassed by a unidimensional scale.

The semantic-differential method

Each of the above approaches measures attitudes by examining the extent to which people agree or disagree with various opinion statements. In contrast, Osgood and his colleagues (Osgood *et al.*, 1957) focused on the meaning people give to a word or concept. A semantic-differential instrument consists of a particular object, situation or event which people then rate on a series of bipolar adjectives, such as good–bad, fast–slow, active–passive and so on.

Extensive research by Osgood and colleagues suggests that most adjectives can be grouped into three categories. The largest number of adjectives, such as good–bad and happy–sad, reflect evaluation. A second group of interrelated dimensions, including strong–weak and easy–hard, reflect perceived strength or potency. The third group, including dimensions such as fast–slow and young–old, is termed activity. The potency and activity dimensions do not relate very closely to attitude research. The evaluative dimension is the one used by most other kinds of attitude scale and, as noted earlier, is the dimension that most definitions of attitude stress as distinguishing between an attitude and a simple belief. The term *semantic differential* refers to the way of measuring several different semantic dimensions, or different kinds of meaning reflected by the different adjective descriptors.

An example of this method used in nursing research is a study which evaluated nurses' attitudes towards patients with AIDS (Cole & Slocumb, 1993; and see Fig. 23.3).

The ten bipolar adjectives expressing evaluative meaning were selected from previous research and subsequent review by nursing experts. Six of the bipolar adjectives were randomly reversed in order to provide a positive–negative/negative–positive balance. To examine whether nurses' attitudes differed according to the manner of contracting AIDS the semantic-differential scale was headed with one of four modes of a male acquiring the virus – that is, through (a) sexual activity with males; (b) sexual activity with females; (c) sharing needles; and (d) a blood transfusion.

As research has established which adjectives express evaluative meaning, semantic-differential attitude scales are easy to construct. However, the task of completing a semantic-differential scale may be seen as rather unusual – we do not normally rate objects, situations or events on scales such as strong–weak or hard–soft.

A male who acquired AIDS through sexual activity with males		
1.	good _____:_____:_____:_____:_____:_____:_____	bad
2.	immoral _____:_____:_____:_____:_____:_____:_____	moral
3.	dangerous _____:_____:_____:_____:_____:_____:_____	safe
4.	clean _____:_____:_____:_____:_____:_____:_____	dirty
5.	unjustified _____:_____:_____:_____:_____:_____:_____	justified
6.	victim _____:_____:_____:_____:_____:_____:_____	perpetrator
7.	trustworthy _____:_____:_____:_____:_____:_____:_____	dishonest
8.	unfair _____:_____:_____:_____:_____:_____:_____	fair
9.	positive _____:_____:_____:_____:_____:_____:_____	negative
10.	guilty _____:_____:_____:_____:_____:_____:_____	innocent

Fig. 23.3   Semantic-differential instrument for one concept (from Cole & Slocumb, 1993).

Assessing attitudes and normative beliefs

In thinking about attitude measurement it is clearly important to link theory with assessment. In research, the need for a clear rationale for conducting the measurement, other than that it is of an intrinsically interesting topic, is important. Unfortunately much attitude research fails to address this issue. One such method of not just measuring but also analysing attitudes, which is referred to as the expectancy-value approach, was proposed by Fishbein & Ajzen (1975). Respondents are asked to rate their beliefs about each item (that is, the 'Value' component) and then the extent to which they believe each dimension applies to the issue being considered (that is, the 'Expectancy' component). Each expectancy is combined with its value to give an overall E–V score. This method can be used to analyse the assumption of the theory of reasoned action (Fishbein & Ajzen, 1975) that overt behaviour in a particular situation is related to the individual's intention to carry out the behaviour in question. As noted earlier, the probability that we will engage in a behaviour is related not only to our beliefs but also to other variables such as our expectations of significant others, that is, normative beliefs, and our perceived control over the behaviour in question.

This theory and approach was used in a study by Nash *et al.* (1993) to assess nurses' attitudes towards and intention to assess patients' pain. Different pairs of questions were used to assess attitudes, normative beliefs, behavioural intention and perceived control. Attitude was measured by subjects' responses to items concerning six identifiable beliefs and corresponding evaluations of those beliefs. Normative beliefs were similarly assessed by examining three sets of beliefs about others and motivation to comply with these expectations of others. Behavioural intention was assessed by two questions concerning the likelihood of conducting pain assessments. Perceived control was evaluated by two questions concerning degree of control over and ease in conducting pain assessment. Each item was rated on a 7-point scale from +3 (indicating whether the item was likely, or desirable, or involved complete control, or was easy) to –3 (indicating whether the item was unlikely, or undesirable, or involved very little control, or was difficult). Examples are shown in Fig. 23.4.

1. Attitude
   (a) Behavioural belief:
       A comprehensive pain assessment will permit a more accurate picture of the patient's situation
       likely _____ unlikely
   (b) Evaluation:
       An accurate picture of the patient's situation is:
       desirable _____ undesirable

2. Subjective norm
   (a) Normative belief:
       Other nurses think that I should conduct comprehensive pain assessments
       likely _____ unlikely
   (b) Motivation to comply:
       I do what other nurses think I should do for patients
       likely _____ unlikely

Fig. 23.4   Examples of questionnaire items assessing attitudes and normative beliefs.

The main advantages of this approach are that it is clearly linked to theoretical assumptions and that it provides the possibility for analysing assumptions behind an overall score.

Other methods

As noted earlier, attitudes consist of a behavioural, evaluative and cognitive component, each of which can be measured. Discussion on this point has focused on the evaluative component. There are numerous occasions when actual behaviour can be assessed as an attitudinal indicator – for example, refusing to sign a petition or to go along with a group decision. In recent years psychologists have also grown more interested in assessing the cognitive component of attitudes. One such technique is *thought listing* (Petty & Cacioppo, 1981). After hearing or reading a message subjects are asked to write down in a specified time (say three minutes) all their thoughts which are relevant to the issue and message in question. Subsequently the thoughts are rated and categorized, for example, according to whether they agree or disagree with the message or issue. From such information it is possible to learn about the beliefs and knowledge underlying attitudes. Similar information can be obtained from content analysis of essays or group discussion.

Research has also investigated whether specific bodily reactions reflect attitudes. Cacioppo & Petty (1987) found small but measurable changes in the activity of facial muscles around the mouth as people listen to and think about persuasive messages. One pattern emerges when the message produces a positive, agreeing response while another pattern occurs with a counter argument.

Given the variety of methods available for assessing the different components of attitudes a legitimate question to ask is whether one measure is more appropriate than another.

Determining the measure to use

Given that different researchers focus on differing aspects of attitudes it seems quite appropriate that different measurement methods should be used. The emphasis in some studies might be on the belief or cognitive component of attitudes while in others it might be the evaluative component. There are other occasions when more than one domain might be assessed – for example, evaluative and behavioural. However, as noted earlier, it is important to bear in mind that there may be a less than perfect relationship between the scores obtained in this way. The measure should suit the aims of the study. If, for example, the aim is ultimately to change behaviour then clearly a baseline assessment of behaviour is required. If it is simply to gauge how people feel about a particular issue, then one of the attitudinal scales discussed could be used.

The question of which scale to use has been partly addressed in previous sections. The Thurstone method is extremely time consuming and the Likert method may be a more appropriate alternative. The Guttman method is relatively straightforward, although it can be difficult to construct a unidimensional scale. The semantic-differential method may seem rather unusual to respondents but allows for the assessment of meaning rather than just opinion. As the results of using different scaling methods to assess attitudes are remarkably similar, the decision about which scale to use is likely to be based on ease of construction of the scale and ease of administering it to respondents.

However, it is important to bear in mind that a major problem with any self-report measure of attitudes is that people may wish to conceal rather than reveal their true attitudes. This may be particularly likely if their views are unpopular or extreme. It is well known that many people wish to make a desirable impression and, rather than give their real views, may respond by giving views they believe the respondent wishes to know. As a result of this problem some researchers have used a technique referred to as the bogus pipeline (Jones & Sigall, 1971). The basic paradigm involves attaching respondents to a machine which they are told measures tiny electrical changes in muscular movements and can hence assess their true opinions. Respondents are then asked attitude questions to which the experimenter knows their views (respondents having been pretested some weeks earlier) and can then 'rig' the machine so that it seems to respond to these attitudes very accurately. Respondents are then asked to express their views on a new set of issues in the belief that erroneous responding will be indicated by the machine. There is some evidence that this technique yields more accurate measures of attitudes (Gaes *et al.*, 1978), although not all findings have been positive (Cherry *et al.*, 1976). In addition, the need for equipment, pre-assessment measures for respondents and the fact that only one person can be assessed at a time, clearly imposes serious practical constraints on the use of such a procedure.

In conclusion, therefore, no method of attitude assessment is completely problem free. In thinking about which scale or method of attitude assessment to use, the most important consideration is that the measure should suit the aims of the study.

References

Aranson, E., Wilson, T.D. & Akert, R.M. (1994) *Social Psychology: The Heart and the Mind*. New York: Harper Collins.

Barclay, J.E. & Weaver, H.B. (1962) Comparative reliabilities and the ease of construction of Thurstone and Likert attitude scales. *Journal of Social Psychology* 58: 109–20.

Bogardus, E.S. (1928) *Immigration and Race Attitudes*. Boston: D.C. Heath.

Bowman, G.S., Thompson, D.R. & Sutton, T.W. (1983) Nurses' attitudes towards the nursing process. *Journal of Advanced Nursing* 8: 125–9.

Cacioppo, J.T. & Petty, R.E. (1987) Stalking rudimentary processes of social influence: a psychophysiological approach. In M.P. Zanna, J.M. Olson & C.P. Herman (eds) *Social Influence: The Ontario Symposium* (Vol 5). Hillsdale, NJ: Erlbaum.

Cherry, F., Byrne, D. & Mitchell, H.E. (1976) Clogs in the bogus pipeline: Demand characteristics and social desirability. *Journal of Research in Personality* 10: 69–75.

Cole, F.L. & Slocumb, E.M. (1993) Nurses' attitudes toward patients with AIDS. *Journal of Advanced Nursing* 18: 1112–17.

Fishbein, M. & Ajzen, I. (1975). *Belief, Attitude, Intention and Behavior: An Introduction to Theory and Research*. Reading, Mass.: Addison-Wesley.

Gaes, G.G., Kalle, R.J. & Tedeschi, J.T. (1978) Impression management in the forced compliance situation: two studies using the bogus pipeline. *Journal of Experimental Social Psychology* 14: 493–510.

Guttman, L. (1944) A basis for scaling quantitative data. *American Sociological Review* 9: 139–50.

Guttman, L. (1950) The third component of scaleable attitudes. *International Journal of Opinion and Attitude Research* 4: 285–7.

Jones, E.E. & Sigall, H. (1971) The bogus pipeline: a new paradigm for measuring affect and attitude. *Psychological Bulletin* 76: 349–64.

Likert, R. (1932) A technique for the measurement of attitudes. *Archives of Psychology* 22: 1–55.

McKenna, H.P. (1994) The attitudes of traditional and undergraduate nursing students towards nursing models: a comparative study. *Journal of Advanced Nursing* **19**: 527–36.

Nash, R., Edwards, H. & Nebauer, M. (1993). Effect of attitudes, subjective norms and perceived control on nurses' intention to assess patients' pain. *Journal of Advanced Nursing* **18**: 941–7.

Osgood, C.E., Suci, G.J. & Tannenbaum, P.H. (1957). *The Measurement of Meaning.* Urbana, Illinois: University of Illinois Press.

Petty, R.E. & Cacioppo, J.T. (1981). *Attitudes and Persuasion: Classic and Contemporary Approaches.* Dubuque, IA: Wm C. Brown.

Thurstone, L.L. (1928). Attitudes can be measured. *American Journal of Sociology* **33**: 529–54.

Wicker, A.W. (1969). Attitudes versus actions: the relationship of verbal and overt behavioral responses to attitude objects. *Journal of Social Issues* **25**: 41–78.

CHAPTER 24

Interview

David Pontin

Most people at one time or another will have taken part in an interview, either as an interviewee (the person being interviewed) or as an interviewer (the person doing the interviewing). Consequently, there is a 'common sense' idea of what occurs at an interview and what it means to be involved in an interview. For most nurses, their experience of interviews – being interviewed and interviewing – is likely to be linked to two main areas: either securing a new job or recruiting staff to their workplace; or the process of assessing clients/patients in their everyday work. As with some of the other research methods outlined in this book (for example, see Chapter 26), there is a difference between such 'everyday' interviewing and interviewing for research purposes.

The difference between everyday interviewing and research interviewing centres on the purpose of the interview and the anticipated outcome. Obviously with job interviewing one person hopes to be successful and to be offered a job, while the other wants to make sure that the right person is selected in terms of her ability to meet the job specification. These factors determine the setting of the interview, the questions that are asked as well as the responses that are given. Similarly, in clinical interviewing the roles of the people concerned are clear – one person wishes, or needs, to receive health care services and the other person is able to provide them to a lesser or greater extent. The provider is aiming to clarify which services are required, those that are necessary, and when they need to be delivered. The receiver of services gives information with the intention of gaining some sort of intervention – although the precise nature of such interventions may not be known at that time.

Interviewing people as part of a research project is likely to be different from the examples given above in terms of where the interview takes place, the reasons people have for participating, the roles of the people involved, how the interview is conducted and the way in which the outcome of the interview is recorded. It could be said that the only similarity between everyday interviewing and research interviewing is that two people communicate with each other directly, at a given time, with a shared understanding that one of them will ask questions of the other and the other may choose to answer!

This chapter is concerned with interviewing as a method of collecting or generating research data about the phenomena which are of interest to nurses, midwives and health visitors. It will also highlight some of the differences that exist when interviewing is used in qualitative and quantitative enquiry.

Characteristics of interview data

Interviews may be included in a wide variety of research designs (see Fig. 24.1) and there are differences between the two main traditions of research in the way interviews are conducted, the precise form of the data generated and what may be said about the phenomena being studied. However, despite these differences there are three main types of data that are characteristically generated from interviews: people's experiences and accounts of events; their opinions, attitudes and perceptions about phenomena; and biographical and demographic details.

Quantitative designs (Cross-sectional and longitudinal)	Qualitative designs (Cross-sectional and longitudinal)
Experiment (Meininger *et al.*, 1998) Quasi-experiment (Rowe & King, 1998) Survey (Kyngas *et al.*, 1998) Case study (Higgins, 1998)	Ethnography (Gates & Lackey, 1998) Phenomenology (Beck, 1998) Case study (Mackenzie, 1997) Ethnomethodology (Mason, 1997) Grounded theory (Williams, 1998)

Fig. 24.1 Different research designs and the use of interviews.

People's experiences and accounts of events

The accounts and experiences which are found in nursing, midwifery and health visiting research tend to be those of clients/patients or of practitioners. Mitchell & Koch (1997) provide a useful account of how they gained the perspective of 32 elderly frail residents and their relatives when conducting qualitative evaluation research in an Australian nursing home. They describe the process they adopted to ensure that the 'voice' of key stakeholder groups were incorporated in the research design by means of in-depth interviewing.

While Mitchell & Koch's research refers to a specific situation and set of circumstances, Smith-Battle & Wynn (1998) give an example of how qualitative interviews may be used in longitudinal work to examine people's experiences over time. They examined key moments and patterns in 13 young mothers' narratives about themselves and their visions for the future. The aim of the study was to generate data that would inform the development of programmes of care and interventions so that they might be better fitted to the realities of the lives and the possibilities the women face as young parents. These young mothers had been interviewed four years previously by Smith-Battle & Wynn, and in this subsequent study they gathered from the women life-history accounts of the inter-vening period, stories of the women's caregiving routines for their children and recent examples of how they coped as parents.

While Smith-Battle & Wynn (1998) interviewed young mothers in order to gain access to their experiences and so shape and change professional practice, Bush & Barr (1997) interviewed 15 critical care nurses about their experiences of caring for patients in the Southwest of the USA. Their aim was to draw out and make explicit the fundamental structure of caring as experienced by critical care nurses. They did this by using a phenomenological research design which included in-depth interviewing and close analysis of the data that were produced. These examples illustrate the breadth of topics that may be investigated as a consequence of using interviews to research people's experiences and accounts of events.

People's opinions, attitudes and perceptions about phenomena

Interviews are a particularly useful way of finding out about people's perceptions or opinions on specific matters. In their study of the role of nurses in health promotion, Haddock & Burrows (1997) evaluated a smoking cessation pro-gramme in surgical pre-admission clinics. They used a quasi-experimental design to randomly allocate 60 patients who smoked to either a control or a treatment group. The control group received routine information, whereas the treatment group were given educational interventions and self-assessment exercises when they attended clinic. Haddock & Burrows used structured interviews as part of the data collection and report that 80% of the treatment group stopped or reduced their smoking prior to admission compared with 50% of the control group. In the interviews, patients perceived the approach of the nurse and the information leaflet prepared for the study as being particularly helping towards changing their behaviour.

Biley & Smith (1998) also focus on respondents' perceptions of an issue, although in this case it is graduate nurses' evaluation of the effectiveness of a problem-based learning programme in preparing them for the realities of pro-fessional practice. Qualitative interviewing techniques were used to interview 12 graduates of the programme so that the categories that were characteristic of their experience could be identified. The categories related to their transition from student to staff nurse ('all of a sudden'), the characteristics which they felt made them different from nurses who followed other programmes ('not an unthinking assistant') and the personal responsibility they felt for their learning and actions ('the buck stops here'). In both of these examples, interviews have been used to provide data on the interviewees' opinions and perceptions of the issues being investigated – nurses' role in health promotion programmes and the preparation of nurses using a problem-based curriculum – but the designs of the two projects have been quite different.

Biographical and demographic details

An example of the collection and use of biographical and demographic details may be seen in the work of Kimble & King (1998). As well as investigating patients' perceptions of the benefits and side effects of percutaneous transluminal coronary angioplasty (PTCA) in the early post-discharge period, they also look for any association between demographic and clinical variables and patient perception. People's sex, age and a history of PTCA were not linked to any benefits (reduced chest pain) or to any side effects (groin discomfort) that were reported. Having reviewed the types of data that interviews may produce, and identified that the interview method may be used in both qualitative and quantitative research designs, it is appropriate to look at the way interview data are produced.

Generating and capturing interview data

At this point, the difference between using interview techniques in qualitative and quantitative research becomes most noticeable. While the types of data may be the same (experiences, opinions/perceptions and biographical/demographic details) the way that these types of data are produced are quite different in qualitative and quantitative research due to the way that knowledge production about the world is conceived (the epistemological traditions of each approach; see also Chapters 2, 12 and 14).

Structured and semi-structured interviews

For those researchers using a quantitative research design, the emphasis when using interviews is on maintaining objectivity, controlling for bias and measuring the opinions/perceptions of the interviewees (Schumacher & Gortner, 1992). The interview process is characteristically ordered and structured in advance so that the same sort of information may be obtained from each person who is interviewed in the same way without it being contaminated by the interviewer. The interview is viewed as a mechanism or a conduit for the untrammelled transfer of facts from interviewee to interviewer (Brink & Wood, 1994). In order to do this, interview schedules are developed which tell the interviewer exactly what words to say when beginning the interview, when asking questions, when probing for specific replies and when closing the interview. Similarly, the responses that interviewees make to the questions are recorded in an orderly and structured manner, in much the same way that a person fills in a questionnaire (see Chapter 25). In fact it could be said that by using structured interviews, researchers are administering a questionnaire rather than letting respondents complete it themselves (Barriball & While, 1994; Nay-Brock, 1984). The use of schedules in this way is an attempt to produce a standardized process for conducting interviews and, consequently, standardized data (Poole & Jones, 1996). However, there are a number of issues that underlie the use of structured interviews and need to be made explicit.

Maintaining reliability and validity when using structured interviews

The main issues of reliability and validity when using structured interviews relate to language and its effect on the motivation of people to answer the questions appropriately. If the language that is used by interviewers is over-complicated or, conversely, too simplistic it will not encourage interviewees to give full and appropriate answers to the questions put to them (Brink & Wood, 1994; Barriball & While, 1994). Thought also has to be given by interviewers to the frame of reference that people use when interpreting the words that are spoken to them. If interviewees are using a different frame of reference to the interviewer (for example, if a person is under the impression that his answers will affect his access to health care services or the quality of the services) then either the interviewees will not be able to understand the question, or the answer they give to the question will be inappropriate and not representative of their usual opinion (Robson, 1993).

The point here is that each question has to mean the same thing to each person to whom it is put if there is to be standardization of data. Therefore, the wording of the questions and the order in which the questions are asked has to allow the best access possible to the variables that are being investigated (see Chapters 2, 14, 30 and 31). This may mean interviewers using different forms of questions – open, closed, two-way (either/or) or multiple choice – to obtain the most appropriate data. Also the effectiveness of the questions in gaining appropriate responses from interviewees has to be tested, as well as the presentation order (see Chapter 3). Therefore, before interview schedules are used in research they have to be piloted so that the reliability and validity may be gauged. This is another similarity between interviews and questionnaires (see Chapter 25; see also Burns & Grove, 1995; Brink & Wood, 1994; Nay-Brock, 1984).

Unstructured, informal or depth interviews

When looking at interviewing within the qualitative tradition of enquiry compared with the quantitative tradition, a different state of affairs is found. Interviewing here is characterized by letting interviewees say in their own words what is relevant and pertinent to them about the topic in focus. The aim of qualitative research is to examine social life by gaining an understanding of the meaning people attach to their experiences and behaviour (Hammersley & Atkinson, 1995; Silverman, 1993; Stanley & Wise, 1993; Tesch, 1990). For nurses, midwives and health visitors using qualitative interviewing, the particular focus of enquiry is on people's experiences of health, illness, disability and health care provision (see Chapters 12 and 13; see also Silverman, 1992; Morse, 1991; Gerhardt, 1990).

By emphasizing the importance of people's lived experience, researchers using qualitative interviewing are celebrating the subjective quality of the data that are generated (Williams, 1998). After all, if you want to understand how it feels to be in hospital and to have to work out different ways of managing your time from those to which you are accustomed, the best thing to do (as Holloway *et al.*, 1998 did) is to ask people about their experiences. By interviewing different people with different experiences categories and themes may be built up which may be used to develop theories about people's experiences of health and illness, and from which analytical generalizations may be made (Rolfe, 1998; Strauss & Corbin, 1990).

Interviewing, then, is not seen as a mechanism but as a dynamic interaction between two people which takes place in a particular set of circumstances for a particular purpose. Although the interaction does not have a rigid, predetermined structure, this is not to say that there is no logic or rationale to the proceedings. Interviewers have a repertoire of strategies and tactics at their disposal which they may use in conversation to gain access to the meanings people attach to their experiences (Morse, 1991). It is fair to say that in most qualitative research carried out by practitioners the general focus of the interview is decided in advance and interviewees give their consent in light of this. However, interviewers using a qualitative approach will be open to unforeseen avenues of enquiry opening up during the encounter with the interviewee. They may follow this new development and ask further questions – testing out what other interviewees have said about things to see if this corresponds with the experience of the person at hand. By doing this they are ensuring that the experiences that interviewees talk about are meaningful to the interviewees and are not those of the interviewer (Hammersley & Atkinson, 1995).

To make sure that all of the data generated from the interview are captured, most interviewers now use audio recordings. This allows interviewers to turn transient data into permanent data that may be analysed carefully over a longer period of time away from the interview site. The recordings include what was said (as well as what was not said), and the way the interviewee spoke about the topic being investigated (i.e. pauses and tone of speech). These data are usually supplemented by recorded observations made by interviewers after the interview. These usually include what they noticed about interviewees during the proceedings and any initial analytical points they wish to make while things are still fresh in their minds. In order to fully comprehend the meaning of what is said during the interview it is important not to lose sight of these circumstances – and this is what is meant by 'placing the data in context' (Silverman, 1993; Tesch, 1990).

The issues about maintaining rigour in unstructured intervie[...] those discussed in the use of observational methods in Chap[...]. problem for readers of research accounts that use unstructured interviews is: How do they know that people have said the things the interviewers claim? (Sandelowski, 1986). Rather than including the complete set of whole interview texts (which probably wouldn't be very helpful to the reader), researchers using qualitative interview techniques include quotes from the transcripts of the audio tapes to illustrate the points they are making (Hammersley & Atkinson, 1995; Tesch, 1990). The main reason for doing this is to allow the 'voice' of the interviewees to come through the text and speak to the reader. A text which allows the reader to 'hear' the interviewee's voice and uses full, illustrative quotes is said to be a 'thick' text. A text which only relies on the researchers' interpretations and does not include the 'voice' of the interviewee is said to be 'thin'. Obviously there are degrees of 'thickness' and 'thinness' and the reader of the text may judge the quality of the work in light of this (Hammersley & Atkinson, 1995; Williams, 1990). The other main device for maintaining rigour is for researchers to produce 'reflexive' accounts of their work (see Chapter 26).

Common issues in maintaining reliability, validity and rigour in interviewing

As well as the specific issues for ensuring the reliability and validity and rigour of the interview work which are discussed above, both qualitative and quantitative interviewing face two common issues: the training of interviewers to meet the requirements of each tradition, and the immediate environment in which interviewing takes place.

Training

For quantitative interviewing the main reason for training interviewers is to reduce bias and to ensure that the interview schedule is adhered to. Where more than one interviewer is used then inter-rater reliability has to be maintained (see Chapter 3) to ensure that the quality of data does not vary between one interview and another (Mullhall, 1998).

In qualitative interviewing, the emphasis in training is to encourage interviewers to let interviewees tell their stories and to avoid predetermining the course of the interview. Interviewers have to be able to listen actively, analyse and probe issues that they may not have anticipated and still allow the interviewees to recount their experiences. This means that the interviewers must possess a repertoire of tactics and techniques to ensure that full and representative data are collected during the interview (Hammersley & Atkinson, 1995; Spradley, 1979).

Environment

In both traditions of interviewing, there are some logistical considerations that have to be attended to. For interviewees to be able to answer questions appropriately, they have to be in a place which allows them to comprehend the questions. This means that the place should be free of distractions such as noise (televisions, radio, other people talking), visual stimuli (events outside the place of interview, work demands, people passing) and interruptions (children, pets or family members, other health care staff providing care, telephones and pagers). Consideration also has to be given to the gender relationships between interviewer and interviewee (Eichler, 1988; Warren, 1988).

As equally important, interviewees have to be in a place where they feel safe enough to provide answers to what may be difficult, awkward or compromising questions without fear of being overheard. Traditionally, most interviewing has taken place 'face-to-face'; however, there is a growing trend to use telephone interviewing in an effort to reduce the amount of travelling involved in interviewing (Armitage & Kavanagh, 1998; Wilson & Roe, 1998). When interviewing patients it is tempting to believe that the 'best' place is in people's own homes. However, interviewers will have less control over the 'home' environment and there is no guarantee that the interviewee will be able to maintain a 'safe' place free from intrusion, interruption and being overheard (Pontin & Webb, 1995, 1996; Webb & Pontin, 1996).

Conclusions

This chapter has examined some of the issues surrounding the use of interviews in research. It has identified the sorts of design in which interviews may be used, as well as the three common types of data that are produced – people's experiences and accounts of events; opinions, attitudes and perceptions; and biographical and demographic details. The different ways in which quantitative and qualitative interviews are used have been highlighted, as well the issues in maintaining the reliability, validity and rigour of the data that have been generated.

Disadvantages in using interviews

From this discussion of the characteristics of generating interview data in quantitative and qualitative research it is possible to identify a number of strengths and limitations. As with any method used in research there are shortcomings and limitations. The main issue for researchers is that they are aware of the disadvantages and design research accordingly. With interviews, given the one-to-one contact involved, it is of no surprise that they are time consuming. This does not just refer to the actual interview itself but also to the travelling which may be involved by interviewers and/or interviewees. For quantitative interviews, the disadvantage of having structured interviews is that valuable information may not be captured for analysis because it does not correspond with the interview schedules that structure the interaction. This raises the issue of how researchers know what to collect in advance of collecting it.

For qualitative research, the disadvantage of allowing interviewees to tell their stories and not wishing to restrict them too rigidly in any one direction, is that they may not tell you anything that is of relevance to your agreed interview topic. Finally, for both traditions, researchers are only collecting data on people's accounts of their experiences of events rather than the events themselves. Similarly, data about the opinions and attitudes and perceptions people have about phenomena only allow researchers to discuss people's perceptions, etc., rather than the phenomena.

Advantages in using interviews

In both forms of interviewing it is possible for interviewers to ask unambiguous questions. With quantitative research this is made possible by testing interview schedules for content validity and piloting schedules in advance of their general use in research (Armitage & Kavanagh, 1998). In qualitative research, interviewers may pitch questions which are appropriate to the setting, the topic in hand, the previous statements made by interviewees and the rapport between them. Both forms of interviewing are able to gain immediate responses from interviewees which allows further questioning or probing on a particular aspect of their replies. It is these particular aspects of the technique that make interviewing so useful.

References

Armitage, S.K. & Kavanagh, K.M. (1998) Consumer oriented outcomes in discharge planning: a pilot study. *Journal of Clinical Nursing* 7 (1): 67–74.

Barriball, K.L. & While, A. (1994) Collecting data using a semi-structured interview: a discussion paper. *Journal of Advanced Nursing* 19: 328–35.

Beck, C. (1998) Postpartum onset of panic disorder. *Image: Journal of Nursing Scholarship* 30(2): 131–5.

Biley, F.C. & Smith, K.L. (1998) 'The buck stops here': accepting responsibility for learning and actions. *Journal of Advanced Nursing* 27 (5): 1021–9.

Brink, P. & Wood, M.J. (1994) *Basic Steps in Planning Nursing Research*, 4th edn. Boston, MA: Jones & Bartlett.

Burns, N. & Grove, S. (1995) *Understanding Nursing Research*. London: W.B. Saunders.

Bush, H.A. & Barr, W.J. (1997) Critical care nurses' lived experiences of caring. *Heart and Lung: Journal of Acute and Critical Care* 26 (5): 387–98.

Eichler, M. (1988) *Non-Sexist Research Methods: A Practical Guide*. London: Allen & Unwin.

Gates, M.F. & Lackey, N.R. (1998) Youngsters caring for adults with cancer. *Image: Journal of Nursing Scholarship* **30** (1): 11–15.

Gerhardt, U. (1990) Qualitative research on chronic illness: the issues and the story. *Social Science and Medicine* **30** (11): 1149–59.

Haddock, J. & Burrows, C. (1997) The role of the nurse in health promotion: an evaluation of a smoking cessation programme in surgical pre-admission clinics. *Journal of Advanced Nursing* **26** (6): 1098–1110.

Hammersley, M. & Atkinson, P. (1995) *Ethnography: Principles in Practice*, 2nd edn. London: Tavistock.

Higgins, P. (1998) Patient perception of fatigue while undergoing long-term mechanical ventilation. *Heart and Lung: Journal of Acute and Critical Care* **27** (3): 177–83.

Holloway, I.M., Smith, P. & Warren, J. (1998) Time in hospital. *Journal of Clinical Nursing* **7** (5): 460–6.

Kimble, L.P. & King, K.B. (1998) Perceived side effects and benefits of coronary angioplasty in the early recovery period. *Heart and Lung: Journal of Acute and Critical Care* **27** (5): 308–14.

Kyngas, H., Hentinen, M. & Barlow, J. (1998) Adolescents' perceptions of physicians, nurses, parents and friends: help or hindrance in compliance with diabetes self-care? *Journal of Advanced Nursing* **27** (4): 760–9.

Mackenzie, J. (1997) 'A thorny problem for feminism': an analysis of the subjective work experiences of enrolled nurses. *Journal of Clinical Nursing* **6** (5): 365–70.

Mason, T. (1997) An ethnomethodological analysis of the use of seclusion. *Journal of Advanced Nursing* **26**, (4): 780–9.

Meininger, J.C., Liehr, P., Mueller, W.H., Chan, W. & Chandler, P.S. (1998) Predictors of ambulatory blood pressure: identification of high-risk adolescents. *Advances in Nursing Science* **20** (3): 50–64.

Mitchell, P. & Koch, T. (1997) An attempt to give nursing home residents a voice in the quality improvement process: the challenge of frailty. *Journal of Clinical Nursing* **6** (6): 453–61.

Morse, J.M. (1991) *Qualitative Nursing Research: A Contemporary Dialogue*. Newbury Park, CA: Sage.

Mullhall, A (1998) Methods of data collection for quantitative research. In B. Roe & C. Webb (eds) *Research and Development in Clinical Nursing*. London: Whurr.

Nay-Brock, R.M. (1984) A comparison of the questionnaire and interview techniques in the collection of sociological data. *Australian Journal of Advanced Nursing* **2**: 14–23.

Pontin, D. & Webb, C. (1995) Assessing patient satisfaction. Part 1. The research process. *Journal of Clinical Nursing* **4**: 383–9.

Pontin, D. & Webb, C. (1996) Assessing patient satisfaction. Part 2. Findings: nursing, the hospital and patients' concerns. *Journal of Clinical Nursing* **5**: 33–40.

Poole, K. & Jones, A. (1996) A re-examination of the experimental design for nursing research. *Journal of Advanced Nursing* **24**; 108–14.

Robson, C. (1993) *Real World Research*. Oxford: Blackwell Science.

Rolfe, G. (1998) *Expanding Nursing Knowledge: Understanding and Researching your own Practice*. London: Butterworth Heinemann.

Rowe, M.A. & King, K.B. (1998) Long term chest wall discomfort in women after coronary artery bypass grafting. *Heart and Lung: Journal of Acute and Critical Care* **27** (3): 184–8.

Sandelowski, M. (1986) The problem of rigor in qualitative research. *Advances in Nursing Science* **8** (3): 27–37.

Schumacher, K.L. & Gortner, S.R. (1992) (Mis)Conceptions and reconceptions about traditional science. *Advances in Nursing Science* **14** (4): 1–11.

Silverman, D. (1992) Applying the qualitative method to clinical care. In J. Daly, I. McDonald, & E. Willis (eds) *Researching Health Care: Designs, Dilemmas, Disciplines*. London: Tavistock/Routledge.

Silverman, D. (1993) *Interpreting Qualitative Data: Methods for Analysing Talk, Text and Interaction*. London: Sage.

Smith-Battle, L. & Wynn, L. (1998) Adolescent mothers four years later: narratives of the self and visions of the future. *Advances in Nursing Science* **20** (3): 36–49.

Spradley, J. (1979) *The Ethnographic Interview*. New York: Holt, Rinehart & Winston.

Stanley, L. & Wise, S. (1993) *Breaking out Again: Feminist Ontology and Epistemology*. London: Routledge.

Strauss, A. & Corbin, J. (1990) *Basics of Qualitative Research: Grounded Theory Procedures and Techniques*. Newbury Park, CA: Sage.

Tesch, R. (1990) *Qualitative Research: Analysis Types and Software Tools*. London: Falmer Press.

Warren, C.A.B. (1988) *Gender Issues in Field Research. Qualitative Research Methods*, vol. 9. London: Sage.

Webb, C. & Pontin, D. (1996) Introducing primary nursing: nurses' opinions. *Journal of Clinical Nursing* **5**: 351–8.

Williams, A. (1990) Reflections on the making of an ethnographic text. *Studies in Sexual Politics*. Monograph 29, pp. 1–60. Dept of Sociology, University of Manchester.

Williams, A.M. (1998) The delivery of quality nursing care: a grounded theory study of the nurses' perspective. *Journal of Advanced Nursing* **27** (4): 808–16.

Wilson, K. & Roe, B. (1998) Interviewing older people by telephone following initial contact by postal survey. *Journal of Advanced Nursing* **27** (3): 575–81.

CHAPTER 25

Questionnaire

Tricia Murphy-Black

Questionnaires are the most common form of instrument for collecting data. They are used for different research designs and have advantages in both audit and research. The researcher's aim is to collect written or verbal responses to specific questions. Different techniques can be used to gather the data and some will be discussed in this chapter. The apparent ease with which questionnaires can be constructed is deceptive. Many questionnaires are distributed that have badly worded or confusing questions, which leave the respondent uncertain, and in such instances the data are probably of dubious value.

Administration of questionnaires

Questionnaires can be used in different ways, ranging from the formal structured questionnaire, completed by the respondents on their own, to the semi-structured interview completed with the researcher face to face. The special skills required for interviewing were described in Chapter 24, but some of the skills in questionnaire design and construction are also needed for the semi-structured questionnaire which can form the basis of a face-to-face or telephone interview.

How questionnaires are distributed and filled in or completed may define them. The most common questionnaire is postal. It may be used to collect information for market research, provision of local services, views or attitudes on a wide range of subjects and may be of intense interest or of no interest. The person receiving it may sit down eagerly to provide the answers or toss it in the waste paper basket after a quick glance.

A questionnaire handed out personally has the advantage that the respondent connects it with an individual or an organization, which may improve the response rate (Sitzia & Wood, 1998). Both the postal and personally distributed questionnaires are self-administered, that is, the respondents are left to answer the questionnaires on their own.

The research instruments with a structured or semi-structured list of questions, used in the face-to-face interview, are usually completed or filled in by the researcher. This type of interview, common in market research, is also used in nursing and midwifery (e.g. Clayton *et al.*, 1998). The questionnaire, also called an interview schedule, has to go through the same development process as the postal questionnaire. One advantage is that it allows for the rephrasing or clarification of a confusing question or range of responses. The major disadvantage is the increased cost in the employment of interviewers. The telephone interview is between the face-to-face interview and the postal questionnaire. The researchers have structured or semi-structured interview schedules from which they read both the questions and the range of possible answers.

Advantages

The advantages of using postal questionnaires to collect data are many:

1. Distribution in large numbers
2. Cheaper than other methods of data collection
3. Ease of administration, especially to a group or by post
4. Designed properly, the analysis can be easy
5. Anonymity
6. No training required
7. Reduced interviewer bias

Disadvantages

The following disadvantages need to be considered:

1. Low response rate.
2. Inability/difficulty in completing questionnaires, e.g. the illiterate, the elderly; the visually impaired; young children; non-native speakers (understand the spoken but not the written word).
3. Forced choice answers not reflecting an individual's experience reducing the willingness to respond.
4. Introduction of bias by reading and/or answering questions out of order.
5. Impossible to clarify or rephrase.
6. Lack of personal contact between researcher and respondent.

Purpose of questionnaires

Questionnaires are research instruments. They need to be designed for their purpose, which is to collect specific information that will provide answers to the overall research question of the study. The data collected, and hence the findings, can only be as good as the questions asked. The most important stage of a project using a questionnaire is the preparation and design of the questionnaire itself.

Audit

Although most of the reference to the use of questionnaires in this chapter has been to research, the techniques used to design and administer questionnaires for research purposes also apply to audit. There is a danger that some might think audit does not require such detailed preparation and development, but this is not the case. If nursing and midwifery are to be evidence based, part of the evidence comes from audit and it cannot be stated too often that the data are only as good as the instrument or tool used to collect them. Meurier (1998) gave an example of the careful preparation of a questionnaire for an audit.

Designing a questionnaire

The first decision to make is the type: will it be a postal questionnaire, used in a telephone interview or a face-to-face interview? The next stage involves the actual questions that will appear on the page. Both of these stages are strongly influenced by the nature of the project, amount of funding, time and people available. During early discussions, all these issues will influence each other, and the initial plans may change considerably.

Designing a questionnaire is the process of deciding:

1. The questions that should be asked: the amount of data required to give the information needed to answer the research question.
2. How the questions should be asked: whether to use open or closed questions, fixed choice, or one of a variety of scales.
3. When questions should be asked: whether before or after an event of interest to the researcher; also the order within the questionnaire.
4. Where the questions should be asked: whether in the street, at home, in hospital, alone, or in a group.
5. Why the questions should be asked: whether these particular questions are more likely to get better answers than a different set of questions.

Exploratory work is useful in the preparation of a questionnaire. This may involve a critical analysis of the literature; group discussion with people similar to the sample; testing of ideas with experts or relevant individuals or groups; or taking account of special needs of particular groups (Meurier, 1998; Murphy-Black, 1989a; Worth & Tierney, 1993).

When planning a questionnaire, the following guidelines are useful:

1. The shorter the question, the better the respondents will like it.
2. The bigger the sample, the more precise the results.
3. The more relevant the topic to the respondent and the more practical it is to answer, the better the response rate.

Length of questionnaire

Despite advice to keep questionnaires short, recent research examining the relationship between the rate of returned questionnaires and the length showed that the response rate was not related to questionnaire length (Sitzia & Wood, 1998) and that responses were similar for the short (4-page) and long (16-page) questionnaire groups (Hoffman *et al.*, 1998).

Content of questions

The content of the questions should relate to the ability of the respondents to answer. The willingness to respond will be enhanced if the questions do not expose ignorance. The people in the sample ought to be able to answer the questions, otherwise they should not be sent the questionnaire. The language needs to be pitched at the appropriate level for the population. Questions appropriate to health care professionals may not be suitable for patients. Testing of the questionnaire may reveal a better choice of words or phrases, appropriate to the group for which it is intended.

Wording

A number of issues are relevant when choosing the words for the questions. Each question should be specific, simple and straightforward. Keep the questions short; long ones, with many different clauses, are difficult enough to follow when written but are even harder when they are spoken out loud as they will be in a face-to-face or telephone interview. (Try reading that last sentence out loud and compare it with the one before it.) Ambiguity – where the question could have two or three meanings – confuses the respondent and results in answers that are confusing. Avoid vague words such as occasionally or regularly. If asking 'How often...?' put the question in the context of frequency within a time limit, for example:

> How often do you shop in the city?   once a month
> once a week
> every day

Never presume (e.g. State the number of children you have); either give options (How many children do you have? Which allows the respondent to say none) or use a filter (e.g. Please answer questions 3–5 if you have children or go to question 6 if you have none). Filter questions can also be used to funnel the replies from the general to the particular, for example:

1. Have you read the remit of the UKCC Commission on Education?
2. Have you been asked to comment?

3. Have you given your views on the Commission on Education?
4. Please give your views below.

Leading questions, which invite certain types of answer, should be avoided (e.g. Are you satisfied with hospital food?). Try instead to give the respondent a range of options (Please indicate how satisfied you are with hospital food: poor, reasonable, excellent). If the project is looking for explanations of behaviour, it may be necessary to ask a number of questions to arrive at the answer. The first question asks about the behaviour, for example:

How often do you exercise?   every day,
                               twice a week,
                               once a week,
                               less than once a week?

Then the next question asks for reasons (e.g. Please give three reasons for your response to the previous question).

Sometimes a hypothetical statement is useful to lead into a question about a difficult, sensitive or embarrassing subject. For instance, the statement: 'Some men are unable to have an erection as often as they want' could lead to a question about impotence, offering a range of answers. By giving 'permission' to have the complaint, the respondents will feel they can answer the questions. Another technique with wording is to use personal language, referring to 'your' rather than 'the', e.g. 'your baby', 'your illness', 'your back' or 'your house', etc.

If the respondents are a homogeneous group such as nurses or midwives or mothers, it may not be necessary to define terms; for instance, most nurses and midwives in the UK will not need G Grade explained to them. If, however, the respondents are a heterogeneous group, from a varied background, and the purpose of the survey is very specific, it may be necessary to explain the terms. A number of definitions or explanations could be placed at the beginning of the questionnaire. If only one or two, then they can be included in the question.

The nature of the question and the type of response will guide the way the question is worded. For example, a factual question like 'Do you wear a watch?' will expect a 'Yes' or 'No' answer and is unlikely to be influenced by other factors. The question 'How much do you spend on beer each week?' is different. The answer can be factual (the actual amount spent each week) or it can be wishful thinking (more than is spent to look generous), less than is spent (to conceal heavy drinking) or vague. If the question is factual but about something that only occurs occasionally, e.g. 'How much do you spend on liqueurs at Christmas?', there can be genuine problems with giving an accurate figure, especially if asked a few weeks or months later. Questions about smoking, drinking and sexual behaviour are ones that are commonly answered in the way the respondents think the researcher wants them to answer.

Types of questions

There are a number of different types of question which have a variety of uses in questionnaires.

1. Closed – where the respondent is expected to answer 'Yes' or 'No'; e.g. 'Have you been in hospital in the last year?' It allows the researcher to direct those who say 'No' to skip a number of questions to reach the next relevant question. A series of closed questions reduces the time it takes to complete the questionnaire.
2. Forced choice – where the respondent has to choose between one of two categories, but is slightly more comprehensive than the closed question. Perhaps the most common is asking the gender of the respondent, but even this requires a little thought. I take great pleasure in answering 'Yes, please' to any questionnaire that expects me to respond to

Sex? _____

3. Multiple choice – or alternative statements: these may specify whether the respondent is to choose only one of the list or more than one. Unless the list is completely exclusive, it is always worth adding 'Other, please specify' at the end.
4. Scales – there are a number of different scales which can be used to obtain data. These may be little more than a closed question, expecting the respondents to 'agree' or 'disagree' with a statement or may give a range of options similar to the multiple choice; for example:

I was discharged from hospital: | | too soon
                                                  | | at about the right time
                                                  | | not soon enough

5. Ranking questions ask the respondents to state their preference. This may be a list provided within the questionnaire; for example:

> From the list of journals please rank them according to usefulness to your work; where 1 is the most useful and 5 is the least useful:
>
> *Nursing Times*
> *Nursing Standard*
> *Journal of Community Nursing*
> *Journal of Advanced Nursing*
> *British Journal of Nursing*

Alternatively the respondents may be asked to provide their own list and then to rank them in order; for example:

Please give three reasons for your choice of professional journal and list below:

Considering the list given above, please rank according to importance to you, with 1 as the most important and 3 as the least important.

6. Likert scales, which have a number of different statements, ask the respondents to choose one of five points between 'strongly agree' and 'strongly disagree' in relation to each statement; for example:

	Strongly agree	Agree	Uncertain	Disagree	Strongly disagree
Nurses and midwives prefer job satisfaction to a high salary					

This scaling method was developed to measure attitudes; specifically all the items were measuring the same dimension (Oppenheim, 1992). Although this looks easy, it is important, however, to develop the items for the scale using the procedure set out by Likert. This involves the development of a pool of statements (also called items) which are subjected to different tests before use in the questionnaire. The original description is in a paper published in 1932 and may not be readily available; details have been published recently (Oppenheim, 1992) and examples are published in nursing or midwifery research, such as Clifford (1996).

7. Open questions ('How do you feel about the birth of your baby?', 'Have you any further comments on your experience of nursing care?') give the respondents the freedom to answer in their own words. This can range from a single word or phrase, to sheets and sheets of closely written text. In designing the questionnaire, it is essential to plan for such a variety of answers. There is a danger, however, that such large amounts of data will never be analysed.

Other issues concerning questionnaires

It is important to give respondents clear instructions. Should they mark certain answers with a tick, a circle or a cross? How should numbers (especially dates) be written? Should all the questions be answered or are some not applicable? Instructions can be given in various different ways (for example, see Marsland, 1995) and these need to be tested in the pilot study.

For a postal questionnaire the covering letter is vital. It makes the first impression on the respondent, good or bad. A decision needs to be made about how personal or impersonal to make the form of address. A letter addressed personally to each individual is more effective than 'Dear Patient' 'Dear Mum' or 'Dear Colleague'. With word processors and a mail merge facility it is easy to put each individual's name on the letter. Anything that requires the respondent to do something has to overcome a natural prejudice; so the opening paragraph should address the respondent rather than tell him about the research or the researcher. 'You have been chosen because' rather than 'I am a nurse or midwife doing research'. The letter should state:

- The reasons for the project.
- What is involved.
- How long it will take.
- If it can be done without checking details.
- Who is to fill it in.
- If it can be passed to someone else.
- If it can be completed anonymously (the researcher need not know who has filled it in).
- If it is confidential (the researcher knows who has filled it in but will not tell anyone).
- Who, if anyone, will be identified in the report.
- How the respondents have been selected.
- Why they should reply.

A strong statement of gratitude is essential as the questionnaire is asking someone to take time and effort to provide data for little or usually no return.

Validity and reliability

A questionnaire that does not measure what it is designed to measure is not valid, and one that cannot measure the differences between two people answering the same questionnaire is not reliable.

Validity

Examination of the validity of questionnaires can be undertaken by the test–retest method (administering the same questionnaire twice to the same sample within a short time frame) to see if the same responses are obtained. A more sophisticated method is to vary the administration – for instance, using the same format for a personal interview, telephone interview and postal questionnaire (Zielhuis *et al.*, 1992).

Sometimes validation of questionnaires can happen by chance. During the second round of testing questionnaires, the spontaneous comments by the elderly subjects reflected the recent cuts in service. This questionnaire was able to show less patient satisfaction while there was no change in the measure of satisfaction with life (Gilleard & Reed, 1998).

Britton *et al.* (1990) tested the validity of a questionnaire designed to elicit symptoms of urological disease. It was acceptable with a completion rate of 99%. Only 3 of 648 answers were changed on the test–retest analysis. In the same study the consistency was checked by both clinicians and patients. The questionnaire successfully identified a high-risk group of patients from the community, requiring further urological evaluation.

Reliability

Checking that a questionnaire is reliable may be done by asking groups with known differences to take part in the testing process. This may compare the sick and the healthy or other groups. For instance, Zielhuis *et al.* (1992) examined the responses from a group of primiparous and then multiparous women.

It is sometimes reported that time constraints make the testing of a questionnaire for validity and reliability impractical (Clayton *et al.*, 1998). This is to be regretted as the findings have to be challenged when there is no supporting evidence that the questionnaire measures what it is designed to measure or demonstrates the differences between different subjects.

Response rates

All quantitative research, which uses a representative sample, is dependent on a good response rate. If low, it can have a significant impact on the usefulness of the findings. Examples of variations in the response rates are given in Fig. 25.1.

Research to find the most efficient way of handling large postal surveys has included anonymity. Reputed to increase the response rate especially where the topic is sensitive, such as knowledge of AIDS, a trial where the questionnaires

Sample	Response (%)	Authors
Nurse teaching staff	51.5	Clifford (1996)
A sample from GPs' age-sex registers	59	Walsh (1994)
Population based study of women who had recently had a baby	30–89	Adams et al. (1991)
Student nurses	87	Marsland (1995)

Fig. 25.1 Variations in response rate.

were randomized to anonymous or numbered groups showed no differences in the response rates (Campbell & Waters, 1990).

Although sending another copy of the questionnaire as a reminder can increase the response rate (e.g. from 51–72%, Campbell & Waters, 1990), it also increases the cost of the survey. If the questionnaires were completed by anonymous respondents, reminders have to be sent to the entire sample as there is no means of knowing who has or has not returned the questionnaire. To see if there was a method of overcoming this problem without compromising on anonymity, Asch (1996) used coded postcards as well as questionnaires in a survey about euthanasia. The respondents were asked to post back the questionnaires and the postcards separately. Although it did appear to lower the response rate, it also lowered the cost and Asch claimed that it did not introduce additional bias.

A personal approach, whether for recruitment alone or for data collection, was associated with a significantly higher response rate compared with recruitment and data collection by post (Sitzia & Wood, 1998). Tai *et al.* (1997) reported that sending reminders by recorded delivery was more effective than telephone reminders.

Partial response

Partial response, where some of the questions have been answered but others are left blank, is irritating. It may not happen frequently and may appear that there is no pattern. It is worth checking the data carefully to see if there are any common features. For instance, there was a relatively high level of non-response to the clinical component of the questionnaire to nurse teachers (Clifford, 1996). In the general population, it is more common in the elderly (Eaker *et al.*, 1998).

Recall

One explanation of partial response is poor recall. Any questions which are asking the respondent to remember events, behaviours or emotions are potentially subject to bias. Even something that focuses on a relatively recent period can be difficult to report accurately. For instance, a question asking for a list of the amount and type of alcohol taken over the last week can be problematic if there is considerable variation. Certain groups, such as the elderly, may have difficulty in remembering details (Worth & Tierney, 1993) while critical life events may be easier. A study to test recall compared information obtained by questionnaire with contemporaneous records of the time it took women to become pregnant. Data from the questionnaire and from these records agreed, for both recent events and those older than 14 years (Joffe *et al.*, 1995).

Non-response

Are those who do not return postal questionnaires similar to or different from those who do return them? As there is always a danger of bias, this is an issue of considerable importance, yet it is not always reported. A meta analysis of 210 studies showed that only 48% of them reported the response rate (Sitzia & Wood, 1998).

Some workers have demonstrated differences between responders and non-responders. This may be due to demographic characteristics, such as young age, male sex and urban residence (Eaker *et al.*, 1998) or health-related behaviour such as smoking (smokers are less likely to return questionnaires – Bostrom *et al.*, 1993). In certain groups, such as mothers of newborn babies, the non-responders may share a number of characteristics. For example, the non-responders were significantly more likely to be unmarried, unemployed, have an unemployed partner, and to have a low birthweight baby, with a low APGAR score one minute after birth (Murphy-Black, 1989a).

The method of collecting data has been associated with different response rates. It is lower for questionnaires than for telephone or personal interviews (Bostrom *et al.*, 1993; Hoffman *et al.*, 1998). Eaker *et al.* (1998) tested various formats and achieved the lowest response (40%) with a combination of no preliminary notification, a long questionnaire, and mention of telephone contact. Sending a postcard reminder was not as effective as sending a second copy of the questionnaire (Hoffman *et al.*, 1998). Receiving a questionnaire just before a weekend did not improve the response rate (Olivarius & Andreasen, 1995). In a study by Choi *et al.* (1990), the use of paper stamps, especially large commemorative stamps, rather than reply-paid format on return envelopes both increased the response rate and reduced the response time, although Murphy-Black (1989b) reported no difference between these two methods – that is, stamps or reply-paid envelopes.

Pilot study

It is important to develop questionnaires, and in more complex studies the piloting may take months. Robinson *et al.* (1998) had an eight-month period for design and testing questionnaires with their pilot cohort, involving a three-stage process where each member is involved in one or more stages. The use of words, the word order, the question order within the questionnaire and the presentation will all benefit from testing before the pilot study. The pilot study is a small-scale version of the main study and is useful to test all the procedures and the feasibility of study. This includes selecting the sample, distributing the questionnaires, checking the returns, and the analysis and examination of the findings to see if the questionnaire provides the data expected.

Conclusions

A questionnaire is a very flexible and versatile method of collecting data. It can be used within a wide range of different research designs and has many advantages for both the novice and experienced researcher. There is much to learn about questionnaire design and this chapter has just given an outline of some of the aspects to consider, which it is hoped will whet the appetite.

References

Adams, M.M., Shulman, H.B., Bruce, C., Hogue, C. & Brogan, D. (1991) The Pregnancy Risk Assessment Monitoring System: design, questionnaire, data collection and response rates. PRAMS Working Group. *Paediatric Perinatal Epidemiology* 5 (3): 333–46.

Asch, D.A. (1996) Use of a coded postcard to maintain anonymity in a highly sensitive mail survey: cost, response rates, and bias. *Epidemiology* 7 (5): 550–1.

Bostrom, G., Hallqvist, J., Haglund, B.J., Romelsjo, A., Svanstrom, L. & Diderichsen, F. (1993) Socioeconomic differences in smoking in an urban Swedish population. The bias introduced by non-participation in a mailed questionnaire. *Scandinavian Journal of Social Medicine* 21 (2): 77–82.

Britton, J.P., Dowell, A.C. & Whelan, P. (1990) Validation of a self-administered urological questionnaire. *British Journal of Urology* 65 (2): 131–3.

Campbell, M.J. & Waters, W.E. (1990) Does anonymity increase response rate in postal questionnaire surveys about sensitive subjects? A randomised trial. *Journal of Epidemiology and Community Health* 44 (1): 75–6.

Choi, B.C., Pak, A.W. & Purdham, J.T. (1990) Effects of mailing strategies on response rate, response time, and cost in a questionnaire study among nurses. *Epidemiology* 1 (1): 72–4.

Clayton, J., Smith, K., Qureshi, H. & Ferguson, B. (1998) Collecting patients' views and perceptions of continence services: the development of research instruments. *Journal of Advanced Nursing* 28: 353–61.

Clifford, C. (1996) Nurse teacher's clinical work: a survey report. *Journal of Advanced Nursing* 23: 603–11.

Eaker, S., Bergstrom, R., Bergstrom, A., Adami, H.O. & Nyren, O. (1998) Response rate to mailed epidemiologic questionnaires: a population-based randomized trial of variations in design and mailing routines. *American Journal of Epidemiology* 147 (1): 74–82.

Gilleard, C. & Reed, R. (1998) Validating a measure of patient satisfaction with community nursing services. *Journal of Advanced Nursing* 28 (1): 94–100.

Hoffman, S.C., Burke, A.E., Helzlsouer, K.J. & Comstock, G.W. (1998) Controlled trial of the effect of length, incentives, and follow-up techniques on response to a mailed questionnaire. *American Journal of Epidemiology* 148 (10): 1007–11.

Joffe, M., Villard, L., Li, Z., Plowman, R. & Vessey, M. (1995) A time to pregnancy questionnaire designed for long term recall: validity in Oxford, England. *Journal of Epidemiology and Community Health* 49 (3): 314–19.

Marsland, L. (1995) Career guidance for student nurses: an unmet need. *Nurse Education Today* 16: 10–18.

Meurier, C.E. (1998) The quality of assessment of patients with chest pain: the development of a questionnaire to audit the nursing assessment record of patients with chest pain. *Journal of Advanced Nursing* 27: 140–46.

Murphy-Black, T. (1989a) *Postnatal Care at Home: A Descriptive Study of Mothers' Needs and the Maternity Services*. Nursing Research Unit, University of Edinburgh.

Murphy-Black, T. (1989b) *Appendix to Postnatal Care at Home: A Descriptive Study of Mothers' Needs and the Maternity Services*. Nursing Research Unit, University of Edinburgh.

Olivarius, N. de F. & Andreasen, A.H. (1995) Day-of-the-week effect on doctors' response to a postal questionnaire. *Scandinavian Journal of Primary Health Care* 13 (1): 65–7.

Oppenheim, A.N. (1992) *Questionnaire Design, Interviewing and Attitude Measurement*. London: Pinter.

Robinson, S., Marsland, L., Murrells, T., Hickey, G., Hardyman, R. & Tingle, A. (1998) Designing questionnaires in a longitudinal study of nurse diplomates' careers. *Nursing Times Research* 3 (3): 195–8.

Sitzia, J. & Wood, N. (1998) Response rate in patient satisfaction research: an analysis of 210 published studies. *International Journal of Quality Health Care* 10 (4): 311–17.

Tai, S.S., Nazareth, I., Haines, A. & Jowett, C. (1997) A randomized trial of the impact of telephone and recorded delivery reminders on the response rate to research questionnaires. *Journal of Public Health Medicine* 19 (2): 219–21.

Walsh, K. (1994) Evaluation of the use of general practice age-sex registers in epidemiological research. *British Journal of General Practice* 44 (380): 118–22.

Worth, A. & Tierney, A. (1993) Conducting research interviews with elderly people by telephone. *Journal of Advanced Nursing* 18: 1077–84.

Zielhuis, G.A., Hulscher, M.E. & Florack, E.I. (1992) Validity and reliability of a questionnaire on fecundability. *International Journal of Epidemiology* 21 (6): 1151–6.

CHAPTER 26

Observation

David Pontin

The English language is littered with phrases which refer to the everyday practice of looking at things in order to find out about the world, and examples such as 'seeing is believing' and 'actions speak louder than words' are familiar to many. I am sure that, given time, readers would be able to generate a fuller list of phrases about looking at things which would reflect the history and tradition of their own culture and locality and also of languages other than English. Looking at things, as a way of finding out about the world, is familiar to us. By looking at things as nurses, midwives or health visitors we make judgements and decisions which inform our actions. The capability to do this is present in most people provided their vision is good enough, and it happens every day without people giving it a second thought. And there lies the issue – people are so familiar with looking at things on a personal level that they might not necessarily think about the differences between everyday observation of the world and the way in which observation is used in research. If it is assumed that the way in which people look at things in their everyday lives is the same as in research, then a grave error will be made. This chapter will look at the way observation as a research method is carried out in nursing research and the differences which exist between the use of observation in quantitative and qualitative enquiry.

Characteristics of observational data

The typical things or phenomena which researchers include as the focus for their observational research are people and their activities, objects and situations or events. There is an overlap between these phenomena and the sorts of things people might look at in everyday life. However, the main difference between them is that researchers use observation methods to examine the world in a systematic way to identify concepts and theories which can then be tested and used to inform practice. While people may use 'everyday-looking-at-things' to make sense of the world they do not necessarily use it explicitly in a systematic way to develop and test theories about the world. So using observational research methods allows researchers to go beyond the everyday (see Fig. 26.1).

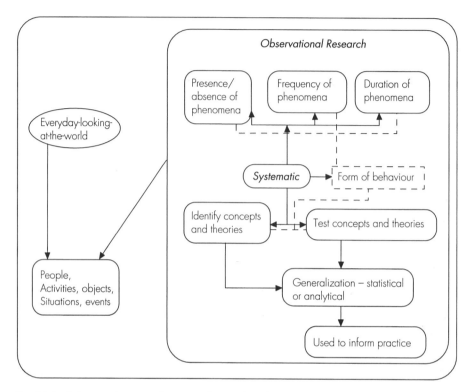

Fig. 26.1   Differences between observational research and 'everyday-looking-at-the-world'.

Interaction

There are a number of particular facets which make observational research systematic. The first is the presence or absence of interaction between people or between people and things, events or activities in a given setting. An example of this can be seen in Watkins & Redfern's (1997) evaluation of a night nursing service for elderly people with dementia. They used the Crichton Visual Analogue Scale (Morrison, 1983) to measure clients' abilities in carrying out activities of living and to assess the degree of dementia-related behavioural problems. They found that clients increasingly spent about 30% of their waking time at the facility in self-contained behaviour. Given that people with dementia often exhibit restless, noisy behaviour, the fact that there was an absence of this behaviour for long periods of time may be interpreted as a positive outcome of the nursing care initiative that was being investigated.

Duration of behaviour

The second systematic facet is the duration or the length of time a particular behaviour is exhibited by people in interactions, events or activities. Cleary (1992) presents a very useful account of the development of a care-by-parent scheme in a children's ward. As part of the research design she records the percentage of time various groups of babies (non-resident-parent, resident-parent and care-by-parent) spent crying. She notes that crying for babies is a way of drawing attention to unmet needs, and while all three groups of babies cried for a large part of their waking time the proportions varied between them. The main difference between them was 'crying alone' – for non-resident-parent babies this was 10.7% of waking time, babies with resident parents but not included in the care-by-parent scheme cried alone for 4.4% of waking time, and care-by-parent babies cried alone for only 2.1% of their waking time (Cleary, 1992).

Frequency of interaction

The third facet is the number of times interactions occur between people or between people and things, or the number of times events or activities happen in a given period. This may be expressed as an absolute number or as a relative number, for example as a percentage. Lundgren *et al.* (1993) describe the frequency of thrombophlebitis in surgical and internal medical ward patients in relation to intravenous cannula size and insertion point, the length of time *in situ* and the care and handling of peripheral cannulae. Their work suggests that the frequency and severity of thrombophlebitis increases with time after cannula insertion, particularly after 24 hours. They also observed that the level of care and handling of peripheral intravenous cannulae decreases with the number of days they are *in situ* and deficient care was noted to be present after the second day.

Form of behaviour

In all the examples given above, the types of behaviour observed do not obviously correspond to an everyday perspective. Elderly clients' self-contained behaviour is used as a positive indicator for a nursing care innovation, 'crying alone' time is used as an indicator of supportive nursing care to parents, and thrombophlebitis is used as an indicator of careful handling and attentiveness by nurses. This final facet of being systematic – the form of behaviour – is the characteristic of observational research which is most different from everyday looking at the world because it links the act of observing to the generation and testing of theory.

Generating and capturing observational data

Structured/formal observation

The way in which observation is used in quantitative research and in qualitative research is different and the difference between them reflects the characteristic paradigm of each tradition (see Chapters 12 and 14). As would be expected from a quantitative research method (see Chapter 14), structured/formal observation is used to provide objective measurements of phenomena. It is a way for researchers to quantify specific behaviours which are being investigated and to produce data which are valid, reliable and replicable. Carrying out structured, objective measurements in this way provides researchers with certain advantages: they can avoid memory recall effects in the production of their data and can adapt the research design to different settings. Perhaps the most notable benefit of this method is that introspection is not required of the people being observed. Therefore behaviour such as babies crying may be observed (Cleary, 1992), or inarticulate people such as clients with dementia (Watkins & Redfern, 1997) may be the focus for investigation.

Schedule of observation

There are many sorts of behaviour which may be observed in this way and taxonomies of behaviour have to be developed to categorize specific types of data which will be collected in advance (Mullhall, 1998). By specifying the types of data to be collected and developing unambiguous definitions of the behaviour to be observed, a schedule of observation may be produced (Endicott, 1994; Pretzlik, 1994). The schedule may then be used by one or more observers in the process of generating data. The data may be generated from live observation of phenomena or from recordings such as video. The advantages of live observation are that researchers are able to take the context of the phenomenon into account when analysing the data. If the phenomenon to be observed occurs as a single event then live observation is an economical way to proceed (Fig. 26.2); however, once the phenomenon has taken place it is lost for ever and may not be re-analysed, whereas a recorded phenomenon is available for re-examination for as many times as the format of the recording allows.

Sampling

An issue to be considered for both forms of data generation is the type of sampling strategy to be used – intermittent or continual. In intermittent sampling the observation will last for a set time, e.g. every 2 minutes, while the continual form is determined by the phenomena being observed, the research design and the

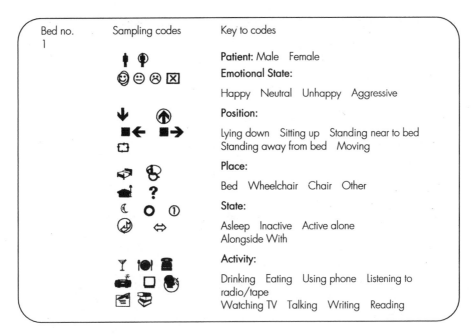

Fig. 26.2   Example of section of observation schedule looking at patient activity.

questions being asked (see Chapter 7). Cheng & Chapman (1997) provide an example of this when they report on their decision-making in modifying an infant behavioural observation record for developmental care. One of the changes they made involved changing the time of observation from every 2 minutes when developmental care was delivered in the observation period to continual observation of the delivery of developmental care by nurses. They then evaluate the validity and reliability of the modified tool in the light of these and other changes.

Naturalistic observation

The purpose of naturalistic observation is different from that outlined above. It does not quantify behaviour but it is nonetheless systematic in its approach to the collection and generation of data (Hammersley & Atkinson, 1995; see also Chapter 12). The point of generating data via naturalistic observation is to develop an account of a 'natural' setting, develop theories and test them through analytic generalization (Rolfe, 1998; Hammersley & Atkinson, 1995; Hammersley, 1992; Williams, 1991). The main difference between structured or formal observation and naturalistic observation is that the latter does not specify in detail and in advance what will be observed and it aims to incorporate the views and perspective of the participants. This is not to say that researchers using naturalistic observation have no idea what they will observe. They have various research questions to be answered, but they are concerned not to exclude behaviour or events which cannot be predicted in advance that may cast new light on particular situations or scenarios (Stanley & Wise, 1993). After all, if you knew everything about a given situation, including exactly what was going to happen in advance, there would be no need for an investigation.

Finding meaning in a situation

Naturalistic observation involves searching for the presence or absence of behaviour, events or activities as well as their duration and frequency. However, it does so in relation to the context in which the behaviour, events or situations occur and is not concerned with quantifying the duration or frequency of such phenomena. In using naturalistic observation researchers are aiming to identify the meaning such phenomena have for people or their understanding of what is happening, so that theories about the world may be developed. Turton (1995), in her account of the development of a community nursing-based service for people with human immunodeficiency virus (HIV) and acquired immune deficiency syndrome (AIDS), describes difficulties in building trust with clients. In particular she describes the effects of junior doctors' actions in not following accepted procedures for the administration of intravenous drugs, such as not using gloves. Because Turton was new to the unit and followed the public protocol of using gloves, the doctor's actions affected clients' ability to develop trusting relationships with her because they felt that her use of gloves reflected her attitude towards them. It would have been impossible for Turton to know in advance that the behaviour of junior doctors in such a specific set of circumstances could have an effect on her own efforts to build trust with clients, but by being open to the circumstances in which she was researching she was able to observe such behaviour at first hand.

Field role

This raises the issue of how to carry out observation in natural settings, or 'the field' as it is often known. One of the major considerations for researchers when using naturalistic observation is what role they will take in the field – observer or participant or somewhere in between. Junker (1960) and Gold (1958) carried out early work on delineating the different sorts of roles available to researchers in naturalistic observation research. Junker (1960) identifies a continuum of roles with four main staging points which reflect the degree of involvement or detachment that researchers have with the settings being observed. These roles are complete-participant, participant-as-observer (involvement), observer-as-participant, and complete-observer (detachment). Nurses have taken a number of roles in naturalistic observation research, however, in practice the demarcation between these positions often changes during the life of the research project (Webb *et al.*, 1998). Titchen & Binnie (1993) have maintained both participant-as-observer and complete-observer roles in their work on nursing developments by separating out aspects of the research design and functioning as a research partnership. However, Binnie acknowledges that there were times when her role was more participant-as-observer, such as when she was in practice as a senior nurse. When she and Titchen discussed issues relating to the project, she changed her role once more to observer-as-participant. Pontin (1997) describes the process of changing his fieldwork roles in response to changes in the day-to-day running of an action research project investigating primary nursing where there were personnel changes in the development worker role. He moved from being an observer to observer-as-participant, to participant-as-observer and back to observer again. Similarly, Waterman (1998) discusses how she changed her behaviour as an ophthalmic nurse depending on the context. When she was in the treatment room of the outpatient department she participated fully as she was confident of her clinical skills and her understanding of the setting. Yet in the consulting and waiting area of the clinic she took on more of an observer-as-participant role because she did not understand the clinical functioning well enough to participate safely.

Ethics of field roles

It is very unusual for nurses to adopt a complete participant role as this involves an element of deception by researchers with the people in the research setting. In these circumstances people are said to be carrying out covert research and they do not inform other people present in the setting under study that they are researchers. Field (1989) describes covert work which investigated the way dying patients were nursed by having researchers work as health care assistants in order to collect data unknown to patients and nurses. It is argued that covert research is necessary where physical access to a setting is not given or may be difficult (Homan, 1980). However, these designs are only useful if researchers are not discovered. It is unlikely that covert nurse researchers would be physically harmed if they were unmasked, but Johnson (1992) points out that it is professionally unethical for nurses to act in such a way. Hammersley & Atkinson (1995) also make the point that covert research may limit the scope of the research project because researchers have to stay 'in role' and cannot ask the naive questions which 'outsiders' are allowed to ask. If you are a nurse then you are expected to know about nursing; if you constantly ask questions about what people are doing they will quickly suspect that either you are not a nurse or you are 'spying' on them. Consequently, the behaviour observed will then be that of people who suspect they are being spied on.

Recording data in the field

The way in which data from naturalistic observation work is usually generated is by writing down observations in a field journal, or by using a tape recorder, as the event happens or as soon as possible afterwards – the interval between the event and the record depending on the field role taken by the researcher. In overt research, where the people in the research setting know that research is taking place, it may be appropriate for the researchers to record events as they happen. Alternatively, they may wish to move away from the event to write up their notes without distraction. Covert researchers have a problem: they have to record the events in their field diary in such a way as not to attract attention to what they are doing, stay true to the setting and avoid memory effects. There are only so many trips to the toilet people can make without attracting attention to themselves and arousing suspicions. As well as writing descriptions of interactions, events or situations, researchers using naturalistic observation will also write analytical notes to themselves when they are in the field. Analytical notes are records of their own thoughts and feelings about what is happening in the setting and include phenomena which they were not expecting or things which surprised them, This helps researchers to understand what they are seeing and perhaps to focus their observation work in the future to test whether such phenomena are important for the research project. It is important to differentiate analytical material from observed material to ensure that they do not become mixed up as they are different forms of data. One way of doing this is to use the left-hand page of the notebook for analytical notes and the right-hand page for observed material.

Rigour

The field observations form the foundation of descriptions of events, situations or interactions which are often combined by researchers with interview data (see Chapters 12, 24 and 32) to produce an account which is faithful to the setting they have been observing (Hammersley & Atkinson, 1995). However, how do readers of field work accounts know that the events described actually took place and that the interpretation presented by researchers is 'trustworthy'? (Sandelowski, 1986; see also Chapter 3). One way of demonstrating 'trustworthiness' is to include *reflexive* elements in the work.

Reflexivity is an acknowledgement that researchers are shaped by their experiences of the particular time and moment of the world in which they live. Rather than try to standardize research procedures (as quantitative research does) or become a cultural 'sponge' soaking up all aspects of culture, these presuppositions about the world should be made as explicit as possible (Hammersley & Atkinson, 1995). The fact that the presence of researchers will change the settings being researched need not be a 'problem' – it is possible to minimize people's reactivity to researchers or to monitor the extent of their reactivity. More interestingly, it is also possible to exploit the fact that people react to the presence of researchers. Pontin (1997) describes how, during his fieldwork of observing the implementation of primary nursing on a rehabilitation ward, patients would approach him in full knowledge of his role as a researcher and engage him in detailed conversations about their experiences of being patients on the ward,

'Jack, a patient, asked me what I was doing. I explained that I was monitoring staff actions to let them know if the innovations that they were carrying out were successful or not. He asked if it was "time and motion!" I said no, but that I was looking for change over time.

'He told me that there were things that "need[ed] to be looked at from the patients' point of view". The wardrobe and dressing table unit was a right-handed one but on the left hand side of his bed. This meant he could not "get at anything on the dressing table when [he was] in bed". He had asked if he could "swap with a gentleman opposite who had the same problem". He was told that he couldn't swap because of the need to disinfect the equipment. To overcome the problem of left- and right-hand units he suggested having push-through units and front and rear doors for the wardrobe. Also, that nurses should consider which side patients are affected by weakness before placing in the ward. This interchange took place in the ward with a lot of staff about, as well as patients.

'He approached me again later as I was carrying out the activity sampling. He pointed out that his wardrobe obscures the plug sockets. This meant that he couldn't use his electric razor. Also, because his bed was adjacent to the aisle, he couldn't put a urinal in the holder on the bed frame. As the dining table was inaccessible, he had to use his side table where his water jug and glass were kept. Fieldwork Journal 2 page 35.' (Pontin, 1997)

This extract from a fieldwork journal shows that it is difficult for researchers to predict accurately what will happen when they are in the field and that by recording the effects they have on a setting, a useful adjunctive form of data may be generated.

Strengths and limitations of observational research methods

Advantages

The main advantage of observational research methods for nurses, midwives and health visitors is that they can be used to analyse direct care giving in real life situations (Robson, 1993). Researchers are able to study interactions, events or situations as they occur in everyday settings and identify the antecedents and consequences of these phenomena. In this respect observational research methods, particularly naturalistic observation, demonstrate a high degree of 'ecological validity' (Hammersley & Atkinson, 1983). Ecological validity may be achieved by studying people in natural settings and recognizing that people's behaviour changes depending on the context in which it occurs. In this way researchers are more likely to access 'real world' behaviour rather than 'experimental laboratory' behaviour. Observational methods may also be used by researchers to match what people say they do to what they actually do. Matching words to deeds helps to develop a finer picture of how people behave and react in settings and also their understanding of their everyday world. Finally, by using observational methods, researchers can identify the situational factors which bring about, influence or hinder interactions, events or situations relevant to the phenomena being studied.

Disadvantages

One of the main limitations to using observation methods as the sole method of enquiry is the problem of gaining access to the meaning which people attribute to events, behaviour or situations. Within naturalistic enquiry it is common for researchers to include interviews with participants in the research, as mentioned above, but in using structured/formal observation it is not. This is mainly to prevent corruption of the research design and to ensure the reliability and validity of the data that have been collected (see Chapter 3). Another limitation which has to be considered is the amount of time it takes to collect observation data in real-life settings. Researchers cannot just go out and 'observe'; they have to negotiate access to the research setting (see Chapter 11), develop working relationships with the people concerned and observe what goes on. This may have consequences for the research design as researchers then have to decide whether to develop a serial design or use a parallel form of observation with more than one observer, which raises the issue of inter-rater reliability.

Conclusions

In this chapter the differences between everyday-looking-at-the-world and observational research methods have been explored. Observation methods are ways of investigating people, things or situations and looking for the presence/absence, duration and frequency of interactions, events and activity. Depending on the questions being asked, researchers may use structured/formal observation techniques or systematic naturalistic fieldwork. Reliability and validity are maintained in the former by developing taxonomies of behaviour, constructing observation schedules, piloting them and checking inter-rater reliability and using sampling strategies. In naturalistic fieldwork, researchers maintain the rigour of their work by being systematic in their collection and generation of data, and by providing reflexive accounts of their work. Both forms of observation demonstrate ecological validity although naturalistic fieldwork does more so. Their strength lies in studying nursing, midwifery and health visiting in the 'real world', seeing what actually happens and identifying situational factors. Their limitations when used alone are difficulty in accessing people's meanings for their behaviour and the amount of time it takes to generate and collect data.

References

Cheng, C. & Chapman, J. (1997) Assessment of reliability and validity of the behavioural observation record for developmental care. *Nursing Research* **46** (1): 40–45.

Cleary, J. (1992) *Caring for Children in Hospital: Parents and Nurses in Partnership.* Harrow: Scuatri.

Endicott, R. (1994) Objectivity in observation. *Nurse Researcher* **2** (2): 30–40.

Field, D. (1989) *Nursing the Dying.* London: Routledge.

Gold, R. (1958) Roles in sociological fieldwork. *Social Forces* **36**: 217–23.

Hammersley, M. (1992) *What's Wrong with Ethnography?* London: Routledge.

Hammersley, M. & Atkinson, P. (1983) *Ethnography: Principles in Practice.* London: Tavistock.

Hammersley, M. & Atkinson, P. (1995) *Ethnography: Principles in Practice*, 2nd edn. London: Tavistock.

Homan, R. (1980) The ethics of covert methods. *British Journal of Sociology* **31** (1): 46–59.

Johnson, M. (1992) A silent conspiracy: ethical issues of participant observation in nursing research. *International Journal of Nursing Studies* **29** (2): 213–23.

Junker, B (1960) *Field Work.* Chicago: University of Chicago Press.

Lundgren, A., Jorfeldt, L. & Ek, A. (1993) The care and handling of peripheral intravenous cannulae on 60 surgery patients and internal med patients: an observation study. *Journal of Advanced Nursing* **18**: 963–71.

Morrison, D. (1983) The Crichton visual analogue scale for the assessment of behaviour in the elderly. *Acta Psychiatrica Scandanavica* **68**: 408–13.

Mullhall, A. (1998) Methods of data collection for quantitative research. In B. Roe & C. Webb (eds) *Research and Development in Clinical Nursing.* London: Whurr.

Pontin, D. (1997) *The effect of primary nursing on the quality of nursing care: an action research study of nursing development work.* Unpublished PhD thesis, University of Manchester.

Pretzlik, U. (1994) Observational methods and strategies. *Nurse Researcher* **2** (2): 13–21.

Robson, C. (1993) *Real World Research.* Oxford: Blackwell Science.

Rolfe, G. (1998) *Expanding Nursing Knowledge: Understanding and Researching your own Practice.* London: Butterworth Heinemann.

Sandelowski, M. (1986) The problem of rigor in qualitative research. *Advances in Nursing Science* **8** (3): 27–37.

Stanley, L. & Wise, S. (1993) *Breaking out Again: Feminist Ontology and Epistemology.* London: Routledge.

Titchen, A. & Binnie, A. (1993) Research partnerships: collaborative action research in nursing. *Journal of Advanced Nursing* **18**: 858–65.

Turton, A. (1995) *Developing a community nursing service for people with HIV disease: an action research project incorporating ethnographic methods.* Unpublished PhD thesis, University of Manchester.

Waterman, H. (1998) Data collection in qualitative research. In B. Roe & C. Webb (eds) *Research and Development in Clinical Nursing*. London: Whurr.

Watkins, M. & Redfern, S. (1997) Evaluation of a new night nursing service for elderly people suffering from dementia. *Journal of Clinical Nursing* 6: 485–94.

Webb, C., Turton, P. & Pontin, D. (1998) Action research: the debate moves on. In B. Roe & C. Webb (eds) *Research and Development in Clinical Nursing*. London: Whurr.

Williams, A. (1991) Practical ethics: interpretive processes in an ethnography of nursing. In J. Aldridge, V. Griffiths & A. Williams (eds) *Rethinking: Feminist Research Processes Reconsidered*. Feminist Praxis, Monograph 33. Sociology Dept, University of Manchester.

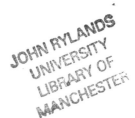

CHAPTER 27

The critical incident technique

Desmond F. S. Cormack

The critical incident technique is a set of procedures for collecting direct observations of human behaviour in such a way as to facilitate the solution of practical problems. An incident relates to any observable human activity that is sufficiently complete in itself to permit inferences to be made. This data-collection technique was popularized by Flanagan (1954), an American psychologist, who wrote one of the earliest comprehensive descriptions of it.

The use of this technique by researchers in the 1940s demonstrates how it was applied during the early stage of its development. Although the situation and problems described below are clearly not related to nursing or midwifery, the same principles apply irrespective of the situation being researched. The problems facing the researchers towards the end of the 1939–45 war related to establishing those factors (incidents) which enabled United States Army Air Force crews to achieve success during their combat flying missions. Following each mission, crew members were asked to report incidents observed by them which were effective or ineffective in terms of achieving a successful flying mission. The questions put to the crew members related specifically to the activities of the officer leading the mission; they were asked, 'Describe the officer's action' and 'What did he do?'. Analysis of several thousand responses (critical incidents) from crew members enabled the researcher to describe what the officer leading such a mission would have to do to achieve success and what he should not do to avoid failure.

It is possible to see how such a technique might be used in nursing and midwifery to establish the factors that relate, for example, to giving a good report. In this example, potential respondents who receive reports may be asked to describe activities (critical incidents) which result in an effective report being given by the person in charge of the ward. Examples of responses to that question are: 'The ward sister gave *all* staff a report' or 'She gave us a report on *all* patients' or 'The report was very clear and specific'. A question relating to ineffective reporting might get replies such as: 'Sister is very vague when she tells us about the patients' or 'She occasionally forgets to tell us really important things' or 'Only the senior staff get the report'. Analysis of respondents' responses will enable the researcher to compile a description of effective and ineffective report-giving.

The use to which the researcher puts the information collected using the critical incident technique, depends on the purpose of the research. For example, the analysed critical incidents may be used when teaching students how to give reports, or they may be used when assessing the ward sister's ability to give a report. As a result of having effective/ineffective report-giving analysed in this way, the teachers or assessors are able to have specific and critical elements of the report-giving process in mind when teaching or assessing. In short, they will no longer teach and assess in terms of what they *think* is important from a highly personal and often biased viewpoint. Rather, they will teach and assess in terms of specific criteria arrived at as a result of having applied this technique. Figure 27.1 shows how the critical incident technique may be used to improve the quality of report-giving.

A major advantage of the critical incident technique is that it depends on descriptions of *actual* effective events, rather than on descriptions of things as they should be. Thus the technique is more concerned with the real rather than the imagined world, and is able to take account of the constraints and limitations under which we all live and work.

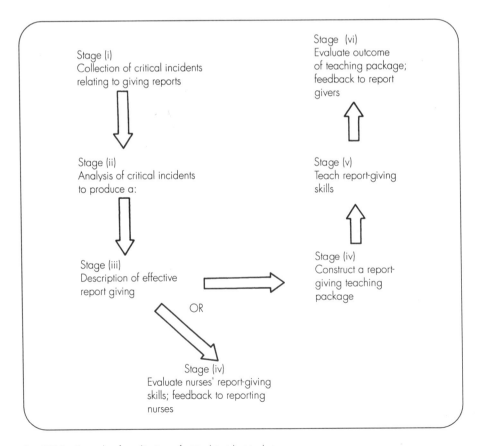

Fig. 27.1 Example of application of critical incident technique.

Use of the critical incident technique

The critical incident technique, as a means of collecting research data, has been widely used in the USA for over 30 years. It has been used, for example, to identify the role of the private duty nurse, to identify criteria for the evaluation of students, and to develop an evaluation procedure for assessing trained staff. Two early seminal reference works on the use of the technique in the USA are those by Fivars & Gonsell (1966) who used it to identify problems in nursing, and the major work by Jacobs *et al.* (1973) who undertook a nationwide study of the work of the psychiatric nurse.

Researchers in the UK are increasingly using the critical incident technique (see Norman *et al.*, 1992 and Cox *et al.*, 1993).

The versatility of the critical incident technique is considerable, and it is particularly effective in obtaining data relating to actual activities which are considered to reflect effective or ineffective education, management or clinical work. One disadvantage of this technique is that it relies on the memories of respondents, their ability to distinguish between effective and ineffective functioning, and their ability to recollect specific and concrete examples. However, the advantages considerably outweigh the disadvantages.

Application of the critical incident technique

Having decided that this particular data-collection technique is most suited to your needs, you can then proceed through a series of six phases, as shown in Fig. 27.2. (These phases are in addition to those described in other chapters relating to the research process in general.)

To illustrate the application of this technique, it will be assumed that you are seeking to obtain incidents which will enable you to describe the work of staff nurses in a particular hospital.

Decide who should provide critical incidents

First, identify the group or groups of people who will be able to give an informed description of effective/ineffective nursing. It is often useful to include a range of

1. Decide who should provide critical incidents.
2. Consider the number of critical incidents required.
3. Design a data-collection form.
4. Decide where to collect critical incidents.
5. Collect critical incidents.
6. Analyse critical incidents.

Fig. 27.2 Application of the critical incident technique.

respondent groups who are close to the work of the nurse. Bearing in mind that the work of nurses may include patient care, relating to other staff members, communicating with relatives, and working with other staff groups, all of these may be considered as potential respondents.

Clearly, the range of respondent groups will vary considerably from setting to setting. It may be impossible to include patients who are extremely ill, but possible to include those who are relatively well. Similarly, in those settings where the work of nurses takes them into contact with other staff groups such as physicians, occupational therapists, physiotherapists, social workers and psychologists, it may be appropriate to invite those groups to contribute. In short, decide which groups to include on the basis of their knowledge of the work of the nurse, and which groups to exclude because of their lack of contact with, or knowledge of, them.

Consider the number of critical incidents required

There is no way of knowing in advance how many incidents need to be collected to answer the question being researched. As a general guide, the less complex the subject being researched, the smaller is the number of incidents required; and the more complex the subject, the greater the number of incidents required. For example, if you are only concerned with the work of the nurse as it relates to student teaching, far fewer will be required than if you are concerned with all work carried out by the nurse. Even so, there is no way of predetermining the number of required incidents.

As a general rule, begin by collecting critical incidents without having any specific number in mind, and collect the minimum number which will provide an answer to the question being asked. This can be achieved by continuing to collect and analyse critical incidents until the last one hundred incidents fail to provide new information about the work of the nurse. Only then can you be reasonably sure that the collection of further incidents would add nothing new, and that the incidents already collected contain a reasonably comprehensive description of the subject being researched.

Design a data-collection form

The data-collection form is used to give instructions to respondents and to record their responses. It may also be used to contain additional information such as the grade of the respondent, and the grade of nurse being described in the incident. As with all data-collection tools, only information which is needed should be collected.

The form on which the critical incident is to be written will, in most instances, be accompanied by written information giving the respondent additional information such as the purpose of the study, the promise of anonymity and confidentiality, or both. An example of a data-collection form relating to effective incidents is shown in Fig. 27.3.

Please recall a time when a nurse did something which you think should be ENCOURAGED because it seemed to be very EFFECTIVE. Please give your answer in five parts as follows:

A. Grade of nurse being reported on. _____

B. What were the events leading up to the activity? _____
_____
_____
_____

C. What did the nurse do that seemed so EFFECTIVE? _____
_____
_____
_____

D. Why was the activity so EFFECTIVE? _____
_____
_____
_____

E. Grade of respondent. _____

Fig. 27.3   Sample form for collecting effective critical incidents.

In most instances, it is also of value to collect critical incidents which describe activities which are ineffective – that is, the behaviours which should be avoided in order to achieve effective functioning. Figure 27.4 presents an example of a form for collecting examples of ineffective critical incidents.

Decide where to collect critical incidents

The setting in which incidents will be collected depends largely on the purpose and scope of the study. If you are concerned only with the work of nurses within a single ward of one hospital, then only incidents from respondents who are familiar with the work of nurses in that particular ward are collected. Alternatively, to describe the work of nurses in six surgical wards within a hospital, the source of critical incidents must be extended accordingly. Finally, if you are interested in describing the work of nurses in a group of hospitals, a sample of respondents who are familiar with the work of nurses in that group of hospitals will be recruited.

Collect critical incidents

Two methods of collecting critical incidents, which resulted in very different response rates, were used by Cormack (1983). First, groups of potential nurse

Please recall a time when a nurse did something which you think should be DISCOURAGED because it seemed to be very INEFFECTIVE. Please give your answer in five parts as follows:

A. Grade of nurse being reported on. _____

B. What were the events leading up to the activity? _____

_____

_____

_____

C. What did the nurse do that seemed so INEFFECTIVE? _____

_____

_____

_____

D. Why was the activity so INEFFECTIVE? _____

_____

_____

_____

E. Grade of respondent. _____

Fig. 27.4 Sample form for collecting ineffective critical incidents.

respondents were personally given appropriate forms and instructions and asked to use the internal mailing system to return the completed critical incidents to him. The response rate using that method was 2.45%. Second, groups of nurse respondents were given the appropriate form and instructions and asked to complete them in his presence. The response rate using that method was 79%.

It is probably best to gather potential respondents in small groups and ask them to participate by giving appropriate information about the study, what is required of them, and answer questions they might have. Cormack (1983) asked his nurse respondents to provide two effective and two ineffective critical incidents.

Analyse critical incidents

Although all critical incidents will relate to the same general subject – the work of the nurse, for example – they will describe differing aspects of that work. Some incidents may relate to administrative tasks, others to patient care or to teaching, for example.

Analysis of data usually takes the form of inductive classification of incidents. This means that a classification system is constructed as the data are being analysed, rather than before. If the first incident relates to 'Physical nursing care', then one part of the classification will relate to 'Physical nursing care'. If the second incident relates to 'Teaching learners' this clearly does not fit into the only existing part of the classification system, therefore a second part must be created. This process continues until all incidents have been classified within the system which is being created as a result of the classification. The incidents may well be classified using a two- or three-tier system which starts with a fairly general description and progresses to an increasingly more specific one. The classification system may contain a number of general areas, one of which is 'NURSING CARE', a category of which may be 'Physical nursing care', and which contains a sub-category such as 'Gives bed bath'. In using critical incidents to describe the work of psychiatric nurses, Cormack (1983) created a classification system with four major areas, each with a number of categories, with each of these having a number of subcategories. An adaptation from that classification system (shown in Fig. 27.5) will demonstrate its structure.

If the critical incidents relate to the work of the nurse, you now have a description of the work of that group, and can proceed beyond this point according to the purpose of the research. If a description of the work of the nurse is all that is required, the analysis need go no further. If the aim is to establish what nurses require to be taught in order to be effective nurses, the description of the work of that group might be converted into an in-service or continuing education syllabus which will form the basis of the nurses continuing/in-service education.

A full description of the application of the critical incident technique, and the means of analysing and classifying data, is given in Cormack (1983).

Conclusions

As with all data-collection techniques, the collection of critical incidents requires careful preparation, planning and practice. It is heavily dependent on the ability of respondents to provide specific examples of the activity or work being researched, and their ability to distinguish between effective and ineffective practice. These are skills which may not come easily to potential respondents, particularly some respondents who may have little recent experience in exam-ining and describing their work in this way. However, the researcher who chooses this data-collection technique can, with sufficient effort, skill and understanding, minimize the problems which respondents will undoubtedly have.

The provision of ineffective critical incidents, crucial to understanding some aspects of effective nursing and midwifery, may be difficult for some respondents. Some may be afraid that by describing examples of ineffective functioning, they may be seen as 'telling tales' or 'letting the side down'. Bearing in mind that an understanding of what a work group should not do is as important as the knowledge of what it should do, it is essential that you enable the respondent to provide critical incidents without fear of reprisal or criticism from colleagues or senior staff. In this respect there is much to be done to ensure that the responses are confidential and provided anonymously.

AREA A: STAFF INITIATED THERAPEUTIC INTERVENTION
Categories
(1) Uses self as a therapeutic tool
   Sub-categories:
   (i) Makes self available to patients
   (ii) Provides opportunities or encourages patients to talk about their problems,
       etc. etc.
(2) Makes therapeutic use of the environment
   Sub-categories:
   (i) Encourages patient-patient understanding and relationships
   (ii) Encourages or facilitates patients playing an active part in their treatment,
       etc. etc.
Note: AREA A had a total of 5 categories

AREA B: ADMINISTRATIVE ACTIVITY
Categories:
(1) Ensures availability of non clinical patient data
   Sub-categories
   (i) Is aware of identity of patients
   (ii) Is familiar, when necessary, of the location of patients,
       etc. etc.
(2) Protects and secures patients' property
   Sub-categories
   (i) Arranges for, or offers, security of patients' property
   (ii) Shows respect and concern for patients' property,
       etc. etc.
Note: AREA B had a total of 3 categories

AREA C: PROVIDES, PLANS FOR OR MONITORS PHYSICAL CARE
Categories:
(1) Administers medication
   Sub-categories:
   (i) Administers medications carefully, accurately, and as prescribed
   (ii) Ensures, by observation or assistance, that medications are taken,
       etc. etc.
(2) Gives physical care
   Sub-categories:
   (i) Monitors physical health of patient
   (ii) Selects or initiates appropriate physical care,
       etc. etc.
Note: AREA C had a total of 2 categories

AREA D: PERSONNEL FUNCTION
Categories:
(1) Maximizes staff contribution
   Sub-categories:
   (i) Encourages, accepts, and uses appropriate staff suggestions
   (ii) Arranges work load or routine to maximize staff effectiveness and/or patient care,
       etc. etc.
Note: AREA D had a total of 2 sub-categories

Fig. 27.5 Classification of critical incidents (example).

References

Cormack, D. (1983) *Psychiatric Nursing Described*. Edinburgh: Churchill Livingston.

Cox, K., Bergen, A. & Norman, I.J. (1993) Exploring consumer views of care provided by the Macmillan nurse using the critical incident technique. *Journal of Advanced Nursing* 18: 408–15.

Fivars, G. & Gonsell, D. (1966) *Nursing Evaluation: The Problem and the Process*. New York: Macmillan.

Flanagan, J.C. (1954) The critical incident technique. *Psychological Bulletin* 51 (4): 327–58.

Jacobs, A., Gamel, N. & Brotz, C. (1973) *Critical Behaviors in Psychiatric Mental Health Nursing*, vols 1, 2 and 3. American Institutes for Research.

Norman, I.J., Redfern, S.J., Tomalin, D.A. & Oliver, S. (1992) Developing Flanagan's critical incident technique to elicit indicators of high and low quality nursing care from patients and their nurses. *Journal of Advanced Nursing* 17: 590–600.

Further reading

Allery, L.A. (1997) Why general practitioners and consultants change their clinical practice: a critical incident study. *British Medical Journal* 314 (7084): 870–74.

Buckley, T.A. (1997) Critical incident reporting in the intensive care unit, *Anaesthesia* 52 (5): 403–9.

Callery, P. & Smith, L. (1991) A study of role negotiation between nurses and the parents of hospitalized children. *Journal of Advanced Nursing* 16: 772–81.

Care, W.D. (1996) Identifying the learning needs of nurse managers. Application of the critical incident technique. *Journal of Nursing Staff Development* 12 (1): 27–30.

Cheek, J. (1997) Using critical incident technique to inform aged and extended care nursing. *Western Journal of Nursing Research* 19 (5): 667–82.

Davidson, M. & O'Brien, D. (1997) Humour in midwifery. *Modern Midwife* 7 (4): 11–14.

Minghella, E. (1995) Developing reflective practice in mental health nursing through critical incident analysis. *Journal of Advanced Nursing* 21 (2): 205–13.

Parker, D.L., Webb, J. & Dsouza, B. (1995) The value of critical incident analysis as an educational tool and its relationship to experiential learning. *Nurse Education Today* 15: 111–16.

Perry, L. (1997) Critical incidents, crucial issues: insights into the working lives of registered nurses. *Journal of Clinical Nursing* 6: 131–7.

Rosenal, L. (1995) Exploring the learner's world; critical incident methodology. *Journal of Continuing Education Nursing* 26 (3): 115–18.

von Post, I. (1996) Exploring ethical dilemmas in perioperative nursing practice through critical incidents. *Nursing Ethics* 3 (3): 236–49.

Wilde, V. (1992) Controversial hypotheses on the relationship between researcher and informant in qualitative research. *Journal of Advanced Nursing* 17: 234–42.

CHAPTER 28

Physiological measurement

Paul Fulbrook

Measurement

To measure is to determine the size or range of something. The result is a measurement that is accorded numerical significance to characterize the quantity of the object or thing measured. The tools that are used for measuring are described as instruments and are standardized to enable accurate comparison of measured things.

Physiological data

The measurement of physiological data may be performed for many reasons in nursing, midwifery and health visiting research.

Description

Data may be collected for statistical analysis in order to provide statistics about a group of patients being studied. Mean body weight or blood pressure might be appropriate measurements to make. This type of information helps to give the reader of the research a clearer picture of its relevance to his or her own practice. In other words it assists with the reader's judgement of the generalizability of the findings.

Relationship

Physiological statistics might be further analysed in relation to other data collected and the group of subjects studied. For example, a group of 40-year-old men might be studied over a period of several years in relation to heart disease. By analysing body weight and blood pressure in relation to those who do eventually develop heart disease it might be possible to identify an *at-risk* group on the basis of either their weight or blood pressure, or a combination of the two.

Response

Often physiological features are measured as a means of indicating the response to a controlled action. For example, heart rate and blood pressure changes might be measured in response to a standardized period of rest and used to indicate levels of relaxation. In a *controlled* situation the rest period would be described as the *independent variable* and the heart rate and blood pressure changes as the *dependent variables* (because it is theorized that they depend on the independent variable to produce a change).

Comparison

Physiological measurements may also be used to enable comparison of 'like with like' which would be necessary if, for example, control groups were required for a clinical trial. Using the same examples of body weight and blood pressure – this time as a measure of success – a researcher might compare an innovative nursing strategy with a conventional nursing practice. An example is Naylor & Roe's (1997) research with renal patients requiring continuous ambulatory peritoneal dialysis. They compared two methods of catheter exit site dressing. Although the study was limited by the sample size (making statistical analysis inappropriate), they did obtain a clinically significant difference in colonization rates between the control and experimental groups. (This type of research is still valuable, however, as it adds to the body of knowledge – in this case, justifying the need to do further research in the area.)

A similar, hypothetical example would be a nurse on a medical ward caring for patients following myocardial infarction who felt that her ward's rehabilitation programme lacked adequate dietary information. Although it may only be a 'hunch', a dietary information booklet might be introduced to the rehabilitation programme of an experimental group of 30 patients with high blood pressure and obesity. Its effect might be measured and compared to a control group of 30 patients with statistically similar blood pressure and weight undergoing the conventional rehabilitation programme only. It may also be relevant to record other factors, such as age and gender, since there may be differences within these groups. These factors, which are not always controlled, are described as *subject variables*.

The degree of success of introducing the dietary information booklet would be judged according to the ability of statistics to suggest that the addition of the booklet had a greater effect.

Controlled situations

It is important to note that the clinical setting rarely produces a controlled situation, since there may be many other phenomena occurring at the same time.

These independent factors are described as *extraneous variables*. For example, during a period of rest in a ward environment such as that described in the 'response' example given at the top of p. 338, there may or may not be a lot of noise, the patient in the next bed might be using a commode, or the subject may have slept very badly the night before. All of these factors might affect the person's psychological status, possibly affecting his cardiac response.

Unless the researcher collects an inordinate amount of *possibly* relevant environmental data (extraneous variables) it is impossible to state that heart rate and blood pressure changes (dependent variables) were in response to the rest period (independent variable) alone. Thus the scientific approach is to remove the subject from a relatively uncontrolled setting to a situation, such as a laboratory, where the environment can be better controlled. This approach is also limited, since the fact that the independent variable has an effect under laboratory conditions does not prove that it has the same effect in other circumstances. Thus, laboratory findings may or may not be generalized.

Assumptions

There is also a danger when making physiological measurements that the researcher will fail to measure all relevant physiological parameters. It is possible that the rehabilitation study may find that the booklet was effective in producing a more significant weight loss. However, patients having lost weight might also be suffering from lethargy and general weakness as a result of eating much less, but since there was no mechanism in the research design to account for these phenomena they were not measured and might therefore go unnoticed.

There are clearly many research situations that require the measurement of physiological parameters. The importance of considering the environmental factors has been outlined, but equal importance should be accorded to both the method of measurement and the instruments of measurement. The researcher needs to know that the measurement procedure is appropriate and that the instruments used are accurate and measure what they purport to measure.

Measurement procedures

This section details the process of making physiological measurements.

In vitro and *in vivo* measurements

Physiological measurements may be made either *in vitro* or *in vivo*. *In vitro* measurements are made away from the subject. An example of *in vitro* measurement is given by Smárson *et al.* (1997). They investigated abnormal production of serum nitric oxide in pre-eclamptic women. The sample was tested after it was obtained. In this study, the process of collecting, storing and analysing the serum samples is meticulously described. *In vitro* measurements are frequently made in a laboratory, as was the case in this research example.

An *in vivo* measurement is made directly from the patient, and a value obtained at the time of measurement. Berry *et al.*'s (1996) study examined respiratory muscle strength in older people. Based on *in vivo* measurements they assessed: respiratory muscle strength (measuring forced expiratory volume in 1 second and forced vital capacity); fat free mass (measuring skin fold thickness and bio-electrical impedance); and hand grip strength (measured using a dynamometer). By comparing the results between younger and older subjects they were able to provide evidence that respiratory muscle strength declines with age.

The issues raised in this chapter are generally relevant to both *in vitro* and *in vivo* measurements. However, most nurses are likely to be more familiar with *in vivo* measurements, and may therefore be drawn to these types of measurements in their research. Some common examples of *in vitro* and *in vivo* measurements are given in Fig. 28.1.

Physiological parameter	Measuring instrument	Type of measurement
Blood pressure	Sphygmomanometer/stethoscope	In vivo
	Arterial catheter/transducer	In vivo
	Automated cuff machine	In vivo
Blood sugar	Glucose stick/glucometer	In vitro
Urine volume	Jug/weighing scales	In vitro
	Ultrasound	In vivo
Oxygen saturation	Pulse oximeter	In vivo
	Arterial blood gas machine	In vitro
	Indwelling arterial oximeter	In vivo
Tidal volume	Wright's spirometer	In vivo
Sputum culture	Culture plate/microscope	In vitro
Calf girth	Tape measure	In vivo
Nerve conduction	Peripheral nerve stimulator	In vivo
Plasma potassium	Laboratory machine	In vitro

Fig. 28.1   Some examples of physiological measurements.

There are several research aspects in relation to *in vitro* measurements of which the nurse researcher should be aware. *In vitro* measurements usually involve the taking of a sample from a patient for analysis under laboratory conditions, although many such measurements may be made within the clinical area. Frequently the researcher will be taking samples of body fluids such as blood or urine; therefore, all necessary precautions should be taken to reduce the risk of infection and cross-infection to both the researcher and the patient, and possible contamination of the sample by the researcher.

The integrity of the sample must also be safeguarded. Samples should be taken according to a standardized protocol, correctly labelled and stored, properly transferred and correctly tested (see Ware *et al.*, 1993, for an example of such a procedure). Each step of the journey from patient to laboratory has the potential to render the sample useless for research, due to either deterioration or con-tamination.

Once the sample has arrived at the laboratory the researcher must frequently place trust in the laboratory technicians who handle and test the sample. This trust may also have to be extended to the reliability of the laboratory equipment since researchers may be denied access to the laboratory. To overcome potential problems in the laboratory it is advisable to seek advice and support from the laboratory manager who can ensure that samples are carefully managed and that measuring instruments are accurate and properly calibrated. He should also be able to provide information regarding the specifications, reliability and validity of the measuring instruments, which should be quoted in the research write-up.

Many potential problems can be avoided by maintaining control of samples taken for *in vitro* measurement. As soon as the sample passes from the researcher's hand it is out of her control and the potential for error becomes greater. To ensure the integrity of the sample the researcher should take responsibility for as much of the process as possible. This should include trans-porting samples to the laboratory and, where possible, testing them herself.

It should not always be assumed that laboratory equipment is the most accu-rate and it is well worth the researcher investigating alternative measuring instruments which can be used at the bedside. For example, there are many *dipstick* products that could be used as an alternative to sending samples to the laboratory. Many bedside instruments have been researched and validated and a frequent bonus, such as that found by Newman (1988) researching blood sugar levels, is that such instruments are more cost-effective than laboratory services.

The basic steps of making physiological measurements are summarized in Fig. 28.2.

Variables

When considering the design of a research project it is vital for the researcher to consider all the variables that might affect the physiological parameter being measured. This is particularly difficult when conducting research within the clinical setting of nursing practice because there are so many factors (extraneous and subject variables) which have the potential to influence the dependent vari-able. Examples of subject variables frequently recorded by researchers are age and gender. These are attributes of the research subjects that cannot be changed.

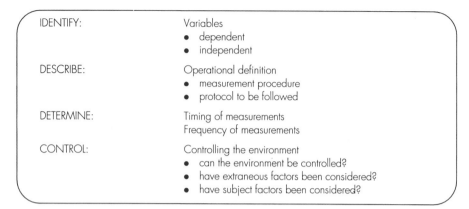

Fig. 28.2 Making physiological measurements.

However, when a researcher introduces an independent variable (such as the information booklet in the hypothetical cardiac rehabilitation study), its content or the frequency of its use might be varied.

A good research example that illustrates the value of recording multiple variables is given by Ware *et al.* (1993) in their study of illicit drug-taking mothers. In their study drug-taking was assessed by measuring drug levels in the urine of neonates. Age, race, residential area, type of delivery, previous number of pregnancies, gestational age of the neonate and several other factors were also recorded. Analysis of the data enabled the researchers to develop a profile of drug-taking mothers that subsequently helped to identify at-risk neonates.

Operational definition

When the researcher has decided which physiological measurements to record, the next stage is to give each one an operational definition. An *operational definition* is one that, for the purpose of the research study, describes what is meant by the variable term and how it is to be measured. An example of an operational definition is (Fulbrook, 1997):

> 'Axillary temperature: temperature is obtained from the sensor matrix of a single-use, disposable clinical thermometer placed high in the axilla against the torso and parallel to the patient's body for a period of 3 minutes with the arm firmly positioned to the side.'

Operational definitions are then used as a framework to guide the research process and to ensure a standardized approach. As such they are also very important for subsequent researchers wishing to replicate the study, and to enable readers of the research to apply the findings to their nursing practice. If, for example, the duration of thermometer placement had been excluded from the above operational definition, neither would be possible.

Timing and frequency of measurement

When taking both *in vitro* and *in vivo* physiological measurements it is vital to ensure that they are taken at the appropriate time and frequency.

Timing of measurement

It is particularly important to consider the measurement of the dependent variable in relation to the independent variable. For example, in the hypothetical study above which measured physiological parameters following a period of rest, there may well be an effect measurable in the cardiac response, but the duration of the effect is unknown. It might be that following a one-hour period of rest, heart rate and blood pressure do indeed fall. However, the duration of this effect might only be 20 minutes, after which the heart returns to its pre-intervention status. All measurements recorded after this time will therefore show no change. A faulty research design that specifies physiological measurements 30 minutes following the rest period will fail to identify any effect. In this respect the importance of a pilot study cannot be over-emphasized. A pilot study can save time and energy by helping to identify the appropriate timing of measurements.

A whole range of factors could affect the validity of physiological measurements if inadequate consideration is given to the timing of their recording. Additionally it may also be necessary to take repeated measurements over a period of time in order to demonstrate consistency of findings.

Frequency of measurement

The frequency with which physiological measurements are taken may itself affect the range of responses obtained, particularly if the research subject finds the measurement stressful. The recording of blood pressure is a familiar example, since blood pressure might be temporarily elevated during a stressful event. Gruber's (1974) study is a similar example. Because there was a documented potential for parasympathetic slowing of heart rate in response to rectal thermometer insertion, she undertook a study of rectal temperature measurement. Contrary to expectations she found, in fact, that her subjects' heart rates tended to increase, probably in response to the embarrassment and anxiety caused by the procedure rather than the procedure itself.

Frequency of physiological measurements should also be planned so that they do not coincide with other events which could affect them. It would be unwise to measure respiratory rate, peak flow and tidal volume on an emphysemic patient only five minutes after he has walked back from the bathroom, unless the walk back from the bathroom was the independent variable under investigation.

Sometimes physiological measurements are taken to compare the accuracy of a variety of measuring instruments, or possibly to compare a physiological parameter measured at different sites. The researcher, for example, might wish to compare the accuracy of blood pressure measurements using a conventional sphygmomanometer with an indwelling arterial line and a non-invasive automated instrument (see Norman *et al.*, 1991, for a comparable example). Another example is that of Fehring & Schlaff (1998), who compared three different methods of predicting/detecting ovulation: assessment of cervico-vaginal mucus (colour, stretch and consistency); detection of luteinizing hormone (using a self-test urine dipstick); and vaginal electrochemical assessment (using an electrical monitor). Following their research they were able to state that the electrical monitor (which they were seeking to validate) was as clinically reliable as other more traditional/conventional methods.

Ideally such measurements should be performed simultaneously to ensure that the conditions under which all measurements are taken are identical. It is also ideal to repeat measurements over a period of time, which enables the researcher to demonstrate reliability of findings and adds to the validity of the research.

Another reason to take repeated measurements is to demonstrate that the findings are consistent under a variety of conditions such as sleep and wake or day and night patterns. In particular, several physiological parameters are known to be affected by circadian variations (Clancy & McVicar, 1994). A single cluster of measurements taken in isolation has little validity compared to repeated measurements taken over a period of time.

Controlling the environment

As described in the introduction, it is very difficult to control the environment when research is carried out within a non-laboratory setting, such as a clinical ward area. The scientific approach is to reduce the potential for unpredictable factors that may affect the research findings; therefore, the easily controlled environment of the laboratory is deemed the most suitable. However, within the clinical setting it is often more appropriate to try to consider all the factors which may impinge on the phenomenon being investigated. When designing a research study the researcher must therefore make a decision in this regard, and the number of variables that require measurement or recording should be determined in advance.

Since nursing, midwifery and health visiting are professions which concern themselves with caring for patients it is very difficult to remove patients from the health care setting and study them in isolation. Most clinical research will probably (and desirably) be carried out in the context of the situation in which it is likely to occur. As such, rather than attempt to control the environment, the researcher should attempt to take into account the environmental factors that might affect the measurement of physiological parameters.

There are many environmental factors that could affect the physiological variable being measured. For example, ambient temperature will affect skin temperature, as might recent exertion. Also, intrinsic psychological stressors such as anxiety or extrinsic psychological stressors such as those produced by excessive noise and other noxious stimuli, such as strong smells, might induce a degree of stress that affects the cardiac parameter being measured. Simple investigations such as pupil diameter may vary in response to changes in light intensity. Thus it is important for the researcher, who is most likely to be found investigating phenomena within the health care setting, to consider environmental influences on the variable being measured. Because it is rarely possible to standardize the environment of nursing practice, variations in environmental factors should be noted at the time and subsequently taken into account.

The potential for environmental influence on a dependent variable is given in the following hypothetical example. An early study of cardiac output in shocked patients suggested that it correlates with great toe temperature (Joly & Weil, 1969). More recently a small study has challenged this, stating that it is irrational to base therapy on this measurement (Woods *et al.*, 1987). An intensive care nurse decides to do a more up-to-date study and records the great toe temperature of a series of clinically shocked patients. She is careful to ensure that her research design is sound and does in fact make very accurate recordings of both cardiac output and great toe temperature. Subsequent statistical analysis indicates a relationship between the two variables whereby great toe temperature falls when cardiac output falls. The nurse is quite pleased with her findings and is considering trying to get her research published. A colleague asks whether she recorded room temperature and also points out that some patients' feet were covered by blankets whereas others were not. The nurse is suddenly aware that there were other factors that might have influenced great toe temperature. Unfortunately she omitted to record them and realizes that, because she cannot categorically state that the temperature changes were solely as a result of cardiac output changes, the validity of her findings is severely limited.

There is clearly a potential for environmental factors to influence both the accuracy and the meaning of physiological measurements. The nurse researcher should attempt either to negate their influence or to ensure that their presence is recorded and considered with respect to the data analysis. Often there may be factors which, on their own, have no measurable effect on the dependent variable, but when they occur in combination with two or more other factors do exert an effect.

Measuring instruments

This section describes issues related to the use of measuring instruments, and is summarized in Fig. 28.3. The strength of measuring instruments lies in their accuracy and objectivity; that is, their ability to quantify a phenomenon. Arguably machines reduce the potential for human error. Therefore, when two or

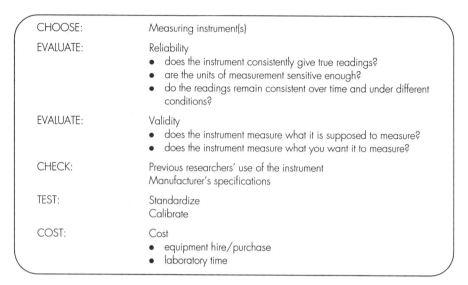

Fig. 28.3 Measuring instruments.

more researchers use the same instrument of measurement, they are likely to obtain highly similar results.

Reliability and validity

There are two main issues to consider with regard to the use of instruments for the measurement of physiological parameters: reliability and validity. Reliability is concerned with the instrument's accuracy of measurement, whereas validity is concerned with its ability to measure what it is supposed to measure.

Reliability in physiological measurement

Reliability is a measure of the instrument's sensitivity – in other words, its precision of measurement. Precision is important in terms of the accuracy and consistency of measurement. A measuring instrument must be sensitive enough to measure a physiological parameter in question to a satisfactory degree of precision. If, for example, babies' weight gains in response to either breast- or bottle-feeding were to be measured with a set of scales whose smallest increment of measurement was a kilogram, they would quite clearly be of no use to the researcher. Similarly, if a set of scales were used for the same study, but were found to have a variance of plus or minus 5% when a standard weight is placed on them, then they too are *unreliable* and of little use.

The reliability of an instrument is determined by many factors and the researcher would be unwise to accept a manufacturer's specification regarding the accuracy of an instrument, since specifications are usually quoted on the basis of standardized laboratory conditions. Some instruments become inaccurate with prolonged use or wear and tear, whereas others may be more prone to errors caused by the local environment. Electronic instruments in particular are prone to errors caused by electrical interference.

Prior to commencing a research study it is advisable to test the measuring instrument to ensure that it is accurate when in use. A pilot study will usually highlight any errors or inconsistencies. Some instruments are supplied with their own testing instruments and, whenever possible, these should be used. Occasionally it is not possible to test some equipment before use, for example sterile equipment. In such circumstances the reliability must be accepted from the manufacturer's specifications.

Validity in physiological measurement

Just because an instrument is reliable does not mean that it is valid. A researcher might obtain a highly accurate measure of body length using a tape measure but it would not be *valid* if the researcher wishes to know the weight of the person.

The researcher needs to address the issue of how appropriate the measuring instrument is for measuring the physiological parameter in question. Some instruments do not actually measure the parameter for which they give a value. For example, tympanic thermometers *predict* core body temperature on the basis of infrared light emitted from the tympanic membrane. It may not therefore be as reliable in measuring as an electronic temperature sensor placed in the pulmonary artery measuring *actual* core body temperature.

It is frequently helpful to refer to previous research studies that have either used the same instrument or evaluated its reliability and validity. A lot of time and energy can be wasted trying to test instruments which have already been scrutinized by previous researchers.

Cost

Another issue to consider with respect to measuring instruments is that of cost. Electronic machines in particular are very expensive, both to purchase and maintain. It is always worth trying to enlist the instrument manufacturer's support for the research study. Because it is in their interests to promote their products they are frequently amenable to lending or even donating equipment for research purposes.

In summary, the nurse researcher must carefully consider the appropriateness of any instrument used to measure physiological parameters for a research study. While the issue of cost must be considered, it should not be at the expense of instrument reliability and validity. Finally, it should not be assumed that a machine is any more capable than a human of measuring a physiological parameter. The more complicated a measuring instrument, the more potential there is for both researcher handling error and internal malfunction.

For an overview on reliability and validity of measuring instruments see Giuffre (1995a, 1995b).

Data collection

Sampling

Sampling procedures are described in Chapter 22. The important factor regarding a sample is that it should be representative of the population being studied. In the context of physiological measurements, sampling merits some consideration.

Data collectors

If, for example, the nurse researcher wishes to know the mean weight and blood pressure of patients admitted to a medical ward, she has a choice: she can measure the above parameters of *all* the patients admitted over a certain period of time, or she can select a sample. What decision she comes to in this regard may depend on what is most convenient for her to do, since time is often a major factor. Should she decide to take measurements from all patients, then her presence, or that of other data collectors, is required throughout the 24-hour period for the duration of the study, which is not usually a practical option. While ensuring that all patients are included, this also introduces the potential for variation in the measurements recorded due to slightly different techniques. The advantage of the nurse researcher taking all the measurements herself is that she is sure, and can therefore state, that a uniform technique was used on every occasion.

Standard technique

If colleagues are enlisted to gather data it is vital to ensure that they are all briefed in the measurement technique required and are fully conversant with the operation of instruments used to obtain measurements. Chan (1993), who compared ultrasound estimation of bladder urine volume with its actual measurement following catheterization, described such a procedure. In order to ensure that the method was correct, nurses had first to be trained in the use of ultrasound techniques.

Pilot study

A pilot study is necessary prior to commencing the main study to test the ability of the research assistants to obtain accurate data.

It is all too easy to assume that nurses, by virtue of their everyday role, are more than capable of taking physiological measurements. Even a simple procedure like taking a patient's blood pressure is fraught with potential problems, which may lead to inaccuracies and inconsistent techniques between data collectors. For example: Was the patient sitting up or lying down? How long had he been in this position? Where was the sphygmomanometer placed in relation to the patient? Where was the cuff placed on the upper arm? Was the cuff the correct size? Was the cuff correctly applied? How was the degree of cuff inflation determined? Was the rubber tubing in good condition? Was the fourth or the fifth Korotkov sound used to determine diastolic pressure? Was the patient relaxed? The list may be very long, but each step of the procedure should be considered to ensure standardization.

Ethical issues

In any research study there are many ethical issues which require consideration. These are addressed in detail elsewhere in this book, but there are some specific ethical issues which should be considered in relation to the measurement of physiological variables.

Foreseeable harm

No foreseeable harm should come to the subject as a result of physiological measurement. The researcher must therefore make a judgement in this respect. Virtually every procedure imaginable carries with it a degree of risk, however small. This degree of risk must be balanced with the need to carry out the research, but always with the balance tilted in favour of the research subject. It should also be remembered that it is not just physical harm that may be caused; there may also be a psychological effect, which might be as simple as embarrassment or loss of dignity.

Abnormal findings

The researcher must also consider in advance what she will do if her findings are such that there is a threat to the patient's health. For example, what course of action should she take if she finds that one of her subjects has an abnormally elevated blood pressure? Again, the principle is that the patient should not come to any harm as a result of the research study. Quite clearly, in such instances, the researcher's priorities must be with the research subjects. All decisions must be made in their best interests, even if this means modifying or abandoning the research study.

Conclusions

Physiological measurements may be taken by researchers for a variety of research purposes, and provided that several basic rules are followed, highly reliable and valid data will be obtained for analysis.

In the first instance the researcher should determine what measurements are necessary for the study. This should be considered from the point of view of both independent and dependent variables and in the light of the potential for environmental factors to affect their reliability and validity. The measurement technique should be carefully thought through and standardized. This is particularly important if more than one researcher is collecting data. Any instruments used to measure physiological parameters should be carefully considered in terms of reliability and validity and ideally should be tested for accuracy prior to commencement of the main study. As with all research, ethical issues must be carefully thought through in advance and permission obtained as appropriate.

References

Berry, J.K., Vitalo, C.A., Larson, J.L., Patel, M. & Kim, M.J. (1996) Respiratory muscle strength in older adults. *Nursing Research* 45 (3): 154–9.

Chan, H. (1993) Non-invasive bladder volume measurement. *Journal of Neuroscience Nursing* 25 (5): 309–12.

Clancy, J. & McVicar, A. (1994) Circadian rhythms 1: Physiology. *British Journal of Nursing* 3 (13): 657–61.

Fehring, R.J. & Schlaff, W.D. (1998) Accuracy of the Ovulon fertility monitor to predict and detect ovulation. *Journal of Nurse-Midwifery* 43 (2): 117–20.

Fulbrook, P. (1997) Core body temperature measurement: a comparison of axilla, tympanic membrane and pulmonary artery blood temperature. *Intensive and Critical Care Nursing* 13 (5): 266–72.

Giuffre, M. (1995a) Reading research critically: assessing the validity and reliability of research instrumentation: Part 1. *Journal of Post Anesthesia Nursing* 10 (1): 33–7.

Giuffre, M. (1995b) Reading research critically: assessing the validity and reliability of research instrumentation: Part 2. *Journal of Post Anesthesia Nursing* 10 (2): 107–12.

Gruber, P.A. (1974) Changes in cardiac rate associated with the use of the rectal thermometer in the patient with acute myocardial infarction. *Heart and Lung* 3 (2): 28–92.

Joly, H.R. & Weil, M.H. (1969) Temperature of the great toe as an indicator of the severity of shock. *Circulation* 39: 131–8.

Naylor, M. & Roe, B. (1997) A study of the efficacy of dressings in preventing infections of continuous ambulatory peritoneal dialysis catheter exit sites. *Journal of Clinical Nursing* 6 (1): 17–24.

Newman, R.H. (1988) Bedside blood sugar determinations in the critically ill. *Heart and Lung* 17 (6): 667–9.

Norman, E., Gadaleta, D. & Grirno, C.C. (1991) An evaluation of three blood pressure methods in a stabilised acute trauma population. *Nursing Research* 40 (2): 8–9.

Smárson, A.K., Allman, K.G., Young, D. & Redman, C.W.G. (1997) Elevated levels of serum nitrate, a stable end product of nitric oxide, in women with pre-eclampsia. *British Journal of Obstetrics and Gynaecology* **104** (5): 538–43.

Ware, S., Liguori, R., Jamerson, P., Weiner, V. & Joubert-Jackson, C. (1993) Prevalence of substance abuse in a midwestern city. *Journal of Pediatric Nursing* **8** (3): 152–8.

Woods, I., Wilkins, R.G., Edwards, J.D., Martin, P.D. & Faragher, E.B. (1987) Danger of using core/peripheral temperature gradient as a guide to therapy in shock. *Critical Care Medicine* **15** (9): 850–2.

D: Data handling

The preceding phases of the research process will have taken full account of the need for data to be stored, analysed, presented and reported. When planning a study, particularly when considering data-collection methods and the quantity and type of data to be collected, the researcher will have taken account of how the collected data will be handled. The handling of data collected during the pilot study will determine whether or not the data can successfully be handled; if there are problems, then the data-collection methods can be adjusted in a further pilot study.

Data handling has three distinct elements: storage (see Chapter 29), analysis (see Chapters 30 to 33) and presentation (see Chapter 34).

Data storage

Desmond F.S. Cormack and David C. Benton

The preceding six chapters have presented a selection of means of collecting research data. As the data are being collected, or at the end of their collection, they will have to be stored and subsequently analysed. Data storage has three basic related purposes: first, to ensure that no data are lost; second, to enable information to be contained in a way which makes it reasonably accessible; third, to enable the researcher to analyse the data.

Nurses and midwives are no strangers to information collection and storage, much of their time being used to record and store clinical data. Usually, however, it is stored in a way which would make an analysis of large quantities difficult. For example, in relation to each of the 600 patients in a given hospital, information relating to all patients' clinical status will be recorded daily, if not more frequently. However, if a nurse, midwife, administrator or researcher wishes to establish how many patients had been incontinent each day during a specific one-week period, this may prove difficult if not impossible to ascertain. The reason for this difficulty is that episodes of incontinence, if they are recorded, are recorded in relation to individual patients and not in a way which would allow easy access, or which would enable overall calculations to be made. Alternatively, a researcher may well collect a large amount of data which, in their original form, are difficult to store and analyse. For example, in relation to the national census, the original data would consist of many millions of census forms. Clearly, it would be difficult, although not impossible, to analyse the data by making a manual count of the many millions of forms involved. However, a better approach is to store the data in such a way as to make such analysis easier – for example, in a computer. The purpose of this chapter is to illustrate two commonly used methods of storing data: storage in original form, and storage using a computer. As with all phases of the research process, those stages which precede data storage must take account of the proposed data storage method. Similarly, the choice of data storage method will have implications for the next phase of the process, data analysis.

The means and ease by which data can be stored partly depends on whether they are of a qualitative or quantitative nature. Qualitative data are not readily transferable into a numerical format; in addition, they are often generated as a result of open questions. An example of an open question is: 'What do you find interesting about nursing?'. Responses to this question may include a verbal reply lasting up to five minutes along with a considerable amount of additional non-verbal information such as gesture, sound inflection and pace of expression. Such responses recorded on paper may occupy two or three pages and are relatively difficult to store in anything other than the original form. However, technology has advanced to a stage whereby various computer programs can take such dialogue and analyse it for the presence of common words and concepts (more information is given on this in Chapter 33). The problem with this approach is that it can disassociate the verbal content from the non-verbal material.

In contrast, quantitative data, which are often generated as a result of closed questions, are relatively easily stored in a non-original format. An example of a closed question is, 'Are you a registered nurse?', responses being 'Yes' or 'No' or 'Don't know'. The data generated as a result of such a question, answered by 100 respondents might be:

'Yes'	24
'No'	75
'Don't know'	1

Storage in original form

Data are usually recorded initially in writing and occasionally by means such as tape or video recordings. Invariably, but not necessarily, data collected by means other than in writing are transferred into written form. However, new digital storage techniques have enabled video and sound recordings to be stored, copied and disseminated using state of the art computer approaches.

It is appropriate for some forms of data to remain (and to be stored) in writing and subsequently to be analysed directly from that format. For example, if data are qualitative in nature, they might be difficult to store in any other than the written form. One instance might be when the data were produced as a result of semi-structured interview in order to determine patients' perceptions of 'being hospitalized', and the researcher feels that analysis is best done by reading and re-reading transcripts of the interview; maintaining data in their original form might then be the preferred option. Alternatively, the data might be sufficiently compact to require analysis in the original form – for example, a single case study. Finally, data may be of the quantitative type but be of a small enough volume to be handled manually – for example, in the case of 100 questionnaires, each with five questions. A limiting factor is, however, often the level of analysis to be carried out. If complex analytical processes are to be undertaken then the advantages of using computer technology as opposed to manual calculation become self-evident. Not only is time saved but invariably accuracy is increased when large data sets are involved.

Data, therefore, can be legitimately stored in, and subsequently analysed from, their original form. Storage of data in anything other than their original form is only undertaken if there are advantages in using some other means of storage and subsequent analysis. When storing data in their original form, ensure that each piece of data is clearly recorded. For example, long-hand notes taken hurriedly during an interview might have to be rewritten and possibly typed. Second, ensure that each answer, or the reply from individual subjects, is discrete and that you can clearly identify and separate each respondent's response generally, and individual questions in particular. Third, ensure that the response from each respondent is clearly labelled – for example, nurse 1, 2, 3, and so on. Fourth, scan all data immediately after recording and ensure that the record of responses is complete. Finally, make a second copy of all data, storing each copy in a separate location. Indeed, this applies to all forms of data storage. Occasionally something catastrophic, such as a fire, can occur and without a duplicate copy many weeks, months or even years of work can literally go up in smoke. With the advent of electronic storage media and ready access to the internet it is now possible to store material in digital vaults. These vaults are in effect nothing more than another computer that will offer you the opportunity to store your data for a small charge. For further information of this type of service readers should access the following web page: http://www.dantz.com.

The remainder of this chapter will be concerned with storage of quantitative data. However, bear in mind that qualitative data can be converted into quantitative data by counting the number of occasions that a particular item appears in the qualitative data. For example, you might count the number of times respondents refer to 'working with people' when describing what they find interesting about nursing.

The most commonly used means of storing data, other than in the original format, is on a computer system; this will be discussed using data collection on a four item questionnaire as an example (Fig. 29.1).

For larger quantities of data, perhaps in excess of 500 questionnaires, and for data which will be analysed using inferential statistics, the use of a computing system becomes rather more necessary although still not absolutely essential.

Computers

A variety of computer systems can be used to facilitate storage and analysis of data. Networked systems are commonly available in many organizations and universities. Stand-alone personal computers, either desktop or laptop, are readily available and can be used to store and analyse a wide variety of data. In addition, a variety of palm-top devices can also be used. All three types may be likened to very sophisticated electronic calculators, with computers having the added ability to store data and accept new programs to enable them to function in a variety of ways.

Please place tick ☑ against appropriate reply/replies to each question			Do Not Write In This Margin
Q1 Sex	Male	☑	1 2
	Female	☐	☑☐
Q2 Qualifications	RM	☐	1 2 3 4 5
	HV	☐	☐☐☑☐☐
	RN	☑	
	RNT	☐	
	Other	☐	
Q3 Work Status	Full time	☑	1 2
	Part time	☐	☑☐
Q4 Shift	Day	☑	1 2
	Night	☐	☑☐

Fig. 29.1   Sample questionnaire (filled in to illustrate data to be stored).

The physical components of a computer – the parts which can actually be seen and touched – are referred to as *hardware*. Thus, if you purchase a computer, you are purchasing hardware. The programs which exist within a commercial computer, or are written by a programmer and placed on it, are referred to as *software*. Computer users can either write their own software (programs), buy them from a company selling specialist software packages, or use the services of a computer programmer. The languages used by computer programmers are many and varied and may only be of passing interest to the researcher since most researchers will use existing programs. Only if you have very specialized analysis requirements will it be necessary to write your own programs. Although the option of writing programs is available, most researchers would not choose to do so since the time required to do so is, for most researchers, excessive. With this point in mind it is important to remember that it is not necessary to understand how a computer works, or how to write programs, in order to make full use of computers. However, if you do not personally have appropriate computer skills and knowledge, you must have access to someone who does.

Networked systems

These are large, usually quite expensive systems that link together anything from a few to several thousand computers distributed over an entire, often multi-site, university campus or hospital. These systems can easily cost in excess of several hundred thousand pounds, and will clearly be beyond the budget of all but very large-scale, long-term research projects. However, access to networked computer systems should be considered, even in relation to the most modest piece of research. In principle, researchers employed within the

National Health Service have reasonable access to such resources, as do staff working in universities and other higher education institutions. These networks will have, in addition to the computers, a wide range of other additional hardware such as printers, input and storage devices. Because of the fact that a network provides contact between a number of computers it is possible to have a number of researchers simultaneously inputting data and/or working on the analysis of large data sets.

In addition to access to the system, nurse researchers should also negotiate access to computer programming and support staff, and to NHS employed statisticians who may be required to give advice regarding data analysis. Thus, the nurse researcher should negotiate, where appropriate, the same access to computing and related facilities as is available to other researchers: medical staff and psychologists, for example.

Personal computers

An average personal computing system can now be bought at relatively low cost, which is invariably within the range of even the modest research budget. Figure 29.2 illustrates the normal system configuration which includes:

1. A personal computer with visual display
2. A typewriter style data input facility (keyboard)
3. Printer and supply of print-out paper
4. Disk drive and supply of disks

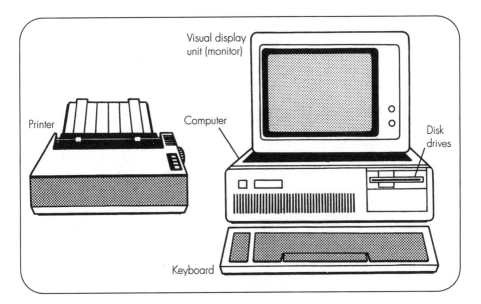

Fig. 29.2 Schematic diagram of personal computer hardware.

At present, an increasingly large range of personal computer systems are available, and you will profit from consulting someone experienced in computing systems before buying one.

The advantage of a personal computer lies in its relatively low cost, its portability, and the ease with which it can be installed and maintained in any domestic style environment that has an electricity supply. With today's technology, the storage capacity of the system, although smaller and less flexible than a networked system, can in real terms be sufficient for all but the largest studies which involve national data sets. Even in these circumstances, with the advent of compact disk storage systems that hold phenomenal amounts of data, personal computers are in effect the preferred choice. For example, some single compact disks can contain the equivalent of about 20 feet of library shelving. For smaller studies, disks which may be as small as three and a half inches in diameter can hold considerable quantities of data. They are easily stored and can be marked to identify the data they contain.

As with the network system, commercial software packages are available, and these will enable you to make full use of the personal computer even if you have limited or, as is usually the case, no programming skills and do not have access to specialist programmers. Such programs include some which enable descriptive and inferential analysis and specialized data presentation. For a full description of the application of computers to data analysis, turn to Chapter 33.

Hand-held systems

Over the past few years a wide range of hand-held devices have become available. These systems can be used to record data direct onto electronic storage devices. Because of their portability and flexibility, data can be recorded immediately as part of the data-collection process. These systems can use miniature keyboards or often a special stylus (pen) to enter the data.

Use of computers

Computers have been designed to enable large quantities of data to be stored and quickly analysed. Not all data, however, are suitable for computer application, but most can be converted into a form which is suitable. Data of the quantitative type are most suitable; qualitative data are less suitable but may be converted into a form suitable for computer storage and analysis (Chapter 30). Figure 29.1 illustrates how a four-item questionnaire might be constructed in order that the resulting data can be stored in a computer.

The sequence of events in the collection of data on the questionnaire – which would obviously be accompanied by detailed instructions and a letter of explanation – is as follows:

1. The respondent places a tick in the boxes which correspond to his answer.
2. On receipt of the questionnaire, the researcher records each of the four answers on a selected single box located at the right margin of the questionnaire.
3. Responses are transferred to a means by which the data can be placed into a computer (see Chapter 33).

Data for network systems, personal computer and hand-held devices can be entered in a wide number of ways. For example, and most commonly, computer systems data can be typed in using a keyboard similar to that on an ordinary typewriter; some systems can use bar codes that can be scanned in a similar way to the systems used in some supermarket checkouts; flatbed scanners, which look like an automatic feed photocopier, can also be used if large quantities of data are to be entered.

Coding

Data that have a fixed number of responses will require to be coded for entry into the computer system of your choice. For example, in relation to question 1 of the questionnaire (sex), the answer is 'male', indicated by a tick in box 1.

The answer to question 1 is subsequently coded using the numerical value that equates to the response given; for example, 1 equals male, 2 equals female. You may also have to agree a value for missing data.

In collecting data for storage and subsequent analysis in a computer, the important point is to collect the data in a format that is suitable for transfer to a computing system. Provided that this is done – usually with advice from someone with an understanding of computing systems – the data can then be transferred into the computer by someone with the requisite specialist knowledge. Thus, if you ensure that data are in a computer-compatible format, then using the computer to store and analyse them will not present problems. The essential points are:

1. Give each subject an individual code number, e.g. 001, 002, 003, etc.
2. Give each question an individual code number, e.g. 0.1, 0.2, 0.3, etc.
3. Give each potential response an individual code number, e.g. male = 1, female = 2; yes = 1, no = 2, don't know = 3.
4. Remember to allocate a specific code for missing data.
5. Try to identify any responses for one question that can be used to identify incompatible responses in a subsequent question.

The need to give each subject an individual and unique code is particularly important if, subsequently, relational database techniques are to be used. This is where data can be gathered from a subject on several occasions and, by use of the unique identifier, all data linked for more complex analysis such as time series techniques.

Some computer programs can be set up to detect incompatible response options between specific questions. For example, a general health questionnaire might include questions on sexual health, and if a subject responds to a question on gender indicating that the subject is female, then questions relating to testicular examinations should be blank. If this is not the case then the anomalous responses are highlighted and the researcher can check the original questionnaire, the coding frame and transcription entry for accuracy.

State of the art solutions

Before deciding which method of data storage to use, consider available alternatives and their relative strengths and weaknesses. The advice of researchers who have used data storage techniques, and of those with experience of computing systems, should be obtained during the planning phases of the research.

Increasingly researchers are using integrated software and hardware systems. For example, a questionnaire can be designed on screen using software that will then generate a data storage structure capable of receiving the information from individual respondents. Respondents may, for example, sit down at a portable personal computer such as a laptop or use a hand-held device and type in the answers to the questions posed. These can then be coded automatically, ready for analysis. Alternatively if a large sample of subjects that are geographically dispersed is being researched, the questionnaire can be printed out and distributed via the mail. Returned questionnaires that have been clearly completed, usually using a soft pencil or black ink pen, can be read into the computer using a flatbed scanner. The scanner essentially locates the ticks made and codes them automatically. The advantage of this approach is that the risk of error resulting from having to have a data entry clerk, or the researcher code, transpose and enter the data is significantly reduced.

Although not readily available, some systems can now use electronically generated speech to ask questions. Provided the responses are limited and the respondent answers clearly, they can be recorded and coded by the computer. Speech recognition is currently progressing rapidly but as yet is only able to deal with quantitative data collection. Often it is necessary for the respondent to pronounce a series of words or phrases to enable the computer to become familiar with the subject's speech pattern (accent). Although this is very much tomorrow's technology some of it is already in use and may well be available to a researcher who cultivates links with higher educational establishments.

Large volumes of qualitative data

Up to this point the majority of data being discussed have been of the quantitative type. However, with the advent of digital cameras and sound recording it is possible to store directly onto electronic computer media, video or audio sequences of data. For example, the clinical practice associated with a nurse offering psychosocial interventions can be recorded. Subsequent analysis can then examine both verbal and non-verbal aspects of the intervention. There are a variety of standard formats that can be used to store video and audio sequences, however these kinds of data, particularly in the case of video, require large amounts of space.

Even with modern computer systems that have large hard disk storage capacities it is normal to use additional high-volume storage devices such as recordable compact disks or digital video disk recording devices. The cost of these devices is reducing all the time but for the neophyte researcher additional advice from both experienced researchers and computer experts should be sought before embarking on a study that requires this sort of data storage approach.

Conclusions

Various approaches can be used for the storage of research data. These range from manual records in original form to a variety of computer-based solutions. The choice of approach should be informed by careful consideration of the relative advantages and disadvantages of storage technique, the volume of data involved and the resources available. Whichever approach is used, the researcher must be confident that the storage will enable the timely and accurate analysis of the data collected.

Researchers can use computers to store both quantitative and qualitative data. Although textual and numeric data are the types most commonly stored and analysed by computer-based systems, the advent of more sophisticated and powerful computers also enables video and audio data to be stored, accessed and analysed.

Further reading

Maintz, J. (1997) Organizing, storing, and analysing qualitative research information in a computer database. *Scandinavian Journal of Primary Health Care* **15** (1): 7–9.

Subramanian, A.K., McAfee, A.T. and Getzinger, J.P. (1997) Use of the world wide web for multisite data collection. *Academic Emergency Medicine* **4** (8): 811–17.

Talacko, P. (1999) Data back-up using the Internet. *Internet Works* **18**: 63–6.

CHAPTER 30

Quantitative analysis (descriptive)

Peter T. Donnan

The following two chapters consider how to go about a quantitative analysis of data. The amount of data collected may be large or small, depending on the purpose of the study. The aims of the study may be either simply descriptive or concerned with making inferences, often involving comparison of groups. In both cases numerical information on a number of individuals will have been collected and these form the dataset for analysis.

One of the main purposes of descriptive analysis is to summarize the data, extracting the salient points from the results, rather than presenting every data item on every subject. Descriptive statistics will form the subject matter of this chapter. This is often thought of as the only purpose of a statistical analysis, but this is only a preliminary stage which leads to the most important purpose, that of drawing inferences from the data.

An inferential statistical analysis is concerned with making judgements and extrapolating results; testing hypotheses about the population of interest based upon the information obtained from a sample of that population. This will be explored more fully in Chapter 31. In practice both approaches are often used as they provide complementary views of the results.

Good design = Good statistics

A good statistical analysis is dependent on good design. A study needs to be well designed in order to provide useful results and conclusions and it is important to consider all aspects of the statistical analysis at the outset. This implies that a well-written plan or protocol is produced at an early stage, giving details of the design, aims, methods and analysis before the data are collected. It is not efficient to consider statistics only after the research has been carried out. Instead, it is necessary to set out the study in such a way that the research is more likely than not to provide the answer sought. It is poor practice to collect data in the hope that it might be useful in the future or concoct the aims of the study after the data have been collected. The most important part of the design process is therefore to state clearly the *aims* of the investigation.

If the aims are stated clearly (see Chapter 7), then all other aspects of design will follow, such as:

(1) the nature of the data;
(2) how the data are to be collected (Chapters 23–28);
(3) the appropriate analysis (Chapter 31).

Assuming a well-designed study, with clearly stated prior aims and with validated data collection, the next step is to consider ways of presenting the results. Communication of the results is a vital aspect of any research. The appropriate use of statistics can provide a systematic means of assessing, summarizing and presenting the findings of such research.

In most research it is usually not possible to obtain all the information from the population of interest because of resource constraints. A *population* is not only a group of people, but, more exactly, is a collection or set of measurements. For example, you might be interested in the proportion of HIV-positive patients who develop full-blown AIDS after a certain period of time. The population consists of all patients who are HIV positive. The data acquired (using the methods of Chapter 22) form a *sample* of this population – one from a single hospital, for example – which it is hoped has characteristics similar to the population from which they were drawn – that is, the data are representative of that population. Simple random sampling (Chapter 22) is used to aid the collection of a representative sample.

Importance of sample size

The size of the sample collected may be outside the control of the researcher. For example, the researcher may be interested in a rare disease and so the number of patients with the disease (those whose records are available) will form the sample. However, in most cases, the researcher will have some choice in the size of the sample to be used. If the questions posed by the study involve the comparison of groups, it is especially important to have an adequate sample size in each group. This is estimated at the design stage. It would be wasteful of resources to sample more than is required, but a more usual error is when the sample is too small, such that the data acquired are not adequate to fulfil the aims of the study. Consider also the ethics of the latter case, especially if the research involves an intervention trial of a new treatment. The topic of sample size is a factor of major importance, although it will not be pursued further here. Textbook formulae are available for use in the calculation of sample size (see Armitage & Berry, 1994 or Lemeshow *et al.*, 1990), and these should be consulted with the aid of a statistician prior to data collection. There are a number of computer packages such as nQuery Advisor® which are devoted to sample size and power estimation.

Types of data

It is necessary to consider the type of data being dealt with in your research since the statistical methods used and the presentation of the data will depend on this. There are basically two types: qualitative (or categorical data), and quantitative data. The qualities and quantities measured are known as variables. Height, for example, is a continuous variable; degrees of pain or satisfaction with care are ordered categorical variables. The term *qualitative* refers to a *type of data* in categories and as such is open to statistical or quantitative analysis. This should not be confused with qualitative *analysis* which is a different approach and method of analysis (see Chapters 12 and 32).

Qualitative or categorical data arise whenever individuals are classified into groups such as sex (male/female), marital status (married/divorced/separated/single) or blood group (A/B/AB/O). There is no numerical relationship between these categories and hence data of this type are known as *nominal* (Table 30.1).

Table 30.1 Types of data

Type	Description		Examples
Qualitative (categorical)	(1)	Nominal: data in separate classes which have no numberical relationship	Types of burn: thermal, chemical, electrical; absence/presence pain (binary)
	(2)	Ordinal: data in separate classes with order relationship	Degrees of pain; social class; degrees of agreement with statement
Quantitative	(1)	Discrete: arise from counts or scales	Number of hospital beds; score on visual analogue scale
	(2)	Continuous measurements: can take any value in range	Height; weight; haemoglobin level; cholesterol level

A special case arises when there are only two categories, such as male and female, which form a binary variable. The outcome of an intervention study is often expressed as a binary variable, for example, satisfied/unsatisfied; hypertensive/not hypertensive. On the other hand, there is sometimes a natural order to the groups, for example, degrees of pain in the categories of none/slight/moderate/severe, and this is referred to as an ordered categorical or ordinal variable. Degrees of agreement with a statement are often found in questionnaires to assess attitudes and feelings on particular topics (Likert scales, see Chapter 25) and these can be treated as ordinal variables.

Quantitative data (Table 30.1) can arise from counts such as the number of hospital beds or the number of angina attacks in a specified time period. These can only have discrete values. Finally, quantitative data come in the form of continuous measures such as weight or blood cholesterol level, and these can take any value in a specified range. These values are only limited by the accuracy and precision of the measuring instrument. Note that there are many variables which lie somewhere between ordinal categorical and quantitative. If the number of ordered categories is large (say 10+) this variable could be treated as quantitative. Values from visual analogue scales or semantic differential scales (Chapter 25) could also be treated as quantitative, where patients are instructed to mark on a line between two extremes or tick in boxes how they feel regarding aspects of their life (Fig. 30.1), which is then given a score using a template.

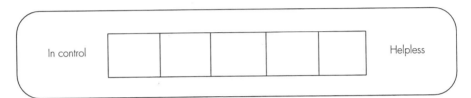

Fig. 30.1   Example of semantic-differential scale.

As well as being useful for presentation purposes, this classification also moulds the way in which the data can be analysed. Discrete and categorical variables lend themselves to comparisons of proportions in different groups.

Continuous data tend to be summarized by some form of average, the mean or median along with a measure of spread, and these terms will be described fully later. In a nutritional intervention intended to reduce blood cholesterol in one group compared to a control group, for example, the comparison would be made in terms of the difference in mean reduction in cholesterol between both groups.

The distinction made between qualitative (categorical) and quantitative, although essential in deciding how to present and analyse data, is not completely clear-cut. It is possible to convert a quantitative variable into a categorical variable by dividing the range of values into groups. If this is carried further, a variable with two categories can be produced, known as a binary variable. For example, let us initially consider age as a quantitative variable (Fig. 30.2). Note that at each step from left to right information is lost, that is, the measure becomes more coarse. All of these age variables may be useful; the form of the variable chosen depends upon the question the study wishes to address. It would be

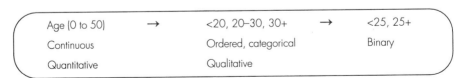

Fig. 30.2   Age as quantitative and categorical variable.

possible to transform in the reverse direction only if the original data were available.

The description of data

Having decided upon the type of data to be collected, and having collected the data (Chapters 23–28), the initial step in any data analysis is to look at the data themselves. In fact, this may be the main purpose of the study: to provide a description of a situation if this is unknown – for example, the extent of knowledge among the nursing profession regarding the condition of AIDS. Even when more sophisticated analyses are planned, looking at the data and the relationships between variables is extremely valuable in deciding what analyses would be appropriate. It is also useful as an aid to interpretation after the analyses have been carried out.

The main ways of presenting data are in the form of tables, pie charts, bar charts/histograms, scatter diagrams, and line graphs. Tables and histograms together can convey the same information, with tables emphasizing particular numerical values, while histograms show overall patterns. All of these can be produced using statistics/graphics computer packages such as SPSS (Norusis, 1993), but although the computer will do most of the tedious work, the researcher needs to consider the purpose and format of these visual presentations and, perhaps more importantly, the relevance of the medium to the presentation.

Tables

A simple table is often all that is required to convey information from a study. Thought should be put into the format, the number of tables, and the type of values to go into the body of the table: counts, totals and percentages. Note that if percentages are to be presented, the number and the total should be stated.

For example, whenever a survey is reported, the first table presented often shows the characteristics of the sample. Table 30.2 shows the characteristics of two groups of childbearing women from the records of the Royal Women's Hospital in Brisbane, Australia; one group from 1986 and the second from 1992 (East & Webster, 1995). The purpose of this study was to determine the trend in incidence of perineal outcomes, including episiotomy.

Such a table is a formal presentation of a number of descriptive statistics such as the mean with a measure of spread (standard deviation), or counts and percentages in groups (which will be described in detail later). Tables of this type are also often used to present the main results of a study. Table 30.3 shows the characteristics of the circadian patterns of systolic blood pressure (SBP) for a group of heart disease patients compared to a similarly aged comparison group (Dunbar & Farr, 1996).

Table 30.2   Characteristics of childbearing women at RWH in 1986 and 1992

Characteristic	1986 (n = 451)	1992 (n = 502)
Maternal age (years)		
Mean (SD)	27 (4.9)	28 (5.2)
Range	14–42	16–47
Gestation (weeks)		
Mean (SD)	39.3 (1.8)	39.2 (2.4)
Range	29–43	23–43

SD = standard deviation

Table 30.3   Characteristics of SBP rhythms

Characteristic	Cardiac (n = 22)	Comparison (n = 18)
Number with 24-hour rhythms	8 36%	6 33%
Mean (SD) amplitude	16 (6)	10 (3)
24-hour mean SBP (SD)	142 (16)	150 (22)

SD = standard deviation

Be wary of any table which only gives percentages, especially if small numbers are involved; a 100% increase from an initial value of 1 is 2! Huff (1988) explores in a light-hearted way some of the more common misuses of statistics in tables and plots.

Line graphs

Line graphs are most frequently encountered in displaying the changes in variables over time, often in different groups. Figure 30.3 shows a measure of immune function, the percentage CD3–/CD57+, in two groups of postpartum women on low- and high-fat diets. The line graph shows that immune function was diminished in women with high-fat diets at both 1 month and 4 months postpartum (Gennaro *et al.*, 1997).

Pie charts

A pie chart consists of a circle representing the total data or 100%, with each slice of 'pie' being proportional to the percentage in a particular category. Thus, a pie chart can convey the information in a table at a glance. Figure 30.4 shows the proportions of a set of new patients attending a geriatric day hospital with dif-

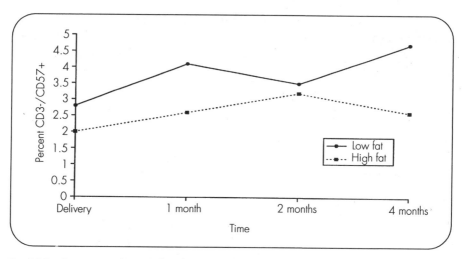

Fig. 30.3 Comparison of immune function in postpartum women with high-fat and low-fat diets (Gennaro *et al.*, 1997).

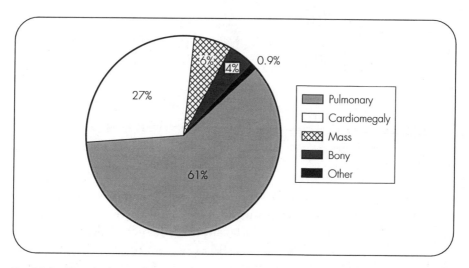

Fig. 30.4 Clinical indication for group of new geriatric day patients (Logan *et al.*, 1997).

ferent clinical indications for a chest x-ray, with 61% presenting with pulmonary abnormality (Logan *et al.*, 1997).

Beware of three-dimensional pie charts which, because they show volume, are misleading in that it is the size of the 'slice' in two dimensions which represents the proportion.

Histograms

Histograms can display the changes in scores in different groups over time. Rothert *et al.* (1997) designed a randomized three-group intervention trial to assess whether an educational intervention for menopausal women would increase knowledge, decisional conflict and satisfaction with their health care provider. The data on knowledge over time from a line graph presented by Rothert *et al.* (1997) can also be presented as a histogram, with columns representing the mean score in the three intervention groups at different time points, showing that knowledge increased in all three groups but by a greater amount in the intervention groups compared to the control group who received the brochure alone (Fig. 30.5).

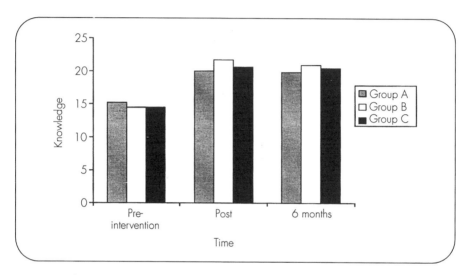

Fig. 30.5 Change in mean score for knowledge in three groups of menopausal women: A = brochure only; B = lecture discussion; C = personalized decision (Rothert *et al.*, 1997).

Histograms are also an effective way of presenting the counts of the number of cases in each category of a qualitative (categorical) variable showing the *distribution* of the data. The count in each category is known as the *frequency* of that category. As well as displaying qualitative (categorical) data, histograms can also be used to display continuous variables, such as age or scores, by dividing the range into equal-sized intervals.

Figure 30.6 shows the distribution of patient satisfaction scores following discharge from hospital of a group of patients (Pound *et al.* 1993). The area of each column represents the absolute count in each category. The frequencies in different categories can be directly compared if the size of each interval is equal. However, the frequency in each category is meaningless in itself; instead the *relative frequency* or proportion in each category is calculated by dividing the number in each group by the total number in the sample. If the proportion in each category is calculated, the full set of possibilities is known as a *frequency distribution*.

The histogram of this would be the same as that shown in Fig 30.6, except that the vertical axis would be the relative frequency or percentage. For this histo-

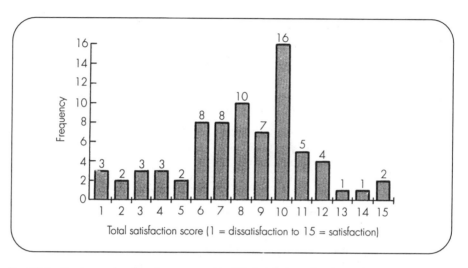

Fig. 30.6 Distribution of total satisfaction scores (n = 75) after discharge from hospital (Pound *et al.*, 1993).

gram, the total area of the columns must represent 100%, assuming that all possible categories are described, and so the area of each column must represent the proportion in each category, or the *probability* of being in that category. Since the proportion in the satisfaction category of 12 is 5.3%, the probability of a member of the sample being in that category is 5.3% or 0.053. This combined set of probabilities is also known as a *probability distribution*.

For continuous data, the actual size of interval is arbitrary; trial and error will show which is most appropriate for a particular dataset, although between 10 and 20 intervals are generally used. Most computer packages will plot histograms with the facility of adjusting the interval width (e.g. SPSS – Norusis, 1993). A histogram can also be computed by hand for small sample sizes by tallying the data.

Normal distribution

As stated above, the set of all probabilities forms a probability distribution. This example was from a sample, so let us assume that we have a complete population. This would also form a probability distribution and if the size of the interval for the histogram were to become smaller and smaller, a curved line would eventually be produced. We would then have the *probability density function* of the population. The probability of lying between any two values can then be calculated as the area under the curve between the two values and, as for the histogram described above, the total area under the curve represents the probability of 1.0. Thus, if you wanted to know the probability of, say, having systolic blood pressure of 130 mmHg or above, you could calculate the area above this value from the frequency distribution of blood pressures. It would, however, be difficult to calculate the area under a curve each time this was required. Expressed mathematically, you would have to know the equation for each distribution and use integration to obtain the probability of lying between two values. Fortunately, there is one particular probability distribution which approximates to reality in a large number of cases, and for this reason the areas under the curve have been tabulated extensively – this is known as *normal* or *Gaussian* distribution.

The normal curve is bell-shaped with most of the values clustered around a central value, with smaller and smaller frequencies moving further and further from the centre. The distribution is symmetric with equal proportions on either side of the centre. The property of symmetry is extremely useful. As noted above, the probability of lying between any two values can be calculated as the area under the probability density curve between these two points. If the probability of one area in one half is known, then, since the normal distribution is symmetric, the total probability for the two tails is twice this value. The normal distribution is often a useful approximation to reality. Returning to the distribution of the sample of satisfaction scores, a normal curve has been superimposed on the histogram (Fig. 30.7) showing a reasonably close fit, despite the anomalous peak at a score of 10.

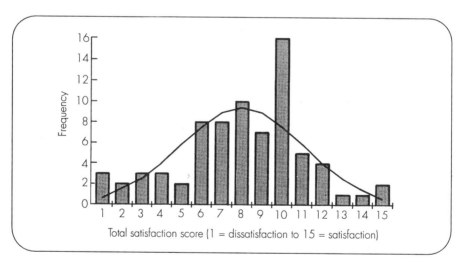

Fig. 30.7 Normal curve superimposed on distribution of satisfaction scores.

The shape and location of a normal distribution is characterized by two values known as *parameters*, the mean and the standard deviation. The mean gives the central point of the distribution while the standard deviation determines the spread; the larger the standard deviation, the more spread out will be the distribution. A special case is when the mean is 0 and the standard deviation is 1, the *standard normal* distribution. Figure 30.8 shows that for this distribution, 95%

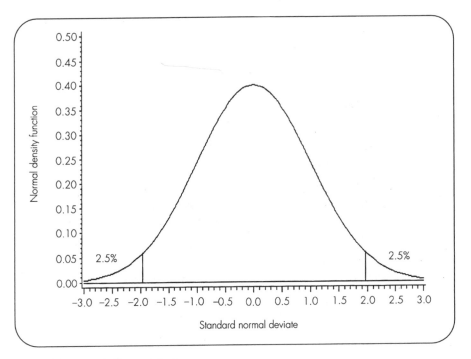

Fig. 30.8 The standard normal distribution.

of the observations will lie between 1.96 standard deviations on either side of the mean. The mean satisfaction score for Fig. 30.7 was 8.1 with a standard deviation (SD) of 3.2, so that 95% of the satisfaction scores lie between 1.8 and 14.4 on this scale, assuming a normal distribution.

Skewness

Whenever a greater proportion of cases fall at one end of the tail, the distribution is said to be skewed. Positively skewed data are often found in research; for example, the number of units of alcohol consumed per week is usually positively skewed. Figure 30.9 shows a positively skewed distribution of depression scores from a sample of 112 hysterectomy patients (Jacobsen *et al.*, 1996). A negatively skewed distribution is the opposite of this, with most of the data to the right of the centre. The normal distribution is clearly *not* a good approximation to these distributions.

Scatterplots

These are used to represent the relationships between pairs of quantitative variables. They consist of one axis for each variable and usually a point (although any symbol will do) representing each data value; this is placed a distance

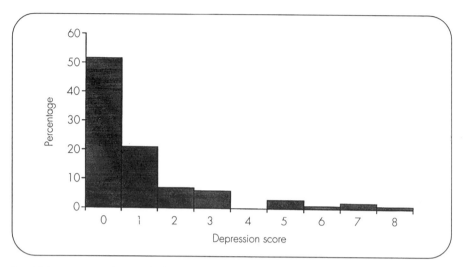

Fig. 30.9   Histogram of positively skewed depression scores (Jacobsen *et al.*, 1996).

along each axis corresponding to the values in these two dimensions. The ways in which these relationships can be explored will be discussed in Chapter 31. Figure 30.10 shows the relationship between changes in left ventricular mass and changes in serum IGF-I concentrations in a scatterplot from a RCT of human recombinant growth hormone in patients with chronic heart failure (Osterziel *et al.*, 1998).

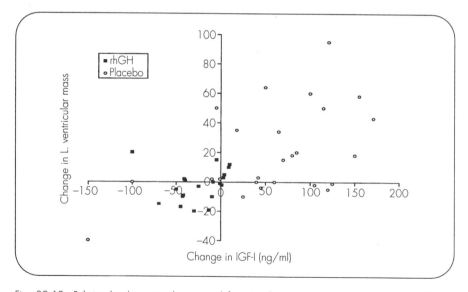

Fig. 30.10   Relationship between changes in left ventricular mass and changes in serum IGF-I concentrations (Osterziel *et al.*, 1998).

Summary statistics

In presenting results, it is unwieldy for the reader to have to consider all the data each time the evidence is examined. It can be more helpful to be given a few numbers which concisely convey the gist of the results, in other words, *summary statistics*. The most common of these are measures of the centre of the distribution of the data, or measures of central tendency, such as the *mean, median* and *mode*. The use of the common term *average* is not advised as it is often not clear what is meant. Often these are presented along with measures of spread or variation such as the standard deviation, semi-interquartile range, and range.

The mean ($\bar{x}$) is simply the sum of all the observations divided by the number of observations. The mean of the numbers 6, 5, 8, 5 is $(6 + 5 + 8 + 5)/4 = 6$. The mean is most useful when the histogram of the distribution looks symmetrical. It has useful mathematical properties and is incorporated into many analyses. The formula for the mean is written thus:

$$\bar{x} = \frac{\sum x}{n}$$

where n = the total number of observations and the Greek capital letter sigma ($\sum$) indicates the sum of all values of x. The mean is a very useful summary statistic. For example, the mean age for childbearing women in 1986 in Table 30.2 was 27 years. The mean has the disadvantage that it is very sensitive to extreme values or outliers and so would not be used to summarize positively skewed distributions such as the number of cigarettes smoked, for example.

The *median* is the centre of the distribution whenever the observations are placed in order or *ranked* so that 50% of the observations lie above and below it. This measure is most useful whenever the distribution of the data is skewed, but it can also be used with a symmetrical distribution. In fact, it is highly misleading to quote the mean when the data are skewed. Consider a report stating that the mean salary for nurses is £20,000! This is misleading if the population of nurses includes clinical nurse managers, and so the distribution of salaries is therefore skewed; the median salary may be much less than this. The main drawback of the median is that it is not so easily mathematically manipulated as the mean.

If the number in the sample is odd, the median is simply the middle value when they are placed in order. It is the $[(n + 1)/2]$th value. If there are five values, the median will be the third value when the data are ranked.

If the number in the sample is even, the median is the average of the two middle numbers. It is the $[(n/2)\text{th} + (n/2 + 1)\text{th}]/2$th value. This looks complicated but is actually straightforward in practice. The median of four values is the average of the second and third values when the data are ranked, so, for example, the median of 6, 5, 8, 5 is $(5 + 6)/2 = 5.5$.

The mode is the most frequent value and is represented by the tallest column of the histogram of the distribution, and is of limited use. In terms of the normal distribution, it should be noted that the mean, median and mode all coincide, forming the central point of the distribution. Hence, one way of assessing whether a sample is approximately normal is to compare these three measures of central tendency.

Percentiles

The median was calculated as the value above and below which 50% of the data lie if placed in order. A percentile is a value below which a percentage of the observations lie. In terms of percentiles, the median is the 50th percentile. The most commonly used percentiles are quartiles. There are three quartiles, in other words, three values which divide the data into quarters. The first quartile (Q_1) is the value below which 25% of the data lie; the second quartile (Q_2) is the median; and the third quartile (Q_3) is the value above which 25% of the data lie. For example, if heights were recorded for a sample of nurses, then 25% of these nurses would have heights which are greater than the third or upper quartile. These measures are also useful to assess the shape of the distribution of a sample. One visual method of exploratory data analysis consists of the representation of the distribution of a variable in the form of a *boxplot*. In a basic boxplot (Fig. 30.11), the median is represented by a plus, the ends of the box are the upper and lower quartiles, while the maximum and minimum are the ends of the hinges if there are no extreme values (indicated by asterisks). Most statistical packages, such as SPSS (Norusis, 1993) and MINITAB (Ryan & Joiner, 1994) can produce boxplots.

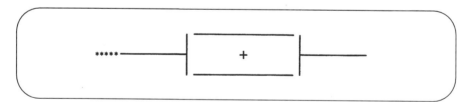

Fig. 30.11 Boxplot (theoretical data).

Measures of variability

As well as these measures of central tendency, some measure of the spread of the data about these points is necessary to fully describe a distribution. The most commonly used measures of variability are the standard deviation, standard error, range and semi-interquartile range.

Standard deviation

This is a measure of the average spread of the data about the mean, assuming that the sample has an approximately normal distribution. The standard deviation (SD) is calculated by squaring the difference between each data point and the mean, summing these squared differences, and dividing the result by one less than the sample size. This is the sample *variance*, denoted by s^2. Finally, taking the square root of this value gives the standard deviation, s. In mathematical notation, this is written:

$$s = \sqrt{\frac{\sum(\bar{x} - x)^2}{n - 1}}$$

For the following data, 6, 5, 8, 5 which has a mean of 6, the standard deviation is calculated as the square root of $[(6 - 6)^2 + (6 - 5)^2 + (6 - 8)^2 + (6 - 5)^2]/3 = 2$. Hence the standard deviation is 1.41.

Figure 30.8 shows the most used percentage point of the normal distribution, with 95% of the observations lying between 1.96 (often rounded to 2) standard deviations above and below the mean. The main drawback of the standard deviation as a measure of spread, is that, like the mean, it is affected by extreme values.

Standard error

The standard error (SE) of the mean is often encountered in the literature in tables and should not be confused with the standard deviation. They are, however, related, but while the standard deviation measures the variability of the *observations* about the mean, the standard error measures the variability of the *mean* of the sample as an estimate of the true population from which the sample was drawn. They are both measures of variability, but of two different distributions. If more samples were taken from the population and the mean calculated for each sample, a distribution of means would be obtained and the standard error would be the measure of variability of this distribution of means. The standard error is easily calculated as:

$$\text{SE}(\bar{x}) = \frac{s}{\sqrt{n}}$$

Thus the standard error is smaller than the standard deviation. This is not a good reason for preferring its use in tables. When the purpose of the table is to compare means, the standard error should be quoted along with the mean. However, if the purpose of the table is to compare the spread of the observations, then the standard deviation should be used. The standard error and the standard deviation, along with the mean, are also used for the purposes of statistical inference and this will be discussed in the next chapter.

Range and semi-interquartile range

The range is simply the difference between the maximum and minimum data values. As such, the usefulness of the range is rather limited and is unduly affected by extreme values, unlike the semi-interquartile range, which is half the difference between the first and third quartiles. It is calculated as:

$$\tfrac{1}{2}(Q_3 - Q_1)$$

All of these summary statistics give slightly different information concerning the characteristics of a distribution and are available in the common statistical packages.

Conclusions

This chapter has described the most commonly encountered ways of describing and summarizing data. The importance of looking at the data in as many ways as possible has been stressed, not only as an end in itself, but also as a means of aiding further analysis.

The chapter that follows moves on to the next step, that of generalizing the results from the sample to the larger population of interest by the application of inferential statistics.

References

Armitage, P. & Berry, G. (1994) *Statistical Methods in Medical Research*. Oxford: Blackwell Scientific Publications.

Dunbar, S.B. & Farr, L. (1996) Temporal patterns of heart rate and blood pressure in elders. *Nursing Research* 45: 43–8.

East, C. & Webster, J. (1995) Episiotomy at the Royal Women's Hospital, Brisbane: a comparison of practices in 1986 and 1992. *Midwifery* 11: 195–200.

Gennaro, S., Fehder, W.P., York, R. & Douglas, S.D. (1997) Weight, nutrition and immune status in postpartal women. *Nursing Research* 46: 20–24.

Huff, D. (1988) *How to Lie with Statistics*. London: Penguin.

Jacobsen, B.S., Munro, B.H. & Brooten, D.A. (1996) Comparison of original and revised scoring systems for the multiple affect adjective check list. *Nursing Research* 45: 57–60.

Lemeshow, S., Hosmer, D.W., Klar, J. & Lwanga, S.K. (1990) *Adequacy of Sample Size in Health Studies*. Chichester: John Wiley & Sons.

Logan, J.A., Vallance, R., Williams, B.O. & Paul, H. (1997) Does a chest x-ray alter the management of new patients attending a geriatric day hospital? *Health Bulletin* 55: 52–7.

Norusis, M.J. (1993) *Statistical Package for the Social Sciences (SPSS)*. *Release 6*. Chicago, Ill.: SPSS Inc.

Osterziel, K.J., Strohm, O., Schuler, J., Friedrich, M., Hanlein, D., Willenbrock, R., Anker,

S.D., Poole-Wilson, P.A., Ranke, M.B. & Dietz, R. (1998) Randomised double-blind placebo controlled trial of human recombinant growth hormone in patients with chronic heart failure due to dilated cardiomyopathy. *Lancet* **351**: 1233–7.

Pound, P., Gompertz, P. & Ebrahim, S. (1993) Development and results of a questionnaire to measure carer satisfaction after stroke. *Journal of Epidemiology and Community Health* **47**: 500–5.

Rothert, M.L., Holmes-Rovner, M., Rovner, D., Kroll, J., Breer, L., Talarczyk, G., Schmitt, N., Padonu, G. & Wills, C. (1997) An educational intervention as decision support for menopausal women. *Research in Nursing and Health* **20**: 377–87.

Ryan, B.F. & Joiner, B.L. (1994) *MINITAB Handbook*. Boston: Wadsworth.

CHAPTER 31

Quantitative analysis (inferential)

Peter T. Donnan

The previous chapter presented various ways of describing the data in a sample. This is fine as far as it goes, but usually the researcher will wish to say something more general concerning the wider target population from which the specific sample was drawn. Often one wishes to assess whether apparent differences between groups could have arisen by chance or represent statistically significant differences. This is achieved through the use of *inferential statistics*.

Consider a survey carried out to discover the satisfaction of mothers with midwifery care in a particular city. The results of this survey will be most useful if the results can be applied to the entire city and so inform the decision-makers of provision of midwifery care in that city. From this sample, one may wish to say something about the population of mothers in the city, that is, inferences are made about the population based on the sample. If the sample is biased, then statistical procedures will not rectify this problem and hence the need for good design in the first place.

Consider also if a midwifery intervention is to be compared to the usual service or the effect of the new service is to be assessed in relation to social class, age or parity. Statistical inference helps to answer these questions.

The answers to these types of question involve the use of various inferential statistical methods. Before expanding on particular methods, it is worth discussing the use of computer packages. It is no longer essential to know the mechanics of calculations since computers are more efficient at this task, as well as being faster. However, some calculations are presented in this chapter, first, and most important, as an aid to understanding; and, second, for those who are interested in the mechanics of the calculations. Although computers are more efficient, the widespread availability and use of computer packages creates a danger of using inappropriate methods, coupled with a lack of understanding of the output. Computers follow the RIRO maxim: 'rubbish in, rubbish out!' What is therefore required is the intelligent use of computers and the knowledge to know when to seek expert advice.

There are many user-friendly packages available for use on personal computers as well as on mainframe computers. Two of the most commonly used are SPSS (Norusis, 1993) and MINITAB (Ryan & Joiner, 1994). See also Chapter 33.

In selecting statistical methods, it is essential to have an understanding of when particular methods are appropriate, what assumptions are being made, when a particular method is chosen and whether these assumptions are valid. Having obtained the result, it is then necessary to know how to interpret the output. Often you will have access to a statistician or find that one is a member of the research team. In endeavouring to manage this part of the research process, it is always worth consulting a statistician.

Inferential statistical methods

There are two main types of inferential statistical methods, known as *parametric* and *non-parametric*. Parametric methods, not surprisingly, centre around estimating parameters of the population – such as the mean – based upon the sample data collected. These methods depend heavily upon making distributional assumptions about the population. On the other hand, there are what are known as non-parametric (or sometimes distribution-free) methods. These methods are applicable to estimation or hypothesis testing when the population distributions are not rigidly specified – that is, they do not have to belong to specific families such as the normal distribution. These methods still have assumptions but these are not as restrictive as those for parametric methods. The pragmatic difference is that non-parametric methods are based upon the ranking of data rather than the actual data itself. For example, the following measurements of haemoglobin levels have ranks 3, 1, 2 and 4 respectively: 13.3, 10.5, 12.6, 14.1.

Faced with a bewildering array of methods, it is tempting to churn out results from as many programs as possible in a statistical package in the hope that some will be useful. A better, more, systematic, approach would be to decide initially between parametric and non-parametric statistical methods.

In deciding between parametric and non-parametric methods the main considerations are:

- *Distributional shape*. Parametric tests depend upon the assumption of normally distributed data for the population of interest. This is often assessed visually from a histogram of the sample. For example, in Chapter 30, the histogram of satisfaction scores (Fig. 30.7) indicates that the assumption of normality would be reasonable. On the other hand, Fig. 30.9 in Chapter 30, which is highly positively skewed, suggests that this assumption would be unwarranted and non-parametric methods are indicated. An alternative would be to transform the data such that the transformed data are approximately normal. For the data in Fig. 30.9 a log transformation is appropriate and parametric methods could be applied to the transformed data. Sometimes there is no simple transformation which 'normalizes' the data and non-parametric methods should be used.
- *Power*. For non-normal data, the *power* of non-parametric tests may be

superior (the power of a test is the chance of detecting a significant difference if it is present in the population).

- *Ease of calculation*. Ease of calculation is greater for non-parametric tests, especially for small sample sizes without the need for calculators or computers.

Many excellent textbooks are devoted to non-parametric methods. If these methods are indicated, a classic textbook is that of Siegel (1988), which is recommended for the details of any test. For a basic introduction, the work by Sprent (1992) is useful.

Parametric methods tend to be more commonly encountered and this chapter will concentrate on these methods. However, in what follows the equivalent non-parametric test will be mentioned alongside each parametric test. The choice of method will depend on the nature of the study and the data collected. Before going into details of the actual tests, it is important to discuss the two complementary approaches to inference: confidence interval estimation and hypothesis testing.

Confidence intervals and hypothesis testing

As discussed earlier, information is obtained concerning the population of interest from a smaller sample. From this sample you may want to say something about the whole population, that is, inferences are made based on the sample.

Assuming an unbiased study, statistical methods can help you to assess whether the result is spurious or not (hypothesis testing). In other words, they evaluate the role of chance as an explanation of the results. In addition, statistical methods also allow calculation of the precision of a given sample estimate such as a proportion or mean (confidence interval approach). In practice, both are used simultaneously to give a comprehensive analysis of the data. For a detailed discussion of the relative merits of these approaches, see Gardiner & Altman (1989).

Confidence interval approach

Consider a proportion or mean, which are population parameters estimated from the data obtained from the study sample. A *confidence interval* is defined as a range of values within which it is reasonably certain (often 95%) that the population value lies. For example, if a painkiller was administered to a random sample of female patients and it was recorded that 60% no longer felt any pain after one hour, the researcher would like to know the precision of this estimate if the painkiller were to be applied to the population in general, that is, to all female patients of the same age range with the same condition. If the confidence interval suggests that the population value could be as low as 20% or as high as 100% then the value of 60% is very imprecise and of little use. If, on the other hand, the confidence interval is from 55% to 65%, then this is a more precise estimate and also more meaningful. You could then make a stronger inference about the effect of the painkiller on the population at large than in the former case.

Confidence intervals are concerned with precision, that is, by how much the sample estimate is likely to differ on average from the 'true' population value. Thus we require an interval defined by two values which has a reasonable chance of containing the 'true' value. This can be represented pictorially as an interval on a number line (see Fig. 31.1).

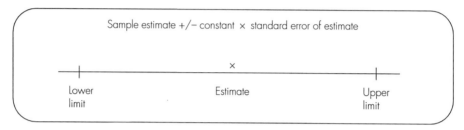

Fig. 31.1 Representation of a confidence interval.

The constant is a number taken from the appropriate percentage point of a probability distribution (often the normal distribution) and the two values calculated are called confidence limits. This defines a confidence interval with a specified chance (often 95%) of containing the true value. Note that this does not mean that the 'true' or population value cannot lie outside the limits; it means that this is less likely. The 95% confidence interval is the one most commonly encountered, but any percentage point is possible; others often used are 90% and 99%.

In Chapter 30 the standard error of the mean was introduced. This can be generalized to any parameter estimate so that if the standard error of a parameter estimate is known, then a confidence interval can be calculated using the equation shown in Fig. 31.1. (See Appendix 31.1 for details of calculations for confidence intervals.)

The size of the confidence interval depends on the size of the standard error and the size of the constant in this equation. In order to emphasize that confidence intervals are concerned with the precision of point estimates, Fig. 31.2 illustrates an estimate with precise and imprecise confidence intervals.

Hypothesis testing

The previous section dealt with the calculations of confidence intervals to estimate the precision of a parameter estimate. This section deals with testing whether or not a particular value of the parameter is consistent with the data; the

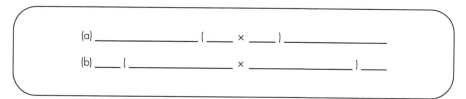

(a) _____ (____ × ____) _____

(b) ____ (_____ × _____) ____

Fig. 31.2 (a) Precise and (b) imprecise confidence intervals.

idea underlying *hypothesis tests*. The outcome of this approach will be a state-ment to say whether a particular value is *statistically significant* or not.

A hypothesis is a statement about the population; it is made prior to data collection and the validity of this hypothesis or assertion is then tested, based upon the evidence from the sample.

The hypothesis to be tested (denoted by H) – for example, whether or not a new intervention is better in the preparation of children for surgery – is couched in neutral terms. In other words, a *null hypothesis* is proposed (the effect of the new intervention is the same as the old regime), and a test is carried out on the sample data. The null hypothesis is analogous to the assumption of innocence of the defendant before a legal trial (Fig. 31.3) and is denoted by H_0. Denote the alternative by H_1. On the basis of this test (examination of the evidence), the null hypothesis is either rejected or not rejected. If rejected, the alternative hypothesis, H_1 is accepted (the new intervention is better or worse than the standard pro-cedure). Note that if the null hypothesis is not rejected, this simply means that there is insufficient evidence to reject the hypothesis, analogous to a 'not proven' verdict in Scottish law (Fig. 31.3). This is not the same as 'no difference' or, in terms of the legal analogy, 'innocence'.

All tests are based on a number derived from the sample values; this is the test statistic. The test statistic often consists of a parameter estimate minus the value

Legal trial	Significance test
Defendant assumed innocent until proved guilty	Null hypothesis assumes no difference in effect between intervention and non-intervention
Examine evidence	Calculate test statistic based on evidence from sample
Either: (1) Accept evidence – proves guilt (2) Accept evidence – does not prove guilt: 'not proven' (Note: not same as innocence)	Either: (1) Accept significant difference and reject null hypothesis (2) Accept evidence – not sufficient to reject null hypothesis: not significant (Note: not same as no difference but evidence failed to demonstrate difference)

Fig. 31.3 Legal analogy to hypothesis testing.

according to the null hypothesis divided by the standard error of the estimate, thus

$$\frac{\text{Parameter estimate} - H_0 \text{ value}}{\text{Standard error of the estimate}}$$

For example, the test of the null hypothesis that the mean is 0 is carried out by dividing the sample mean by its standard error and comparing the resultant test statistic with percentage points of the normal distribution (assuming a large sample size). In summary, the ordering of this procedure is:

Null → Data → Calculate → Accept or reject
hypothesis   collection   test statistic   the hypothesis

The details of the test involve calculating a test statistic and comparing the calculated value to theoretical values from a probability distribution such as the normal distribution. This comparison indicates whether or not the observed value of the test statistic would have been likely to occur if the null hypothesis had been true. If the probability of this happening by chance is sufficiently low (i.e. less than a specified small value called the *significance level* (e.g. 5% or 0.05), the null hypothesis can be rejected and the sample statistic is said to be significantly different from the hypothetical value.

Significance level

Three significance levels or *p-values* (5%, 1%, 0.1%) are in common use, although this is only a convention because of ease of presenting tables (computers now calculate p-values exactly), reflecting generally agreed cut-off points for strength of evidence against the null hypothesis. It is normal practice to quote the lowest of these levels at which one can reject the null hypothesis; for example, the statement '$p < 0.05$' means that you can reject at the 5% level but not at the 1% level. If you cannot even reject the null hypothesis at the 5% level the result is not significant, and so this procedure is often called a significance test.

Types of error

In making any inference about a population there will always be uncertainty. In setting a significance level for the test of the null hypothesis, we are putting a value on the size of that uncertainty. The significance level is the chance of rejecting the null hypothesis when it is true and so represents the probability of an error – a Type I error. With a significance level of 5%, we are accepting a 1 in 20 chance of rejecting the null hypothesis when it is in fact true. Obviously, we wish to render the probability of this error as small as possible, so that the lower the significance level, the lower the probability of obtaining a result by chance.

However, there is another type of error, that of not rejecting the null hypothesis when it is in fact false. This is called a Type II error and is related to the Type I error already mentioned. Often this is larger than the Type I error. It is generally assumed that it is more acceptable to have a higher Type II error than a Type I error. In terms of the intervention trial, we are saying that it is less acceptable to conclude that the intervention has an effect when in fact it does not, than to conclude that there is no effect when in fact there is. Often instead of presenting the Type II error the *power* of a test is quoted. The power is simply 100% minus the probability of a Type II error, and so is the probability of rejecting the null hypothesis given that it is false. Hypothesis tests are often carried out at the 5% level with a power of 90% (or 10% Type II error). The power of any test is a function of the size of the sample; small samples will produce tests of low power. Hence the power of any test is decided at the design stage when the size of the sample is chosen.

Examples

Comparison of two unpaired means: *t*-test

In the comparison between childbearing women in the years 1986 and 1992 (Table 30.2, Chapter 30) interest was centred on the decline in incidence of episiotomy (East & Webster, 1995). This decline in episiotomy was reflected by an increase in the second stage of labour (Table 31.1).

Table 31.1   Length of the second stage in childbearing women at the RWH, Brisbane in 1986 and 1992 (East & Webster, 1995)

	1986 ($n = 451$)		1992 ($n = 502$)	
	Mean	SD	Mean	SD
Duration of second stage (mins)	29	27.5	35	38

The null hypothesis to be tested in this case is that there is no difference between the two means, or the difference between the means is zero. In other words, is the difference of 6 minutes statistically different from zero? A test of this null hypothesis is given by:

$$t = \frac{\text{estimate} - \text{estimate (if } H_0 \text{ true)}}{\text{standard error (estimate)}}$$

$$t = \frac{(\bar{x}_1 - \bar{x}_2) - 0}{s_p \sqrt{1/n_1 + 1/n_2}}$$

where the pooled standard deviation is given by

$$s_p = \frac{\sqrt{(n_1 - 1)s_1^2 + (n_2 - 1)s_2^2}}{n_1 + n_2 - 2}$$

The t-distribution is used in this case, which has a similar shape to the normal distribution but is more spread out, as the combined sample size is less than 100. This value of t is then compared to the theoretical value from t-tables (see Armitage & Berry, 1994) with $n_1 + n_2 - 2$ degrees of freedom. Initially, the calculated value of t is compared to the 5% point of the t-tables, and if the value exceeds the tabulated value, the result is said to be significant at the 5% level. The result obtained is unlikely to have occurred by chance and so the difference is statistically significant. If it exceeds the 1% tabulated value the result is significant at the 1% level, and so on. If the value does not exceed the 5% point, it is said to be not significant (NS). The assumptions being made in this test are that both samples come from a normal distribution and hence have the same standard deviation or variance. This would be checked before carrying out the test by plotting the histograms of the variable in each group. In the example above t is calculated as follows:

$$t = \frac{(\bar{x}_1 - \bar{x}_2) - 0}{s_p\sqrt{1/n_1 + 1/n_2}} = \frac{(35 - 29) - 0}{33.4\sqrt{1/451 + 1/502}} = 2.77$$

Looking up t-tables (see Armitage & Berry, 1994), the value of 2.77 is greater than the value 2.58 for $p = 0.01$ with 951 degrees of freedom. Hence $p < 0.01$ and the result is significant at the 5% level and also at the 1% level. Hence, in 1992 the second stage of labour was on average 6 minutes longer than in 1986, a difference which was statistically significant. The 95% confidence interval for the difference in means can also be calculated using the formula from Appendix 31.1, giving an interval of 2 to 10 minutes. Note that the confidence interval excludes the value zero.

Comparison of two independent medians

As shown in Chapter 30, the median is a better measure of location than the mean for highly skewed data. Consider a study in which Likert scores for two groups on a 4-point scale are collected. The question arises as to whether there is any evidence that these data come from populations differing in median scores. As the data are likely to be highly skewed the assumption that the variables are approximately normally distributed will probably not be met in this case. An alternative to the t-test is a non-parametric test based on the ranks of the data, which tests whether the locations of the two groups are different. The appropriate test in this case is the Mann–Whitney or Wilcoxon Rank Sum test. In order to carry out this test the two samples are pooled and ranked in ascending order, while retaining group membership information. The smallest value is given the rank 1, the next value is rank 2 and so on. If two or more data values are equal they are given their average rank. The ranks are then summed for each group separately so that:

S_A = the sum of the ranks for group A
S_B = the sum of the ranks for group B

Then

$$U_A = S_A - \tfrac{1}{2}n_A(n_A + 1) \quad \text{and similarly} \quad U_B = S_B - \tfrac{1}{2}n_B(n_B + 1)$$

It should be obvious that if the two groups differ in location, the two statistics U_A and U_B should also be different. The test then simply consists of comparing the smaller of the two statistics to critical values in tables. If this statistic exceeds the critical value in the table at the 5% level, then the null hypothesis is rejected and the location of one group is said to be significantly different to the other group.

As a theoretical example, consider the responses to a question on nurses' attitudes to people with HIV/AIDS stating that 'They should be isolated from the rest of the community' posed to one group of nurses who attended a course on HIV/AIDS and a comparator group of nurses who did not. The responses were recorded on a Likert scale with values from 0 = strongly disagree to 5 = strongly agree. The educators would hope that the location of the distribution of scores would be closer to zero in those who attended such a course – that is, they would be more likely to disagree with the statement. The number attending the course was 12 compared to 8 who did not attend. The responses to this question are shown below:

Table 31.2 Scores for attenders and non-attenders on a Likert scale

Attenders (A)	0 0 3 1 1 2 2 3 2 3 5 0
Non-attenders (N)	4 3 2 0 5 4 4 4

Table 31.3 Pooled scores and ranks for attenders and non-attenders

Score	0	0	0	0	1	1	2	2	2	2
Rank	2.5	2.5	2.5	2.5	5.5	5.5	8.5	8.5	8.5	8.5
Group	A	A	A	N	A	A	A	A	A	N
Score	3	3	3	3	4	4	4	4	5	5
Rank	12.5	12.5	12.5	12.5	16.5	16.5	16.5	16.5	19.5	19.5
Group	A	A	A	N	N	N	N	N	A	N

The sum of ranks for the attenders is $S_A = 101$ while the sum of the ranks for the non-attenders is $S_N = 109$. Then $U_A = 101 - \tfrac{1}{2} \times 12 \times 13 = 23$ and similarly $U_N = 109 - \tfrac{1}{2} \times 8 \times 9 = 73$. The lesser value is $U_A = 23$ and this is compared to the 5% critical value in tables, which turns out to be 22, and so the calculated value just exceeds the tabulated critical value and hence the attenders have statistically significantly lower scores at the 5% level. In other words, the attenders tend to disagree more with the statement compared to non-attenders and hence the educators appear to be justified in considering the course successful in this respect.

The measure of location used to report skewed data is the median (see Chapter 30). In the example above the median score for the attenders was 2 compared to a median of 4 for the non-attenders. If you are using a statistical package then a p-value will be given in the output with no need to look up tables. It should be noted that the Mann–Whitney–Wilcoxon test does make some assumptions; namely that the two groups have come from similar distributions with the same variance, but this is a less restrictive assumption than those necessary for a t-test.

Comparison of two independent proportions

Consider the example of a study of attitudes to smoking among Finnish middle-aged men (Koivula & Paunonen, 1998). A 2 × 2 table can be constructed for this dataset concerning the relationship between self-perceived health and smoking status (Table 31.4)

Table 31.4 Association between smoking and self-perceived health among middle-aged men ($n = 81$) (Koivula & Paunonen, 1998)

Self-perceived health	Smokers	Non-smokers	Total
Good or rather good	7 (30%)	49 (85%)	56 (69%)
Average to poor	16 (70%)	9 (15%)	25 (31%)
Total	23	58	81

The table shows that overall 69% of this sample perceive their health to be good or rather good, while only 30% of smokers perceive themselves to have good health compared to 85% of non-smokers. The question is 'Is this difference a chance finding or does it represent a real difference between smokers and non-smokers?'

In order to compare two independent proportions, the chi-squared test is used. This is based on the chi-squared (χ^2) probability distribution which is continuous and approaches the normal distribution for large degrees of freedom. However, in comparing two proportions the χ^2 distribution with one degree of freedom is used, which is highly positively skewed.

In order to facilitate the test, the data are laid out in a 2 × 2 contingency table. The two rows in Table 31.5 represent the two samples, with the column totals

Table 31.5 General form of 2 × 2 contingency table

Sample 1	a	b	r_1
Sample 2	c	d	r_2
	s_1	s_2	n

Note: r_1 and r_2 are the row totals and s_1 and s_2 are the column totals.

being the total number in each sample, and the first row, divided by the column totals, representing the two proportions which are to be compared.

The test compares the two proportions $p_1 = a/r_1$ and $p_2 = c/r_2$. If the proportions in the two populations are the same, then a/b and c/d should be similar and so $|ad - bc|$ should be small. (The symbols $|\ |$ simply mean that the result of the arithmetic between the vertical bars is given a positive sign.) The table can be rearranged so that the columns become the rows if this is more convenient. The test is one of association between the two dimensions which make up the table.

The null hypothesis is that $p_1 - p_2 = 0$ and the test statistic is given by:

$$X^2 = \frac{(ad - bc)^2(n - 1)}{r_1 r_2 s_1 s_2}$$

(X^2 is the sample value which is then compared to the χ^2 distribution).

The value of this calculation is then compared to the theoretical value from chi-squared tables (Table 31.6) with one degree of freedom, and if it is larger the result is significant at that level.

Table 31.6 Critical values of the chi-squared distribution with one degree of freedom (d.f.)

Significance level (p-value)	0.10	0.05	0.02	0.01
Critical value χ_1^2	2.71	3.84	5.41	6.64

A formal test of this difference involves the calculation of the X^2 statistic as described above. The test statistic X^2 is calculated as follows from the data in Table 31.4:

$$X^2 = \frac{(7 \times 9 - 16 \times 49)^2 \times 80}{23 \times 58 \times 56 \times 25}$$

$$= 22.3 \quad \text{with one degree of freedom}$$

This is highly statistically significant as this value is well above the 1% value in tables (6.64) and hence the difference is not a chance finding but represents a real difference between the rates of self-perceived health. This can be written as $p < 0.01$. To further describe the results, a confidence interval for the difference between the percentages, which is 55%, would be calculated. Using the formula in Appendix 31.1 the 95% confidence interval for the difference in proportions is 34% to 76%.

More than two groups

So far, only one variable and a comparison of this measure in two groups (or samples) has been considered. There are extensions of the methods described for comparing more than two groups: for example, one-way analysis of variance for comparison of more than two means and the non-parametric equivalent for comparing more than two medians, the Kruskal–Wallis test, but lack of space prevents their description here and details of these methods can be seen in Armitage & Berry (1994) or Altman (1990).

Correlation

The next step is to consider relationships between two quantitative variables. As an initial step, a scatterplot, as described in Chapter 30, will display this relationship. A summary statistic of the relationship between two quantitative variables is the Pearson correlation coefficient. Table 31.7 shows some of the correlations from a study of work environment scales (WES) and psychological strain in a sample of hospital nurses (Fielding & Weaver, 1994). Note that these have been multiplied by 100 for ease of comparison.

Table 31.7 Pearson correlations × 100 between work environment scales and psychological strain in a group of hospital nurses (n = 67)

Work environment scale	Depersonalization	Emotional exhaustion
Involvement	−29**	−32**
Support	−27*	−26*
Innovation	−25*	−22

* $p < 0.05$; ** $p < 0.02$

   The correlations are all negative, indicating that high levels of one dimension (for example, involvement) are associated with low levels of psychological strain (for example, emotional exhaustion). The p-values indicate that these correlations are not chance findings (i.e. they are significantly different from zero).
   The Pearson correlation is appropriate when the two quantitative variables are approximately normally distributed. The non-parametric alternative is the Spearman rank correlation coefficient (r_S) which is based on the ranks of the data. Melillo et al. (1997) used the Spearman rank correlation coefficient to relate physical fitness scores to self-reported exercise frequency ($r_S = 0.184; p = 0.049$)

as a test of validity. These were 4-point Likert scales and so it would be unlikely that the distribution of scores would be approximately normal and hence the use of the non-parametric Spearman rank correlation.

Linear regression

The correlation coefficient tells us the strength of the relationship between two quantitative variables. On the other hand, the method of regression tells us about the nature of the relationship between any two quantitative variables and precisely how they change numerically together. In regression, one is interested in by how much one variable increases for a given increase in the other. A linear relationship is assumed to model the data. In a study of respiratory dysfunction in chronic heart failure (CHF) the percentage change in minute ventilation was related in a linear fashion to the arterial oxygen saturation as measured by SaO_2 with controlled breathing of 15 breaths per minute (Fig. 31.4).

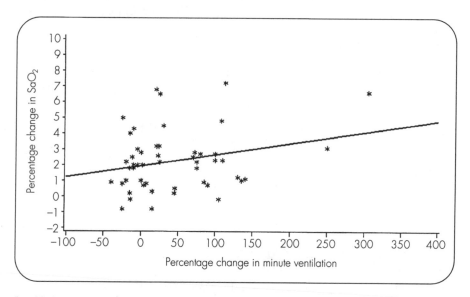

Fig. 31.4   Association between arterial oxygen saturation (SaO_2) and minute ventilation (Bernardi *et al.*, 1998).

One variable is considered as the outcome while the other is known as the predictor, although it is not always obvious which is the outcome. Even though the terms *outcome* and *predictor* are used, as with correlation, causality cannot be assumed.

Multiple linear regression

In reality, there will be many possible predictors or independent variables. In the example of the study of work environment scale and psychological strain after the initial look at the correlations, the next step could be to assess whether the relationship between involvement and emotional exhaustion was still significant, allowing for differences in age, for example. The method of simple linear regression can be extended for this case and most computer packages (such as SPSS – see Norusis, 1993) contain programs which will carry out multiple regression in which the significance of the independent contribution of each variable is assessed simultaneously. In a study to determine the factors that were predictors of psychological distress in chronic pain patients a number of variables were assessed in a multiple linear regression procedure (Walker & Sofaer, 1998). The results are presented in Table 31.8 in terms of the regression coefficient, the t-value and p-value, the latter indicating statistical significance. Positive coefficients such as those for 'fears about the future' and 'regrets about the past' indicate that these factors are associated with increasing psychological distress, while the negative coefficient for age suggests that, allowing for all the other factors which increase distress, increasing age is associated with a decrease in distress. For more details of these methods, see Armitage & Berry (1994) or Altman (1990).

Table 31.8   Results of multiple linear regression analysis with psychological distress as the outcome variable (Walker & Sofaer, 1998)

Variable	Regression coefficient	t	p-value
Fears about the future	4.63	6.1	<0.001
Regrets about the past	2.41	3.6	<0.001
Age	−0.15	−2.9	<0.005
Feeling occupied	1.43	2.0	0.05
Practical help	1.85	2.3	0.02
Personal relationship problems	1.40	2.2	0.03

Conclusions

This chapter has introduced the powerful tool of statistical inference, in terms of estimating confidence intervals and hypothesis testing. These ideas are fundamental, and there are more sophisticated methods (not described in this chapter) which also produce results that generally involve estimation of parameters, estimation of their confidence intervals, and the testing of hypotheses, followed by an interpretation of these procedures.

References

Altman, D.G. (1990) *Practical Statistics for Medical Research*. London: Chapman & Hall.
Armitage, P. & Berry, G. (1994) *Statistical Methods in Medical Research*. Oxford: Blackwell Scientific Publications.

Bernardi, L., Spadacini, G., Bellwon, J., Hajric, R., Roskamm, H. & Frey, A.W. (1998) Effect of breathing rate on oxygen saturation and exercise performance in chronic heart failure. *Lancet* **351**: 1308–11.

East, C. & Webster, J. (1995) Episiotomy at the Royal Women's Hospital, Brisbane: a comparison of practices in 1986 and 1992. *Midwifery* **11**: 195–200.

Fielding, J. & Weaver, S.M. (1994) A comparison of hospital- and community-based mental health nurses: perceptions of their work environment and psychological health. *Journal of Advanced Nursing* **19**: 1196–1204.

Gardiner, M.J. & Altman, D.G. (eds) (1989) *Statistics with Confidence: Confidence Intervals and Statistical Guidelines*. London: British Medical Journal.

Koivula, M. & Paunonen, M. (1998) Smoking habits among Finnish middle-aged men: experiences and attitudes. *Journal of Advanced Nursing* **27**: 327–34.

Melillo, K.D., Williamson, E., Futrell, M. & Chamberlain, C. (1997) A self-assessment tool to measure older adults' perceptions regarding physical fitness and exercise activity. *Journal of Advanced Nursing* **25**: 1220–26.

Norusis, M.J. (1993) *Statistical Package for the Social Sciences (SPSS). Release 6*. Chicago, Ill.: SPSS Inc.

Ryan, B.F. & Joiner, B.L. (1994) *MINITAB Handbook*. Boston: Wadsworth.

Siegel, S. (1988) *Nonparametric Statistics for the Behavioural Sciences*. New York: McGraw-Hill.

Sprent, P. (1992) *Applied Non-parametric Methods*, 2nd edn. London: Chapman & Hall.

Walker, J.M. & Sofaer, B. (1998) Predictors of psychological distress in chronic pain patients. *Journal of Advanced Nursing* **27**: 320–26.

Appendix 31.1: Formulae for confidence intervals

Confidence interval for a sample mean

The standard error for a sample mean $\bar{x}$ is given by $s/\sqrt{n}$, where s is the sample standard deviation. The confidence interval for a sample mean is:

$$\bar{x} \pm t_{(n-1)} \times s/\sqrt{n}$$

where t is the appropriate value from the t-distribution with $n-1$ degrees of freedom.

Confidence interval for a proportion

The standard error for a sample proportion p is

$$\sqrt{p(p-1)/n}$$

The confidence interval for a sample proportion is

$$p \pm 1.96 \times \sqrt{p(p-1)/n} \quad \text{assuming } n \text{ is large}$$

Confidence interval for a difference between two means

The pooled standard deviation is given by

$$s_p = \sqrt{\frac{(n_1 - 1)s_1^2 + (n_2 - 1)s_2^2}{n_1 + n_2 - 2}}$$

where n_1 and n_2 are the sizes of the two samples.

The standard error of the difference $(\bar{x}_1 - \bar{x}_2)$ is

$$SE(\bar{x}_1 - \bar{x}_2) = s_p \sqrt{1/n_1 + 1/n_2}$$

and the 95% confidence interval is given by

$$(\bar{x}_1 - \bar{x}_2) \pm t_{(n_1 + n_2 - 2)} \times s_p \sqrt{1/n_1 + 1/n_2}$$

where $t_{(n_1 + n_2 - 2)}$ is the 5% point of the t-distribution with $n_1 + n_2 - 2$ degrees of freedom.

Confidence interval for difference between two proportions

For proportions p_1 and p_2 the standard error for their difference $p_1 - p_2$ is

$$SE(p_1 - p_2) = \sqrt{p_1(1 - p_1)/n_1 + p_2(1 - p_2)/n_2}$$

and the 95% confidence interval is given by

$$(p_1 - p_2) \pm 1.96 \times SE(p_1 - p_2)$$

(If p is expressed as a percentage, use 100 instead of 1 in the formula for the standard error.)

CHAPTER 32

Qualitative analysis

Sam Porter

What is qualitative analysis?

The uniqueness of qualitative analysis is that it is not primarily concerned with numerical techniques of organizing, describing and interpreting data. It will be remembered from Chapter 12 that the basic premise of qualitative research was that the social world we live in can only be understood through an understanding of the meanings and motives that guide the social actions and interactions of individuals. That sort of understanding cannot be fully gained through the use of quantitative methods. Qualitative analysis is concerned with describing the actions and interactions of research subjects in a certain context, and with interpreting the motivations and understandings that lie behind those actions. This is, of course, a very broad remit, and requires further elucidation.

The problem with attempting to be specific about the nature of qualitative analysis is that it cannot be reduced to a single formulation. Because there is no one method of qualitative analysis, it is impossible to lay down hard and fast rules about the way it should be done. However, there are some general guidelines that can be elaborated.

The place of analysis in qualitative research

Data analysis does not form a discrete stage of the qualitative research process. It is part of the process all the way through from the selection of the research problem to the writing of the final report.

In this section, I will examine the role of analysis in each stage of the research process, illustrating my points with a practical example. Because of my familiarity with the processes involved in it, my own work on interaction between nurses and doctors will be used as a demonstration model. That research was conducted by means of participant observation in an intensive care unit.

Developing research problems

All research begins with the identification of an issue or problem that the researcher feels is worthy of study. This problem often arises out of the researcher's knowledge of previous studies and theories, although it can also derive from personal experience, or the discovery of interesting or surprising facts. It should be borne in mind that to be worth pursuing, research problems need to be both answerable and manageable. The identification of research problems involves focusing upon specific aspects of the social group that it is proposed to examine. These problems are not like scientific hypotheses; they are not designed to be predictive statements that can be verified or refuted by evidence from the data. They are much looser than that – the purpose is to focus the researcher on a general area of enquiry, without compromising the openness of the research by implying answers to the researcher's own questions.

My research into interaction between doctors and nurses began with the identification of a research problem that emanated from two sources – the reading of sociological and nursing literature on the subject, and personal experience as a clinical nurse. This combination led me to identify inequalities in professional relationships as a problem that was worthy of research. Thus, the problem in my research was how power relations affected and were manifested in interactions between nurses and doctors (Porter, 1991).

After research problems have been identified, the next stage is to manipulate them into a form whereby they can be more easily studied in the field, which is usually done by taking a rather general problem and making it more specific.

On thinking about how I should go about observing power relations between nurses and doctors, I decided that this could be most easily done if I restricted my examination to the manifestation of power in decision-making processes. This sharpening of the focus of the research onto a clearly defined type of interaction meant that I could more easily identify, record and analyse pertinent data. However, the increase in clarity involved in this step was bought at the price of excluding other, less obvious instances of the exercise of power; instances that may have been extremely important in the constitution of occupational relations between nurses and doctors. It is well to remember that sharpening the focus of research may mean that the researcher is less sensitive to other important aspects of the research problem. Prior to hardening up research problems, the researcher should think seriously about these alternative avenues, and whether or not they are sufficiently peripheral to be excluded from the research.

A word of warning here. Many qualitative researchers are wary of making up their minds about the social world they are going to examine before they actually get around to examining it. They are suspicious of the sort of hypothesis testing favoured by quantitative researchers because they believe that it encourages researchers to see the world in the image of their own preconceptions, rather than keeping an open mind about what it will be like when they examine it. While it is useful, indeed essential, to have some sort of research problem worked out before entering the field, these problems should not be cased in granite. Be prepared to alter or abandon them in the light of the evidence you will subsequently gather.

The reason for the inappropriateness of definitive hypotheses lies in the subject of qualitative research. Because it focuses on the actions and interpretations of subjects, each social situation examined will have a distinctive character which cannot be totally covered by a general theory. Abandonment of that which is particular to a given situation entails unwarranted distortion. However, it is also the case that there are commonalties between different social situations, the complete rejection of common conceptual formulations would also be inappropriate. A sensible compromise has been offered by Blumer (1954), who advocates using theories as general guides, rather than fixed prescriptions about what researchers should be addressing.

Perhaps the danger of definitive theories can be best illustrated by looking at another study of the relationship between nurses and doctors. Hughes (1988) criticizes previous analysts for taking the concept of the 'doctor–nurse game' (Stein, 1967) as being definitive of the nature of interoccupational relations. To the extent that analysts have accepted a model of interaction which assumes that nurses will invariably be deferent to doctors, Hughes argues that they 'may have been guilty of assuming a homogeneity in the division of labour that is simply not justified by empirical evidence' (Hughes, 1988). Hughes goes on to demonstrate that the degree to which nurses are subservient or otherwise depends upon the specific situation in which they find themselves. In doing so, he does not reject out of hand the concept of the doctor–nurse game; rather, he argues that it is only applicable in certain circumstances.

Even though they are not definitive, the identification of research problems prior to the commencement of qualitative research will guide the collection of data. However, these pre-understandings should not be seen by the qualitative researchers as iron cages. Phenomena that researchers come across and think might be useful, but which fall outside the remit of their preconceptions, should not be ignored. Rest assured that the data will reveal behaviours and ideas that the researcher could not have conceived of prior to entering the field and collecting data.

Reviewing the literature

As can be seen from Hughes's (1988) comments, the degree to which previous work should mould research is a matter of contention within the qualitative research community. My own opinion is that sole dependence on data for the generation of theory, an approach known as induction, leads to a tendency for researchers to continually re-invent the wheel. Previous literature, both descriptive and theoretical, is there to be used. Researchers should make the most of it, without allowing it to predetermine the outcome of their research.

The importance of the literature review to the process of analysis lies in the grounding it gives researchers in the subject area they are proposing to examine. It narrows the field of enquiry by indicating those problems and perspectives that might be appropriate. Examination of the literature will enable the researcher to judge those areas that have not been adequately researched, or, conversely, the conclusions it would be profitable to test in a different setting.

Thus, in my study (Porter, 1991), I used the previous literature on nurse–doctor interactions to further refine the research problem by extracting from the literature four possible ideal types of interaction in decision-making processes: the total subordination of nurses, the use of the doctor–nurse game, informal nursing assertiveness in decision-making, and open and formally sanctioned involvement of nurses in the making of decisions. However, I went into the research consciously trying to avoid any presumption about which concept would be most accurate – the ideal types were simply adopted as frameworks to organize the data. Thus, I was using the literature to generate ideas rather than to help me decide, before empirical examination, what was actually going on. As it turned out, I found examples of all four ideal types of behaviour.

The cycle of data collection and analysis

The process of data collection and analysis in qualitative research is cyclical. The researcher arrives in the field with some conception of the nature of the behaviour and understandings of the people being researched. These theories are then tested on the data, which themselves suggest refinements to the original theories, or even entirely new theories. These new or improved theories, in turn, also need to be tested on the data (Hammersley & Atkinson, 1995).

The cycle of alternating between data collection and analysis can be demonstrated diagrammatically, as shown in Fig. 32.1. It should be noted that Fig. 32.1 is simplified. It is highly unlikely that a single cycle will enable the qualitative researcher to identify patterns of behaviour and meaning, or to discover variations and limitation to those patterns. The terms used in Fig. 32.1 will be discussed in the remainder of the chapter. It is through the cycle of data collection and analysis that the research becomes ever more acutely focused on the problem at hand. On the basis of this analytical discrimination, the researcher is able to construct a theoretical model that can, at least partially, explain the research problem that has been addressed. This process of analytical focusing can be divided into five stages.

1. The first stage involves the qualitative researcher becoming familiar with the situation under study. The researcher will initially be confronted with a mass of undifferentiated information. The process of making sense of this information entails the identification of patterns of behaviour or discourse.
2. Once patterns have been identified, the research can move on to the second

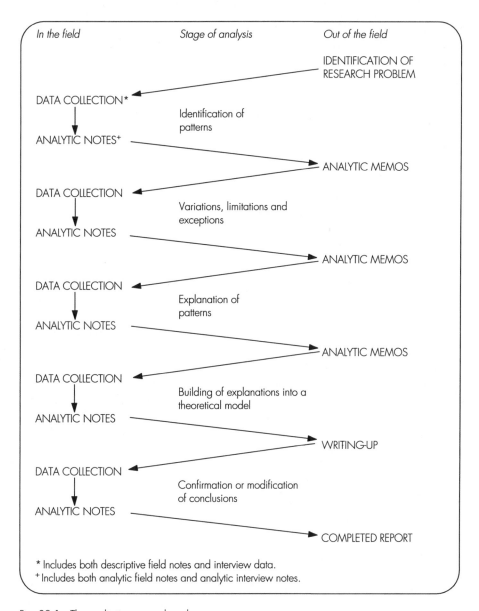

Fig. 32.1 The qualitative research cycle.

stage, which involves fleshing out the data by mapping out variations, limitations and exceptions to the patterns being examined.

3. The third stage of the collection/analysis cycle is concerned with the explanation of patterns that have been identified and elaborated. In qualitative research, this explanation is usually framed around an understanding of the meanings and motives of the research subjects that lay behind their observed behaviour.

4. Having reached the point where patterns have been clarified and explanations for them posited, the next stage of the observation/analysis cycle is the building of explanations into a theoretical model. This involves uncovering the relationship between patterns and tying together the various explanations that have emerged thus far.

5. The final stage involves the confirmation or modification of conclusions that have emerged from the research. This is often accomplished by returning to the field towards the end of the research process.

To illustrate how this process works in practice, I will concentrate on a specific aspect of my participant observation of nurse–doctor relations – namely, the influence of racism upon the dynamics of power (Porter, 1993).

Stage one

I entered the field with a theoretical concept that I had taken from Hughes's (1988) study of nurse–doctor relations. Hughes had noted that white nurses were considerably less deferential in their interactions with Asian doctors than they were with white doctors. Thus the concept with which I arrived was that, to some degree, racism would influence relationships between white health workers and those belonging to ethnic minorities. However, after several weeks in the field as a participant observer, one of the patterns of behaviour that I began to identify was that there was no appreciable difference in the power and status of black and Asian doctors in their interactions with white nurses, as compared to white doctors.

Stage two

Further examination of the behaviour of white nurses revealed that while they were deferent to black and Asian doctors in their open interactions with them, some nurses expressed racist views among themselves in private. Thus, I had identified a variation in the pattern of behaviour of nurses.

Stage three

Given the cycle of observation and analysis that I had thus far conducted, my task was now to explain the variable behaviour of some nurses, taking into account the concept that I had developed from Hughes's study. The explanation evolved around the understandings that nurses had of their occupational situation. I argued that nurses placed considerable faith in the ideology of professionalism. Part of this ideology involved the rejection of irrational judgements. This presented racist nurses with a problem in that racism, by definition, is irrational. Because of the significance of the ideology of professionalism, they were only able to express that racism using an apparently rational pretext. In Hughes's study, this was provided by the cultural unfamiliarity of the Asian doctors observed, which allowed nurses to cloak their racism under the rational veneer of criticism of the doctors' competence. Because the doctors in my study were familiar with the culture pertaining, this avenue of expressing racism was not available to those nurses who were racist.

Stage four

In my study of relations between nurses and doctors, I had noted that, in addition to racism, the quality of interaction was influenced by gender relations and by economic structures. Thus, I had refined three separate theories to help explain the nature of the professional relationship that I was examining. I combined these discrete explanations into a theoretical framework which posited that the actions and understandings of nurses and doctors in their interactions with each other could not be solely understood through examination of factors internal to these occupations or the health care institutions within which they worked. Account also needed to be taken of the powerful influence of wider social structures upon the behaviour of health care professionals (Porter, 1996).

Stage five

In order to test the conclusions that I had come to, I returned to the field several times during the year that followed the initial observation period of three months.

The point of this explanation is to underline the provisional nature of initial theoretical concepts, the requirement to identify the specificities of the social situation being examined and the need to frame qualitative explanations in terms of the understandings of the actors involved.

Having laid out this guide to the stages of qualitative analysis, I should remind readers that it is not a blueprint for every piece of qualitative research. For example, the research might concentrate on a single theme, rendering redundant the final stage of constructing a theoretical model. It is up to each researcher to decide which analytical procedures are appropriate for the research in hand. The only rule is that the researcher should be prepared both to describe and to justify the approach taken.

Triangulation

The key method of ensuring the validity of the processes of qualitative analysis is the use of triangulation, which can be done in two ways. The first method of triangulation involves comparing the outlooks of research subjects. By testing the validity of theories from the different perspectives of different subjects, the researcher can be more confident that the analysis is along the right track.

An example of the use of this sort of triangulation can be seen in research that I conducted into the degree to which the application of ideas emanating from the 'new nursing' has democratized relations between nurses and patients (Porter, 1994). A number of interviewed nurses, who supported the new nursing, claimed that relationships with patients had altered significantly. The danger of sole reliance on these accounts was that they might have led to over-optimistic conclusions about the effectiveness of the new nursing. However, by triangulating these opinions with the responses of subjects who disapproved of the new confidence enjoyed by some patients, but who nevertheless accepted that a degree of democratization had occurred, I was able to improve the validity of my research.

The second method of triangulation involves the collection of different forms of data from the same subjects. If the same sort of results are gained using two or more techniques, then the conclusions that can be drawn are all the stronger. Often triangulation involves the use of both qualitative and quantitative methods. Thus, for example, in an examination of how gender affects nurse–doctor power relations (Porter, 1992), I supplemented qualitative data that indicated that female doctors were more egalitarian in their dealings with nurses than their male colleagues, with some simple statistical analysis. Using the willingness of doctors to tidy up after performing clinical procedures as an indication of egalitarianism, I counted the number of times doctors were prepared to tidy up. I discovered there was a statistically significant association between a doctor's gender and the likelihood of tidying up, female doctors being more likely to do so.

The practicalities of analysis during data collection

The practicalities of data analysis differ according to the method of qualitative research adopted. It will be remembered from Chapter 12 that I identified four major qualitative methods. Here I will concentrate on two – participant observation and in-depth interviews. Because similar techniques are used in in-depth interviews and oral histories, no specific discussion of analysis in the latter method is required. As far as conversation analysis is concerned, the complex technique of breaking down discourse is beyond the remit of this chapter. Readers should consult a specialist text, such as Atkinson & Heritage (1984), if they are interested in pursuing this line of research.

Participant observation

The first thing to note about analysis of material collected during participant observation is that it is dependent upon the quality of data collection. For this reason, the content of the researcher's written descriptions of the situation under study (known as descriptive field notes) should be as full as possible. The recording of speech should be as close to verbatim as the researcher can manage, while non-verbal behaviour needs to be recorded in detail. The context of interactions, in terms of where and when they took place and who was involved, should also be clearly drawn.

Field notes should not simply be descriptive, they should also constitute the first stage of analysis in the data-collection/analysis cycle. Any ideas or comments that researchers have about the situation at the time of observation should be included. These comments are termed *analytical notes*. Because they will subsequently be examined and elaborated upon, analytical notes do not have to be fully worked out, or even consistent. Some will prove to be deadends, but some will supply promising lines of enquiry.

An example of the construction of descriptive and analytical field notes can be taken from qualitative data of the interaction between doctors and nurses of different sexes during aseptic procedures, gathered during my examination into the effects of gender upon occupational relations (Porter, 1992). The first two field notes describe two different social interactions that I observed. In the analytical note that was added to descriptive field note 2, I compare the two interactions and attempt to come to terms with their social significance. The notes remain in the informal language in which they were originally written, although descriptive field note 2 is abbreviated.

Descriptive field note 1 (12/7/89)
'Male SHO and female SN inserting an intercostal drain. Sister has informed staff nurse to prepare. Nurse arrives at bed with trolley, and explains to patient what is going on. Doctor arrives, says nothing to either nurse or patient. Starts procedure. Doctor says nothing at all during procedure except to demand "Gloves!". When he is finished he leaves the bedside without a word, leaving the nurse to clear up his debris.'

Descriptive field note 2 (13/7/89)
'Female SHO and female SN performing intravenous insertion. SHO greets staff nurse and asks if she is free to do it. Both engage in smalltalk... Both nurse and doctor talk to the patient about what is going on, along with smalltalk... Doctor very polite to nurse... SHO "Sorry, would you mind opening these glove for me... Thanks."... On finishing, the doctor tidies away all her waste and thanks nurse.'

Analytical field note (13/7/89)
'Stark comparison between female SHO's actions and those of male SHO yesterday. Two things: (1) She is far more polite, treating nurse and patient with respect. (2) She tidied up after herself and he didn't. Is this an example of gender differences? I could test this by counting whether female doctors tidy up more often than men.'

The main point to be made in relation to field notes is that the participant observer is never only involved in the collection of data. The process of analysis, albeit at a rather crude and spontaneous level, is going on all the time the researcher is in the field. The next level of analysis is the construction of analytical memos. In these, the researcher reviews the research to date, examining the relationship between the data collected and the theories that have been developed. These memos often take the form of short essays, which can be revised, extended or combined as the analytical cycle progresses. In the construction of memos, the researcher calls upon both descriptive and analytical field notes, along with the literature reviewed and analytical memos from previous cycles of analysis. Analytical memos, while involving more reflection than analytical notes, are still provisional pieces of work. However, as the research develops, they will become increasingly sophisticated.

The final analytical stage of writing-up allows researchers to step back, clarify their thinking and organize their ideas more elegantly. Almost invariably, new connections emerge at this stage that were not considered during the period of data collection. For this reason, if possible, it is wise to keep access to the field open, so that these new ideas can be subjected to some empirical testing. As can be seen, the data-gathering/analysis cycle persists to the end of the process of research.

As analytical categories are developed, the researcher will need to code the data collected according to those categories. Coding entails constructing a system whereby all instances of data pertinent to each category can be retrieved. There are a number of methods of doing this. In a grading of technological sophistication, these include the use of card indexes, cutting and pasting on a word processor and the application of dedicated software. The use of computers in qualitative analysis is discussed in Chapter 33.

Interview data

The process of analysis of in-depth interviews is very similar to that of participant observation data. Data collection takes the form of the interviews themselves, while analytical notes can be added immediately after the interviews, while the encounter with the subject is still fresh, or during the process of transcription. Interviews should be transcribed as soon as possible after they take place. The ideal is to transcribe the same day as the interview. This enables the researcher to remember the subtleties of interaction, and perhaps recall unclear pieces of recorded speech. The researcher should listen carefully to the tone and emphasis of respondents, which can often tell a lot.

The same cycle of gathering data and analysing should be adhered to when the data come from interviews. For this reason, researchers should not arrange to conduct all their interviews in a condensed period of time. Spacing out interviews gives researchers the opportunity to use subsequent interviews to retest theories developed both in analytical memos and the writing-up stage.

Reporting qualitative analysis

The variability of qualitative techniques makes the recounting of methods in research reports a lot more cumbersome than it is in much quantitative research. Because of the differences of method between different qualitative studies, it is important that researchers clearly, honestly and comprehensively report the nature of the analytical methods that they use.

An example of good practice can be found in Sherblom et al.'s (1993) examination of nurses' ethical decision-making, where they clearly explain their use of the responsive reader method of analysis. This method of analysing interview transcripts was designed to emphasize the multiple voices of subjects, and indeed researchers, instead of narrowly focusing upon specific issues that the researcher had already decided were important. In Sherblom et al.'s research, the responsible reader method is used to analyse data gained from interviews with nurses in order to show how the concepts of justice and care animate their decisions. Sherblom et al. explain that each interview transcript was subjected to a number of readings. The aim of the first reading was to become attuned with the point of view of the subject. The second reading entailed searching for themes associated with the concept of justice. This process was repeated to identify themes related to caring. A fourth reading highlighted those concerns that did not fit into either the care or justice perspectives. Moreover, in presenting their analysis, Sherblom et al. grounded it in numerous quotations from the nurses interviewed, thus allowing the readers to conduct their own readings of the expressions of the participants.

The painstaking explanation provided by Sherblom et al. means that a reader of that research, who may not have been previously aware of the responsive reader method of analysis, is able to understand clearly the aim and process of the research, and judge its accuracy and utility accordingly.

Conclusions

The reader will now be aware that the process of qualitative analysis is far from being simple or straightforward. The qualitative researcher is largely bereft of the sort of clear guidelines that quantitative colleagues enjoy. To a considerable extent, success depends upon the curiosity, imagination and erudition of the researcher, not to mention the all-important factor of serendipity. This is another good reason for qualitative researchers to include in their written reports a clear description of their analytical procedures. It is only by doing so that they can demonstrate to readers that the path that was taken was a valid one.

One of the consequences of the uncertain nature of qualitative analysis is that it is impossible for textbooks such as this to provide a cookbook recipe for the prosecution of qualitative research. For this reason, anyone considering carrying out a piece of qualitative research for the first time is strongly advised to ensure that she has close supervision from an experienced qualitative researcher, who will be able to guide her through the unexpected pitfalls and opportunities that will inevitably arise. Nevertheless, qualitative analysis, because it involves such close contact with people, is an extremely satisfying way of conducting research work. As such, it has much to commend it to nursing researchers.

References

Atkinson, J.M. & Heritage, J. (1984) *Structures of Social Action: Studies in Conversational Analysis*. Cambridge: Cambridge University Press.

Blumer, H. (1954) What is wrong with social theory? *American Sociological Review* **19**: 3–10.

Hammersley, M. & Atkinson, P. (1995) *Ethnography: Principles in Practice*. London: Routledge.

Hughes, D. (1988) When nurse knows best: some aspects of nurse/doctor interaction in a casualty department. *Sociology of Health and Illness* **10**: 1–22.

Porter, S. (1991) A participant observation study of power relations between nurses and doctors in a general hospital. *Journal of Advanced Nursing* **16**: 728–35.

Porter, S. (1992) Women in a women's job: the gendered experience of nurses. *Sociology of Health and Illness* **14**: 510–27.

Porter, S. (1993) Critical realist ethnography: the case of racism and professionalism in a medical setting. *Sociology* **27**: 591–609.

Porter, S. (1994) New nursing: the road to freedom? *Journal of Advanced Nursing* **20**: 269–74.

Porter, S. (1996) *Nursing's Relationship with Medicine*. Aldershot: Avebury.

Sherblom, S., Shipps, T. & Sherblom, J. (1993) Justice, care and integrated concerns in the ethical decision making of nurses. *Qualitative Health Research* **3**: 442–64.

Stein, L. (1967) The doctor–nurse game. *Archives of General Psychiatry* **16**: 699–703.

Further reading

For readers wishing to study qualitative research in more depth, the following large text is probably the most useful source:

Denzin, N.K. & Lincoln, Y.S. (1994) *Handbook of Qualitative Inquiry*. London: Sage.

The above volume has subsequently been reprinted in three paperback volumes:

Denzin, N.K. & Lincoln, Y.S. (1998) *The Landscape of Qualitative Research*. London: Sage.

Denzin, N.K. & Lincoln, Y.S. (1998) *Strategies of Qualitative Inquiry*. London: Sage.

Denzin, N.K. & Lincoln, Y.S. (1998) *Collecting and Interpreting Qualitative Materials*. London: Sage.

For more specific applications of qualitative research to nursing:

Holloway, I. & Wheeler, S. (eds) (1996) *Qualitative Research for Nurses*. Oxford: Blackwell Science.

CHAPTER 33

Computer-assisted data analysis

David C. Benton

Computer technology continues to advance at a phenomenal rate. It is not long since the only researchers with access to computers were those working for academic institutions or large corporations. However, in the last ten years or so, many households now have their own computer and most health care establishments have a range of equipment available.

The purpose of this chapter is not to describe in detail the technology, hardware and software behind computer-based data analysis, but to look at some of the practicalities. Accordingly, general principles rather than specific details will be explored.

Qualitative and quantitative data analysis

Throughout this text we have considered both qualitative and quantitative research methods. Today's computer technology can assist us in the analysis of data generated by either approach. While computers have been used for many years for assisting researchers in the analysis of quantitative data, their use in analysing and exploring qualitative data is a relatively new phenomenon. It is not the intention to replicate the contents of Chapters 30–32 and therefore the detail of the analytical procedures being used will only be reproduced in this chapter if this adds clarity to the understanding of how computer analysis can be undertaken. Furthermore, reference is made to a number of computer programs throughout this text. In the case of qualitative software a list of contact points for further information is given in Appendix 33.1.

Computerized quantitative data analysis

Quantitative data can be analysed using a wide range of software packages. Some of these packages are specifically designed to conduct statistical analysis, whereas others often offer a limited set of statistical procedures as a feature of a broader specialized program. Programs such as spreadsheets, databases and graphics packages can all offer facilities that will enable statistical analysis to take place.

Spreadsheets, databases and graphics packages

A *spreadsheet* can best be thought of as an electronic data sheet made up of a series of rows and columns. Each row and column is labelled so individual squares can be cross-referenced. Statistical analysis can be undertaken by either writing specific formulae involving the contents of the various rows and columns, or by using predefined procedures. For example, a column of numbers can first be added then divided by the total number of data elements. This would give the mean. Conversely the function MEAN, available on most spreadsheet programs, may be used to perform the same operation.

Databases can contain both textual and numerical information. Databases are in wide use within health service settings. It is often possible for researchers to gain access to data that have been already recorded and stored as part of the patient information system. Researchers can then either formulate queries based on the various information stored within the database and/or take advantage of the wide range of specialized functions offered by the package. Like spreadsheets, databases commonly offer functions such as mean, standard deviation and other basic descriptive statistics.

Graphics packages that can display information in bar, line or pie chart format frequently offer a range of basic descriptive statistical functions that can be applied to the data which generate the graphical output.

In summary, *spreadsheets*, *databases* and *graphics packages* can provide researchers with a restricted range of statistical procedures. On the whole, these non-specialist packages can calculate basic descriptive statistics. However, if more advanced techniques, in particular inferential statistical analysis, are to be conducted then a specialized package is required.

Specialized quantitative computer analysis programs

There are a number of statistics packages available on the market. This chapter will use, for illustrative purposes, one of the most widely used and comprehensive packages available. SPSS* which stands for Statistical Package for the Social Sciences has been developed over the past 30 or so years from a program originally used on mainframe computers to one that is now available on standard desktop personal computers.

A sophisticated program such as SPSS offers a wide range of statistical procedures. Not all of these come as standard and the package consists of a number of modules which can be purchased to meet the specific needs of the researcher. It is important to recognize that even the base package is sufficiently comprehensive

---

* SPSS stands for Statistical Package for the Social Sciences and is the registered trademark of SPSS Inc., 444 North Michigan Avenue, Chicago, IL 60611, USA.

to meet the needs of most researchers unless highly specific and advanced tests are required.

While it is not the intention to give a detailed review of the analytical tools available within this package or the syntax of how the analysis is conducted, a review of some of the basic features is now given. Since personal computers are available to many researchers, rather than examine the mainframe-based version, discussion will be focused around SPSS for Windows. A version which runs under MS DOS, another type of computer-operating system, is also available for older machines. The Windows version is easier to use but does not give the researcher the same level of access to the underlying principles. For those researchers who are less confident with computers, the Windows version certainly requires fewer computing skills.

Starting SPSS

SPSS is a large and sophisticated program. It can undertake both descriptive and inferential statistical analyses, present information in tabular or graphical form, import information from existing data sources such as a database or spreadsheet, and produce output that is ready for inclusion in final reports. In addition to these functions, SPSS can also provide facilities that enable the researcher to create or reproduce on screen questionnaire structures which then can be used for entering data and preparing them for analysis.

Whether using SPSS for Windows or DOS, on starting the system the researcher is faced with a series of menu options. By highlighting one of these options, further related choices can be made. This process of selection from menus continues until the various commands required are reached. Within the Windows version of the package context sensitive help is available at all times and can provide the inexperienced user with easy to follow support.

Preparing data for analysis

It has already been illustrated in Chapter 29 that data can be stored in a variety of formats. SPSS enables data to be entered directly into a template which resembles the original questionnaire, in a spreadsheet format, or as a data list. Figures 33.1, 33.2 and 33.3 illustrate how these would look if such approaches were used. For

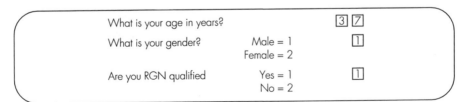

Fig. 33.1 Example of questionnaire entry screen (case 01).

Case No	Age	Gender	RGN
01	37	1	1
02	24	2	1
03	45	1	2
04	32	1	1
05	22	2	2
06	34	2	2

Fig. 33.2   Questionnaire data in spreadsheet format.

```
Data List
/Case 1–2 Age 3–4 Gender 5 RGN 6        }   Describes location of variables
Variable Labels                              within data list
/Case 'Subject Number'
/Age 'Age of Respondent'                 }   Gives labels to variable name
/Gender 'Sex of Respondent'                  which can be printed when
/RGN 'Is Respondent RGN Qualified'           analysis is conducted
BEGIN DATA
013711
022421
034512
043211                                   }   Data (Case, Age, Gender, RGN)
052222
063422
END DATA
FINISH.
```

Fig. 33.3   Questionnaire data in data list format.

illustrative purposes, a very simple questionnaire structure is used. Figure 33.1 illustrates a single set of answers relating to one subject or case. Figures 33.2 and 33.3 illustrate the same case as entered in Fig. 33.1 (case 1) along with the subsequent five cases. A case is the terminology used for the responses made by a single research subject.

Uncategorized data

The examples used in Figs 33.1, 33.2 and 33.3 are all data that reduce to numerical values. That is, the data are either continuous variables such as age or are capable of being categorized and coded, for example yes = 1, no = 2. SPSS can, however, handle uncategorized data. For example, the open-ended question 'What did you enjoy most about your RGN training?' could be stored within an SPSS data file. However, in this case it would be stored as a text string. SPSS would not allow any detailed analysis of this string to take place but could print out all responses to this question so the researcher could then conduct some form of content analysis (see later in this chapter).

Missing data

Sometimes respondents do not complete all questions in a questionnaire. This may be simply a mistake or the respondent may choose not to answer particular questions. Irrespective of the reason, the researcher needs some systematic way of handling these missing responses. It is common practice to allocate a specific code to missing data. When missing data occur, the code can therefore be entered. By examining the percentage of data missing in relation to any particular question, a researcher may gain valuable insights. For example, a lot of missing data relating to a particular question may indicate that the question is poorly structured and therefore respondents are unwilling or unsure as to how to offer a reply. On the other hand, it may indicate a question that respondents find particularly sensitive to answer. Such an example might include 'How much money do you earn?'. Missing data, therefore, may give additional valuable information.

Data entry and verification

As has been seen from Figs 33.1, 33.2 and 33.3, there are a variety of ways of entering data. Chapter 29 illustrated that it is sometimes necessary to code the subject's response into a numerical value. For example, a tick in a particular box might have to be given a numerical coded value. Obviously the more often this has to occur, the greater the chance of an error resulting. SPSS offers a number of ways of ensuring that errors in data entry do not occur. By displaying the information in the spreadsheet format, simple inspection of the layout may reveal errors in data entry. Alternatively the computer can ask you to re-enter perhaps 10% of all questionnaires, comparing the original entry with the subsequent attempt at verification. If a large number of discrepancies are flagged up, then clearly widescale verification is required.

Data cleaning

If the need for widescale verification is identified, then there are a number of ways of 'cleaning' the data – removing errors. SPSS allows the researcher to set certain limits on the types of information that can be entered. For example, if the expected response to the question of gender is 1 for male and 2 for female, any other response such as 3, 4, 5 can be disallowed. This would prevent errors occurring at the data entry stage. It would not, of course, prevent a male respondent being classified as female.

Some conditional responses can also be pre-programmed. For example, if a respondent to a health questionnaire classified himself as male, you would not expect any data to be entered in a section relating to menstruation. Data consistency can therefore be ensured if such rules are entered and applied within individual cases.

Documentation

A piece of research can take anything from perhaps one month to several years to complete. The researcher may after, perhaps, another few years wish to return to the original data to compare it with updated information obtained, or to conduct further analysis. If the data are inadequately documented, then problems can arise. For example, did '1' mean male or female? It is essential that the manner by which data are coded is adequately documented. Some researchers refer to this process as creating a 'data dictionary'. Each variable would therefore have information on the location within a data string, a label attached to the variable which explains in more detail what the information is about, a set of value labels which explain each and every coded response, for example 1 = male, 2 = female, and finally the code that is used for missing data. Only by carrying out such a detailed description can a researcher be assured that mistakes will not occur when she, or perhaps another researcher, explores the dataset in the future.

A worked example In this example, the researcher is trying to identify the barriers experienced by nurses in implementing research into their practice. The questionnaire consists of data from a number of sources – educationalists, community-based nurses, health visitors and midwives. The respondents are asked to give their views on how significant a series of 29 statements are in inhibiting their ability to implement research-based practice. Subjects are then asked to identify what they see as the top three barriers to implementation. Additional demographic information relating to gender, age, highest level of educational attainment is also recorded. Appendix 33.2 gives details of the structure of the data list file and Appendix 33.3, an illustration of the data from the study.

The actual data file contained the responses of 424 respondents. A request to describe the staff group the various respondents came from resulted in the output detailed in Table 33.1. The analysis took less than five seconds to carry out.

Table 33.1 Frequency count of the staff groups of the respondents

Value label	Value	Frequency	%	Valid %	Cumulative %
Educationalists	1	77	18.2	18.2	18.2
Community-based nurses	2	159	37.5	37.5	55.7
Health visitors	3	71	16.7	16.7	72.4
Midwives	4	117	27.6	27.6	100.0
Total		424	100.0	100.0	

Valid cases 424   Missing cases 0

While the above example only illustrates the use of a straightforward descriptive statistic, SPSS can perform a wide range of complex analytical procedures. For each analysis a well thought out layout which presents the results is available – the default format. These default formats, as can be seen from Table 30.1, are of a sufficiently high standard that they can be readily incorporated into the results section of a research report without the need for any modification.

Computerized qualitative research analysis

Computers can be used to assist the researcher in qualitative analysis. As computer technology has become more readily available, qualitative researchers have had at their disposal a new means of supporting the conduct of analysis of interview transcripts, ethnographic field notes and other data sources. These new high-technology techniques are far more sophisticated than the traditional scissors, copier and card indexes traditionally used.

Computers are tools that can undertake repetitive tasks and calculations at incredible speeds and therefore can assist the qualitative researcher by doing anything that it is possible to do on paper, but more quickly, easily and with greater efficiency and precision. Accordingly, the ability of the computer to tirelessly search large volumes of material has enabled qualitative researchers to more easily identify key material embedded within lengthy transcripts. This in turn has made it easier for researchers to find deviant cases and to extract small but significant pieces of information which might otherwise go unnoticed. Computer technology, therefore, provides the researcher with a dedicated assistant that can remove much of the tedium associated with qualitative analysis.

Software available for qualitative analysis

Computer programs for the analysis of qualitative data fall into two distinct types: off-the-shelf and dedicated/specialist programs.

Researchers can make use of generally available software packages such as word processors or database management programs. Both these off-the-shelf solutions offer many of the facilities that can assist the qualitative researcher in analysing her data. In addition, however, there are available a number of specialist programs which have been developed for the qualitative researcher. These fall into three main types: chunking and coding programs, qualitative modelling programs, and expert systems. Both off-the-shelf and specialist package styles are now described.

Off-the-shelf programs

Off-the-shelf programs such as word processors and database management systems can both be used for qualitative data analysis.

Word processors

Standard word-processing packages can be used for the analysis of qualitative datasets. In short, they are ideally suited to identifying words or individual blocks of text. With the advent of more sophisticated packages such as Microsoft Word* Version 8, several files can be searched at once. This could mean, for example, that an interview with an individual subject may be recorded in a single file. By searching all the files, all interviews could be searched for the occurrence of certain word groups or phrases. In addition, such packages can automatically generate an index, detailing the frequency of occurrence and location of the various phrases being searched for.

Database management systems

Relational databases are becoming increasingly sophisticated. Initially they were thought of simply as a means of holding numerical data. However, as each generation of program has been developed, increased sophistication in text management has become a significant feature. Again, like word processors, they can store large quantities of text, search for information and index this for further use.

Specialist packages

While off-the-shelf packages can offer a range of basic analytical tools for more sophisticated techniques, specialist programs are required. Many of these programs have been developed by qualitative researchers who wished to take advantage of the computer's ability to manipulate large quantities of data in a flexible and efficient manner.

Chunking and coding programs

Chunking and coding programs have been specially developed to meet the needs of qualitative researchers and are especially useful in analysing fieldnotes and transcripts. The field notes and transcripts are inspected and codes are then assigned to various segments which are of interest to the researcher. The computer program can then be asked to abstract these various 'chunks' of 'coded' material and display them together with the text with which they are associated. In short, these programs offer little more than the more sophisticated word-processing packages that are now currently available. Programs such as ETHNOGRAPH were developed in the early to middle 1980s when word-processing packages were generally not as sophisticated as the current generation.

---

* Microsoft Word is the registered trademark for Microsoft Ltd, Microsoft Place, Warfdale Road, Winnersh Triangle, Wokingham, Berks RG11 5TP.

Qualitative 'modelling' programs

Qualitative modelling programs try to expose the underlying connections and structures of the data being analysed. Accordingly, many qualitative researchers are wary of these systems since they contend that there is a danger that a mechanical approach to the generation of qualitative theory may result in 'mechanical' solutions. However, if researchers do not blindly accept the connections being suggested but critically consider the material, then the researcher stays in control thereby choosing to either accept or reject the structures being suggested by such programs. ETHNOGRAPH is an example of such a package.

Expert systems

With the increased sophistication of computer technology, expert systems are being developed which can sift through vast quantities of data in such a way as to distil out phrases, their associated linkages and thereby the developing categories and theory. The further development of expert systems could be considered analogous to the computer turning from dedicated clerk to supervised research assistance.

Teaching

Irrespective of the program being used, an added advantage that computerized analysis programs offer is the ability to enable qualitative analysis to be more readily taught. Generally speaking, the principles of qualitative analysis are given to student researchers but it is not until they actually conduct a piece of research that they use the techniques live. With the advent of computer technology, lecturers can offer students the opportunity to analyse existing datasets with the assistance of the various programs available. Since it is the researcher who is controlling the process, this does not mean that all students would necessarily come up with the same or similar analytical solutions, but would at least in a reasonable time frame have had experience of analysing the same data. Accordingly, not only do students gain insight into using the various computer packages on offer, but also via discussion with their peers gain a more comprehensive insight into qualitative analysis.

Software analytical capabilities

While there are significant differences between various qualitative analytical approaches (see Chapters 12, 13 and 32) there are certain commonalities which do exist. These commonalities include:

- locating individual words and phrases;
- creating alphabetic word lists which include the frequency of occurrence of the various words;
- creating indexes (locating the various words within the overall data source);
- attaching key words to segments of text;
- attaching codes or categories to segments of text linking codes to identify and align relationships;
- connecting codes.

Locating individual words and phrases

As already noted, there is no need to buy sophisticated and specialized qualitative analysis packages to enable the researcher to locate individual codes or phrases. The FIND command available in both word processors and database management packages is perfectly adequate for this purpose. In most cases a dialogue box (the way the user requests access to a specific command) is used. Various constraints can be placed on the 'search' – for example, forwards, backwards, finding whole words only or using a phonetic search (that is, finding words that sound like the word being searched for). The computer will then search through the file for all occurrences of the word or phrase being sought. This will then be highlighted and the researcher can view on the screen the various locations. As an illustrative example, Fig. 33.4 displays the output of a search for the word 'research' in a short piece of interview text. Only exact matches, that is, research as opposed to researcher, were sought. Figure 33.4 does not illustrate the use of any particular software program since the syntax varies from one to another and therefore it is only the principles that are illustrated here.

FIND: research

LIMITS OF SEARCH:- WHOLE WORDS ONLY, WHOLE DOCUMENT

While there might have been more lofty aims to do with integrating **research** into practice and all that sort of thing, it was much more about safeguarding nursing. It was about getting influence, I felt that nursing had lost influence when general management came in. Because of the kind of **research** that was put forward I got the feeling that general managers didn't value what was being done. To get any sort of credibility there was a need to take the initiative by getting it right. Playing the game by their rules. Researchers needed to be politically aware if nursing was to progress the **research** based agenda advocated by Briggs and others.

Fig. 33.4 FIND dialogue box and resultant search of an interview text.

Creating alphabetic word list and counting the frequency of occurrence of words

The ability to identify not only the words used by research subjects but their frequency often gives qualitative researchers valuable insights into the vocabulary of the research subjects. Such a tool often provides a basic starting point for content analysis. By comparing the words and their frequency across a number of interview subjects, commonalities can be found. There are a variety of programs that enable this to happen, for example TEXT COLLECTOR, CONCORDANCE and ZYINDEX. These programs allow the researcher to indicate common words such as 'the', 'and', 'he', 'it' which are in effect background noise which can then be discounted. This reduces the total extensive list to a manageable list of words which may provide real insight into the content of the transcript.

Creating indexes

While comparing the vocabulary of one subject to another, or indeed one part of a transcript to another originated by the same subject, it is the ability to locate the occurrences of words within the totality of the document that is important. The production of an index can provide information on several levels. It can identify the source document, the chapter or segment in which the word is located, the page and, perhaps even more importantly for qualitative researchers, the paragraph and line numbers. By comparing the relative location of the occurrences of such words an understanding of the context can be obtained. The key word under consideration can then be placed in the context of the data sources. It may then be possible to identify, for example, that the word 'research' has been mentioned by every respondent and that it typically occurs within the first three paragraphs of the interview conducted. While standard word-processing packages are becoming far more sophisticated in offering such facilities, specialized qualitative research analysis packages do provide a more comprehensive range of options. TEXT BASE ALPHA, a relatively cheap program, excels in this task in that it not only provides all the necessary indexing information but also prints the 30 succeeding and the 30 preceding characters associated with the word being indexed. This obviously gives the researcher significant contextual information upon which to base a more sophisticated analysis rather than simply that which can be derived from location and frequency of occurrence.

Attaching key words to segments of text

It is not always the case that we mention a specific key word when trying to communicate a concept or idea. In Chapter 13 when illustrating memo writing, the category of empowerment was identified. Figure 33.5 illustrates how the key

While there might have been more lofty aims to do with integrating research into practice and all that sort of thing, it was much more about safeguarding nursing. **It was about getting influence**, I felt that nursing had lost influence when general management came in. Because of the kind of research that was put forward I got the feeling that general managers didn't value what was being done. **To get any sort of credibility** there was a **need to take the initiative** by getting it right. Playing the game by their rules. **Researchers needed to be politically aware** if nursing was to progress the research based agenda advocated by Briggs and others.	Empowerment Empowerment Empowerment Empowerment

Fig. 33.5   Illustrating the attachment of key words to segments of text.

word of empowerment is attached to the various segments of text which convey and verbalise this idea.

Attaching codes or categories to segments of text

It is important to note that there is a difference between key words and codes. In short, key words can be considered as one-word summaries of the content of a text segment whereas codes are the abbreviations of category names. Codes can be attached to various chunks of text which then produce or convey a particular category of meaning. Coded text can be overlapping or indeed codes can be nested within existing segments. A search using one of the codes will therefore result in the reproduction of all segments to which that code is attached. Such a search will yield information regarding the location of the segment within the original text. All qualitative analysis programs offer such facilities and QUALPRO is a program that enables the user to segment material, code it, then perform searches.

Connecting codes

If qualitative researchers are truly to understand the nature of the subject under investigation, then it is not simply sufficient to code material but they must gain an understanding of the underlying structures. The ability to link coded sections in a meaningful way provides such a facility. By undertaking this step it is possible then to develop propositional statements or to make assertions regarding the structure of the linkages so that various concepts can be related, thereby enabling the researcher to discover the underlying principles. In short, this feature enables theory-building to take place. Programs such as NUDIST and ATLAS provide the researcher with such facilities. By looking at the pattern of coded segments both within an individual interview and across interviews, it is possible to discover underlying principles and theories. Similarly, by testing for the absence of linkages it is also possible to either confirm or refute the hypothesis being developed.

Conclusions

This chapter has not attempted to provide an in-depth critique of how the various computer programs can be used in both quantitative and qualitative analysis. It has, however, identified some of the basic principles and provided some direction as to how the researcher can take the subject of computer-based analysis further. Extensive texts have been written on this subject, but the selection of these will be dependent on both the hardware and the software resources available to you. Many researchers with links into academia will have ready access to many of the programs described in this chapter; hence, before pursuing the specifics any further, early contact should be made with local research experts and/or computer specialists. A failure to do so may result in much wasted time.

It is important to note that computer technology does not replace the thinking and decision-making required by researchers to analyse and interpret their data intelligently. Computer science only removes the tedium of repetitive calculation and data organization. The time freed from such activities can therefore be applied to data interpretation, hopefully adding to the quality of the research undertaken.

Further reading

Burnard, P. (1994) Searching for meaning: a method of analysing interview transcripts with a personal computer. *Nurse Education Today* 14 (2): 111–17.
Morison, M. & Moir, J. (1998) The role of computer software in the analysis of qualitative data: efficient clerk, research assistant or Trojan horse? *Journal of Advanced Nursing* 28 (1): 106–16.
Ratcliffe, P. (1998) Using the 'new' statistics in nursing research. *Journal of Advanced Nursing* 27 (1): 132–9.

Appendix 33.1: Qualitative software programs

ATLAS	IFP ATLAS Sekr Hab, 6 Hardenbergerstr 28, D-1000, Berlin 12, Germany.
CONCORDANCE	Dataflight Software, 10573 West Pico Blvd, Los Angeles CA 90064.
ETHNO	The National Collegic Software Clearing House, Duke University Press, 6697 College Station, Durham NC 27708.
ETHNOGRAPH	Qualitative Research Management, 73425 Hilltop Road, Desert Hot Springs, California CA 92240.

NUDIST   La Trobe University, Bundoora, Victoria 3083, Australia.
QUALPRO   Qualitative Research Management, 73425 Hilltop Road, Desert
                     Hot Springs, California CA 92240.
TEXT BASE ALPHA   Qualitative Research Management, 73425 Hilltop Road, Desert
                     Hot Springs, California CA 92240.
TEXT COLLECTOR   O'Neill Software, PO Box 2611, San Francisco CA 94126.
ZYINDEX   ZyLab Corporation, 233 Erie Street, Chicago IL 60611.

Appendix 33.2: List of variable definitions, variable labels and value labels for research barrier questionnaire

data list file = "dcb.dat"
/source 1, id 2–4, q1 to q29 5–33, great 34–35, second 36–37, third 38–39, sex 40, age 41, educ 42
variable labels source "Staff Group"
/ID "Questionnaire Number"
/ql "Reports Availability"
/q2 "Practice Implications"
/q3 "Stats Understandable"
/q4 "Practice relevance"
/q5 "Nurse awareness"
/q6 "Implement facilities"
/q7 "Time to read"
/q8 "Research replication"
/q9 "Benefits minimal"
/q10 "Results believable"
/q11 "Methods inadequate"
/q12 "Literature compiled"
/q13 "Authority to change"
/q14 "Not Generalizable"
/q15 "Nurse Isolation"
/q16 "Little self benefit"
/q17 "Reports old"
/q18 "Dr's non-cooperation"
/q19 "Admin non-cooperation"
/q20 "Research value"
/q21 "No stimulus for change"
/q22 "Conclusions not justified"
/q23 "Literature conflicting"
/q24 "Research unreadable"
/q25 "Staff Not Supportive"
/q26 "Unwilling to change"
/q27 "Too much information"
/q28 "Not able to critique"
/q29 "Insufficient time"
/great "Greatest Barrier"

/second "Second Gt Barrier"
/third "Third Gt Barrier"
/sex "Gender of Subject"
/Age "Age of Subject"
/educ "Highest Educational Level"
value labels source: 1 "Educationalists", 2 "Community Based Nurses",
3 "Health Visitors", 4 "Midwives"
/q1 to q29: 1 "To no extent", 2 "To a little extent", 3 "To a moderate extent",
4 "To a great extent", 5 "No opinion"
/sex 1 "Male", 2 "Female"
/Age 1 "Under 25", 2 "25 to 34", 3 "35 to 44", 4 "45 to 54", 5 "55 and over"
/educ 1 "O grade/level", 2 "A level/H grade", 3 "Diploma", 4 "Basic Degree",
5 "Advanced Diploma", 6 "Taught Masters", 7 "M.Phil", 8 "Doctorate", 0 "None"
missing values q1 to q29 sex to educ (9)
/great to third (99).

Appendix 33.3: Sample of data list from barriers to research questionnaire

10772424324551314343231232125533429071513146
10763332432233233343233333222343349282505126
10753342344425244544354211234334431252832
10744333443334344443444243434444433032135
10733334434233344343444335234214415121818134
10721442322434444433333322233349313233135
10713341432442233344155344235333221510515134
10702232431143243243245152445224314905150512124
10694322333322142321231211112223134291201244
...
Continues to end of data file.

CHAPTER 34

Data presentation

Desmond F.S. Cormack and David C. Benton

The dissemination of research has long been, and continues to be, recognized as crucial to the development of a nursing and midwifery research base. However, not only have there been difficulties in gaining access to much of the material produced, but there have also been problems in comprehending some of the material. Data presentation – or, to define it more explicitly, getting your results across and understood by your readers – is a critical element of any study.

By examination of the definition given, it is evident that it is not adequate to simply display results, since they must also be understood. Unless results are comprehended by your audience, there is no opportunity to receive feedback or for readers to consider and reflect on their own practice in the light of new information. It is essential that data are presented in a manner that is clearly understood via an appropriate medium, using an appropriate format, so as to facilitate both individual and our profession's development.

Data can be presented in many ways. The book that you are currently reading is a data source; it has a wealth of information about the research process. Hopefully, the information will be read, reflected upon, integrated into your personal knowledge base and used at some point in the future.

As you can see from this text, in addition to the written word you can also find numeric, graphical and pictorial data, all of which have particular strengths and weaknesses. Before dealing with each of these specific approaches, a number of general issues relating to data presentation are examined.

Data presentation techniques: general issues

The method chosen to present data is obviously dependent on a number of factors such as the type of data, the target readership, and the overall design of your study. In today's technological world, there is an ever-increasing number of aids which can be used to assist in the presentation of material. If communication of results is to be effective, the appropriate use of technological aids must be made.

Whether these aids are used to prepare a scientific paper, a journal article, a book chapter, or an overhead transparency, there are a number of fundamental principles which must be considered.

Computer technology has given the researcher, via the word processor and desktop publishing system, access to a wide variety of means of emphasizing data. Figure 34.1 lists a number of commonly available means of gaining readers' attention.

- Highlighting
- Capitals
- Size of print
- Markers and pointers
- Colour or variations of shading
- Change of colour
- Different fonts
- Indenting – subsections

Fig. 34.1   Approaches to gaining your readers' attention.

There are several means of *highlighting* data so as to enable it to stand out and attract attention. **Bold** and underlining can easily yet effectively help focus attention on a particular point.

Another simple yet effective way of drawing attention to a point, is to use CAPITALS. This can be particularly effective when the rest of the data are presented in lower case.

The ready availability of word processors and desktop publishing systems have given easy access to a number of techniques which were in the past only generally available to printers, graphic artists and designers.

With new technological assistance, it is easy to produce print in a variety of sizes. This feature is particularly useful if you are using overhead transparencies or a poster presentation format. Unless data are presented in large, bold characters, an audience will have great difficulty in seeing and hence interpreting the value of your work.

Markers or pointers in their simplest form may only be an asterisk, and are commonly used as a means of highlighting statistically significant associations (see Table 34.1). However, with the introduction of new technology, much more sophisticated characters can be used. For example, ◆◆□❀●⌘■○.

Table 34.1   Correlation Table demonstrating pointers

	Variable 1	Variable 2	Variable 3	Variable 4
Variable 1	1.000	0.857**	−0.486	−0.403
Variable 2		1.000	−0.777**	−0.692*
Variable 3			1.000	0.820**
Variable 4				1.000

$N = 17$
1 tailed significance level $* p = 0.01$ $** p = 0.001$

With high-technology printers, it is possible to use either colour or variations in shade as a means of enhancing the clarity of data presentation. Colour laser photocopiers can produce material (at a cost) such as photographs or other figures which can add significantly to the quality of a presentation. Consider how effective it is to show a photograph of a wound rather than trying to describe it accurately and succinctly. However, great care must be taken when colour print is used on colour background. If an inappropriate choice is made the colours may clash or, worse still, due to poor contrast, be illegible. As an example, the colour combinations indicated in Fig. 34.2 are acceptable and easy to read.

Text colour	Appropriate background colour
White	Red, blue, black
Yellow	Blue, black
Cyan	Black
Green	Black
Red	White, yellow
Blue	White, yellow, cyan
Black	White, yellow, cyan

Fig. 34.2 Legible text and background colour combinations.

Even the most basic word-processing systems offer the researcher the use of at least two **different fonts**. A font is the term given to a particular typeface in a particular size of print. Commonly a style such as italics is readily available in most basic fonts. Italics are particularly useful for reporting quoted subject material. By incorporating both *italics* and indenting, verbal quotes from subjects can effectively and efficiently be identified from the main text. For example:

'We think new technology offers the researcher a great number of useful and easy to use means of improving the clarity and quality of data presentation.'

Unfortunately, new technology can be seductive and there is a danger that it can be over used. The net result is that instead of enhancing clarity, the effect is one of confusion, resulting in poor data presentation. A good guide is to try to keep the number of techniques you use in any one table, text or figure, to a minimum. Use highlighting techniques to help to get your message across, not just as a means of showing that you have the facility available.

Presenting data as text, numbers, graphs and pictures

Text

The written word is a useful and powerful means of getting views and results across, and is particularly efficient when an individual is attempting to describe a situation or event that is charged with emotion. It also has a potential ability to convey large amounts of data and considerable detail in a relatively compact form. There are times, however, when such an approach is less than ideal. For example, when reporting the results of a survey, it is common to see material presented in the following form:

'A total of 257 questionnaires were distributed of which 204 were returned. Of these, 87, 47, 39 and 31 were received from the Midwifery, Mental Health, Learning Disabilities and Community Services Units respectively.'

Data presented in this form, despite being accurate and factual, are unattractive from the visual and literary view point. More worrying is the point that such a presentation lacks clarity, for it requires considerable concentration and re-reading to ensure that the correct numbers are associated with the correct unit. Furthermore, the use of text to present numerical data gives the reader little visual assistance in relation to identifying trends or differences between groups.

It is not always possible to present data in descriptive formats; equally, it might be extremely difficult to do so. Consider how difficult it would be to describe the layout of your ward or office compared to the relative ease of drawing a plan.

Numbers, graphs and pictures

By using numbers, graphs and pictures as an alternative form of data presentation, you can take advantage of the reader's ability to interpret more visually stimulating material. How often have you flicked through a journal, stopping momentarily to examine an article which catches your eye, usually as the result of an interesting heading, graph, picture, or table.

Visually dynamic data can not only attract an audience, but can also be an efficient method of summarizing large quantities of information in such a way as to illuminate underlying trends. It is not always the case that the researcher takes an either/or decision and quite often will use both textual and graphical data presentation. The use of two approaches can help to clarify the data and also emphasize their importance.

Tabular data presentation

Certain types of data do not lend themselves to textual presentation. Survey data often require the researcher to summarize findings in tabular form. For example, the skill mix of staff working in a hospital can be effectively and clearly displayed by use of a table (see Table 34.2).

Presenting data in tabular form is perhaps one of the most common means of summarizing large quantities of numerical data. Despite the popularity of this approach, it is common for writers to produce tables which are poorly laid out and confusing to the reader. Common mistakes are: inadequately descriptive

Table 34.2 Skill mix of nursing staff, by grade, in medical unit

Grade	Number of staff (N = 47)	Percentage of staff in each grade
G	3	6
F	6	13
E	16	34
D	6	13
C	4	8
A	12	26
Totals	47	100

All percentages are rounded.

titles, misaligned columns, use of abbreviations or units within data columns, omission of totals, totals that do not add up correctly, and omissions of the number of respondents upon which the data are based, detracting from the quality and clarity of the presentation.

With the aid of new technology, many of these mistakes can be avoided and many of the basic problems of layout can be dealt with automatically. For example, the statistical package for the social sciences (SPSS) is now available on micro computer and can present data in tables in an adequate and accurate manner, avoiding all the above flaws.

Tables are extremely useful and relative easy to construct, but care is needed not to overload them with information. Always remember that the primary objective is to ensure that your reader gets the correct, accurate and clear information intended. It is far better to use two or more tables that are effective than one that leads to confusion.

Graphic presentation formats

There are several different ways of presenting data in a graphic form. In the past it has been necessary for writers who wish to present their data graphically to draw the figures by hand and then to physically 'stick' them into their report at the appropriate point. Thankfully, for those with access to new technology, all these steps can be automated. Data can be exported from statistical analysis packages into graphics packages and then electronically 'pasted' into the final report.

There are many programs available which will enable you to perform such activity. The specific program used will be a personal choice which will inevitably be constrained by the type of computer to which you have access and the amount of money you have to spend on the software. In view of the cost of some of these packages, it is recommended that you should attempt to negotiate access to such a facility through your employer. Most Health Authorities or Boards and Trusts will have these resources and people skilled in their use who can advise.

Generally, the types of package that can be particularly useful when presenting data are integrated software packages. These packages incorporate word processors, spreadsheets, databases and graphics. In addition, desktop publishing systems that enable you to paste together the output from other programs such as stand-alone word-processing, statistical analysis, or graphics packages are also available.

Those who cannot gain access to new technology should not despair: all the graphical presentation formats that follow can be produced by hand. The end product can be just as effective, although it does take a little longer.

There are several types of graph that can be used for data presentation. Examples of graphs that can be used include those of line and bar which may or may not be stacked. Furthermore, it is possible to use either two or three dimensions when plotting data, thus further adding to the repertoire of actions available.

Whichever option is selected to present data, it is important that the scales on both axes are chosen appropriately. In most cases it is usual, as in Fig. 34.3, to plot the independent variable, in this case 'months', along the x (horizontal) axis and the dependent variable, here 'shifts lost due to sickness', along the y (vertical) axis. The scale for the dependent variable is extremely important since the scale can over- or under-emphasize any trends present. A small gradual increase in sickness rate can be made to look extremely dramatic if the scale is so sensitive that a single day's sickness is represented by a visually dramatic rise. Great care and common sense are obviously required when selecting the scale.

With the advent of new technology, some graphics packages will automatically scale the data for you and will attempt to emphasize differences on trends – trends

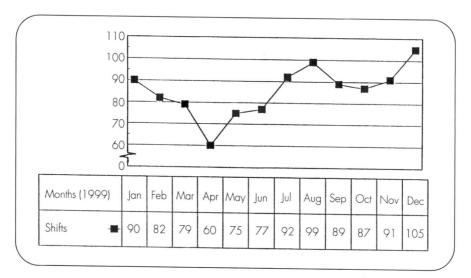

Months (1999)	Jan	Feb	Mar	Apr	May	Jun	Jul	Aug	Sep	Oct	Nov	Dec
Shifts	90	82	79	60	75	77	92	99	89	87	91	105

Fig. 34.3   Shifts lost due to sickness during 1999.

are the tendency for a set of observations to increase, decrease or remain static in relation to time or some other variable. However, because of this feature sometimes these differences of trends are over-emphasized. Under such conditions it may be necessary to over-ride the automatic scaling. The omission of the source of the data is also a frequent error and prevents the interested reader from checking it.

Certain issues are specific to the construction of various types of graph and these are dealt with in the following paragraphs.

Line graphs

Line graphs are particularly useful for displaying changes and are ideal for showing recurring patterns over time; it is important, however, to ensure that the timings along the horizontal axis are equal. A common error seen in graphical data presentation in line graph format is the omission of any discontinuities in the scale. That is, if the first scale point is, for example, '60' then the discontinuity between 60 and 0 should be indicated, as shown in Fig. 34.3.

There is no real limit to the number of points that can be shown on a line graph; indeed, the greater the number, the more accurate any interpretation between points. However, for clarity, it is advisable to limit the number of lines (variables displayed) on any one graph to five or six, particularly if the lines frequently cross.

Bar graphs

This type of graph is one of the most commonly used in the presentation of data. The bar graph is particularly useful when trying to convey the concept of 'leader' or there are preset targets, since such an approach clearly demonstrates those who are meeting the goals and those who are not (see Fig. 34.4). Unlike line graphs, it is unusual to have discontinuities in the y axis since it is then necessary to show the discontinuity in each of the bars.

When drawing a bar graph, it is extremely important to keep the widths of the bars constant since it is in fact the area of the bar which conveys the information. Although Fig. 34.4 illustrates the presentation of variation along the x axis, it is more usual for the y axis to be used. That is, variations in the height of the columns, rather than their length, convey the information.

Bar graphs are often 'stacked' when the most important feature is to convey the total magnitude of the dependent variable being measured. For example, there may be some interest in the breakdown of the component parts of the variable and it is then that the total magnitude can be shown as a sum of a number of elemental parts (see Fig. 34.4). It is importnat to note that, as in Fig. 34.4, it is necessary to illustrate the meaning of the elements by the inclusion of a legend.

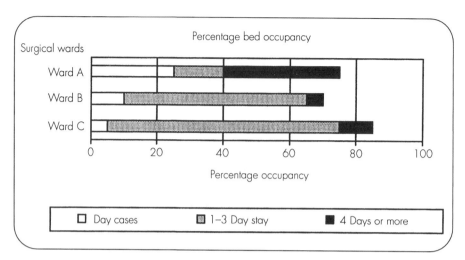

Fig. 34.4 Surgical unit bed occupancy for August 1999.

Pie charts

Pie charts, as the name suggests, are circular in format. The overall circular structure is divided into segments which proportionally represent, by area, data to be presented. Many computer packages will generate the pie chart automatically, but if such a facility is unavailable, the researcher will require a pair of compasses to draw the circle and a protractor to divide the circle into segments.

As an example, the data previously presented in Table 34.2 is displayed in the form of a pie chart in Fig. 34.5. The entire 'pie' represents 100% of the data (47

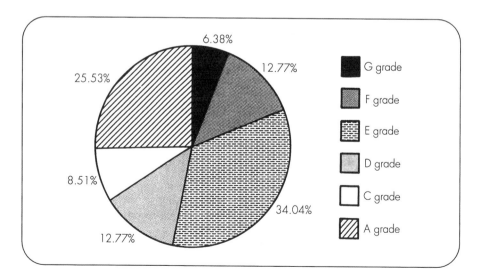

Fig. 34.5 Skill mix of 47 nursing staff by grade: medical ward.

members of staff). Since it is necessary to rotate compasses through an angle of 360° to fully describe the circumference of the circle, 1% of the data is represented by a segment with $360 \div 100°$ at the centre. Therefore, every 1% of the data is multiplied by 3.6° to enable the segment to proportionally represent the percentage fraction of the data.

When using pie charts to display results, it is important to consider the visual impact. If there are too many divisions, the pie chart will become cluttered and small segments will be difficult to interpret. With these points in mind, it is best to limit the number of segments to less than ten and ensure, if possible, that no segment represents less than 5% of the data.

Since the pie chart is designed to enable data to be presented in percentage form, it is common to note that some researchers neglect to state the total number of subjects upon which the data are based.

Pie charts are labelled in several ways. First, it is possible to label each segment within the circumference – that is, to superimpose the labelling upon the specific segments if both the segments and the pie chart are big enough. Second, it is common to have labelling attached to, or placed just outside, the circumference of the circle. Third, it is possible to use different types of shading and then use a suitable legend to define the various areas. Figure 34.5 uses two of these techniques: percentages are placed outside and adjacent to the various segments, but a legend is also used to define the meanings of the shades used.

Sociograms

Sociograms are particularly useful in the display of interactions between a number of individuals. Not only can they visually represent who talks to whom, but they can also be used to analyse the types and quantity of each member's contribution over a certain time period.

From the sociogram (Fig. 34.6), it is possible to identify those individuals who dominate group conversation (subject L), those who did not contribute (subject H), and those who form a subgroup (subjects E and F). Any communication directed to the group as a whole is indicated by an arrow which goes to the centre of the figure.

Problems can arise with researchers who use too long a sampling time period, causing the sociogram to become cluttered and extremely difficult to interpret. Similarly, if the technique is being used by an observer to record the interactions of a very vocal group, it can be extremely challenging to ensure that all conversations occurring are noted.

Organizational chart

The purpose of an organizational chart is to demonstrate the (usually formal) managerial relationship and lines of responsibility between individuals or posi-

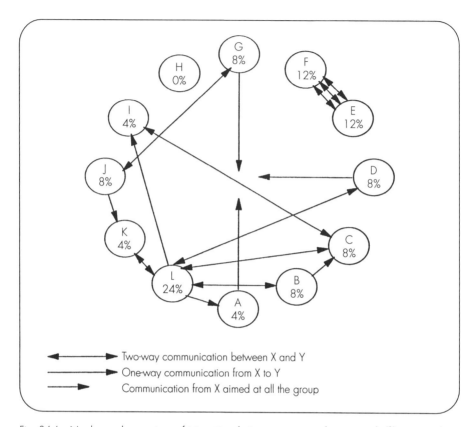

Fig. 34.6   Number and percentage of interactions between group members over a half-hour period.

tions in various parts of an organization. Traditionally, health service provision is managed by means of a hierarchical management structure, although this has started to change significantly since the introduction of the NHS reforms. Figure 34.7 illustrates the use of the organizational chart as a means of succinctly representing the formal lines of communication within a functional unit of a health provider.

Although these charts are frequently used to illustrate lines of communication, it is important to note that these are the 'official' or 'formally' recognized paths. In many cases these will not be the actual paths along which information flows and this can cause problems and mislead naive researchers who take things at face value.

Geographic mapping

This technique is frequently used when a researcher wishes to show the distribution of a variable in relation to a geographic area. A geographic area can be an entire country, a county, or even a postal code zone. Figure 34.8 shows the

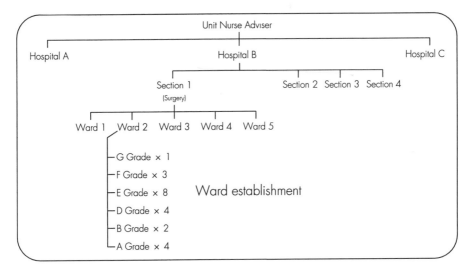

Fig. 34.7 Formal lines of communication in an acute unit.

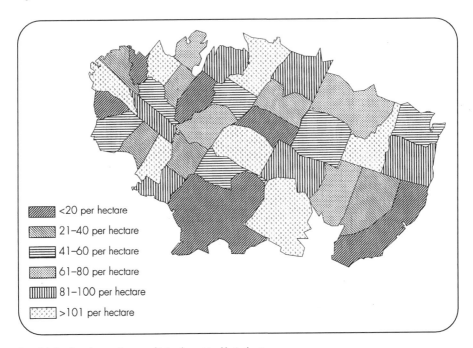

Fig. 34.8 Population density of Nowhere Health Authority.

population density of individuals as identified from census data in a Health Authority area, and, as can be seen, increased population density is represented by increasing darkness of shading. Such a mapping can be produced by hand, but with new technology it is possible to translate data directly from data files into the format by means of a suitable software package.

Flowcharts

Originally, flowcharts were used by systems analysts as a means of interpreting and representing the actions required to guide the development of computer software production. However, many researchers have recognized the utility of this approach for succinctly conveying to readers the relationship and sequential direction of ideas, concepts or propositions. Although it has a use which is, strictly speaking, often different from actual presentation of data, it remains a very useful and powerful tool for the researcher. The flowchart in Fig. 34.9 represents the phases in complaints handling.

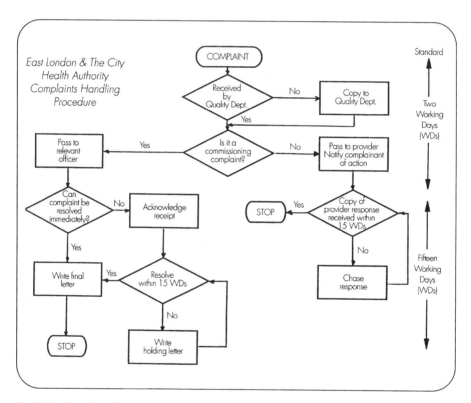

Fig. 34.9 Flowchart of complaints handling process.

Flowcharts should have definite start and end points which are clearly defined, enabling readers to understand how the sequence of events is triggered and completed. The layout of flowcharts is extremely important if clarity of information flow is to be ensured. The best and most easily understood charts should read from top to bottom, with feedback loops going in the reverse direction. Specific activities or processes should be included in rectangular boxes and decision points in diamond shapes.

Common errors seen in the production of flowcharts include:

- the omission of decision conditions – that is, the requirements that have to be met before the particular path is followed;
- the omission of arrows to guide the reader through the chart;
- the cross-over of feedback paths over preceding sections of the chart.

Photographs

Both black/white and colour prints can be used as a means of presenting data which would be extremely difficult to show by other means. For example, photographs are an ideal medium to demonstrate pictorially 'before and after' views of some treatment such as the effects on posture of an intensive exercise programme on a child with multiple physical handicap.

Although the cost of producing the original photograph may be relatively inexpensive, the researcher, if planning to publish the material, should note that not all journals will accept photographic plates; equally, they may require a special size or type of negative. It is therefore essential if considering submitting work for publication that you should enquire about such points at an early stage. However, in recent years with the advent of sophisticated scanning equipment, it is now relatively straightforward for such material to be processed and integrated into reports and publications.

One positive point to bear in mind is the fact that most medical, nursing and midwifery colleges may have an illustrations department which may be quite willing to help with the production of photographic prints. These departments are usually small and over-worked, so it is important to give sufficient warning if you require assistance. The production of monochrome or colour prints can be achieved by means of suitable photocopying machines, but although colour is perhaps more striking, it is also far more expensive. You should therefore assess the benefits versus the cost of using colour.

Blueprints – scale drawings

Blueprints or scale drawings are used to portray size, contents, position and spatial relationship of an item or area such as a hospital, ward or room. Figure 34.10 is an example of such a blueprint. If the blueprint requires to be drawn to scale, each of its parts must be carefully calculated, measured and drawn. While a scale drawing may be essential in some instances, it may not always be needed. The reader, however, must be informed whether it is or is not a scale drawing.

Only items which are necessary should be included in the blueprint. If a major point of the presentation is to indicate the position of each of the rooms in the ward, it would obviously be inappropriate to include individual beds, hand wash basins, and windows.

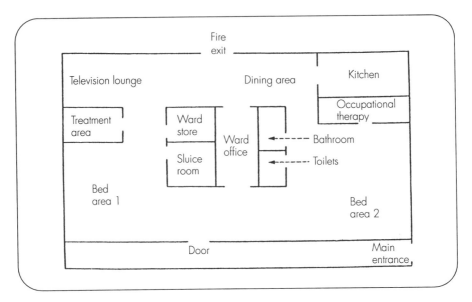

Fig. 34.10 Blueprint of Ward 1 layout (not to scale).

Scatter diagrams

Before the development and ready availability of computers, researchers who wished to examine data for correlations used the initial technique of plotting a scatter diagram. By plotting the value of the independent variable against the dependent variable, it is possible to visually determine whether there is likely to be a statistically significant correlation between the two variables. The decision can then be taken as to whether a statistical calculation should be performed. Examination of the overall shape of the data distribution pattern can reveal such information as positive, negative or no correlation between the variables. The closer the data pattern resembles a straight line, the greater the degree of correlation between the variables. It is common practice to encompass the data points so as to highlight the overall data pattern (Fig. 34.11).

Due to the increased availability of computers and statistical analysis packages, there is now less need to use scatter diagrams, but they are nevertheless a useful way of demonstrating to an audience who have limited understanding of statistical techniques the correlation between two variables under examination.

Contour plots

Perhaps the most readily recognized contour plot in the United Kingdom is that of the air pressure over the British Isles, displayed by the weather forecasting service on television. In that plot, points of equal air pressure are connected, thus displaying a series of contour lines.

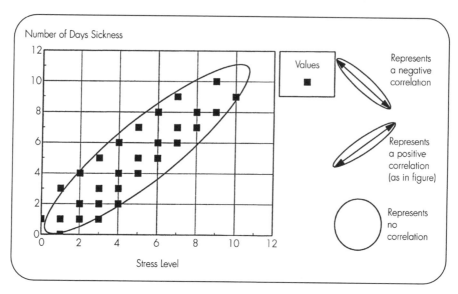

Fig. 34.11   Correlation between stress and days lost due to sickness.

Contour plots are frequently used in diagnostic medical physics departments where the emissions of radioactive isotopes are recorded as a means of identifying, for example, vascular lesions. However, researchers can put the technique to use for far less technologically based applications. For example, if you are interested in the effect of a new treatment on the granulation of a decubitus ulcer, it might be useful to plot the outline of the wound at specific time intervals. It then would be possible to calculate the rate of wound granulation for the patient. The technique would provide an objective, accurate, visual record, over time, of a healing process. Figure 34.12 illustrates the technique.

Cause and effect diagrams

Cause and effect diagrams can be used to identify and illustrate the relationships between an effect or problem and possible causes or factors that contribute to it. Researchers can therefore use this tool to display results that are frequently conceptual or thematic. Cause and effect diagrams are sometimes called fishbone diagrams and have been used in the field of quality improvement for many years.

Conclusions

Many techniques are available for the presentation of data, and if results are to have optimum impact then great care must be taken to ensure that an appropriate method is selected. Unless results are presented in a clear and visually dynamic format, readers may have difficulty in interpreting findings, or, worse still, they

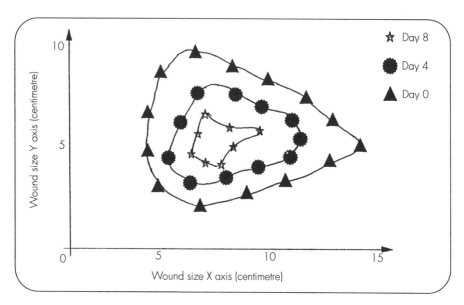

Fig. 34.12   Contour plot of outline of granulating wound.

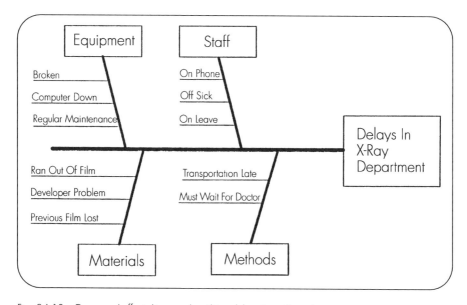

Fig. 34.13   Cause and effect diagram describing delays in an X-ray department.

may not read it. New technology offers a wide variety of aids which can enhance the standard of data presentation and reduce the time taken to prepare material. Nevertheless, remember that the purpose of the presentation will affect many of the choices you make in deciding the most appropriate format. Do not use inappropriate approaches just because they happen to be readily available to you.

With the advent of readily available new technology, computer software can provide considerable assistance – and further assistance is available for the enthusiastic reader by pursuing the entry in the 'Further reading' section.

Finally, throughout this chapter, specific specialized methods of data presentation have been illustrated and, perhaps more importantly, a number of general points have been emphasized. These points can be easily remembered by use of an acronym VACUME. That is, is the format Visually stimulating? Are the results Accurate, Clearly Understandable and Meaningful? Is the format chosen the most Efficient means of getting the message across? If the answer to all these questions is 'Yes', then it is likely that you have made the correct choices.

Further reading

Aitken, P., Fulton, J. Plumley, S. & Wempen, F. (1997) *Microsoft Office 97 Professional 6 in 1*. Indianapolis, QUE Corporation.

Part III

The use of research

The main reason for undertaking research is that it be used by practitioners, educators and managers. The final two chapters in the this book will be helpful to those who make use of, and facilitate, research in practice, education and management (see Chapter 36). This can only be done if the researcher produces a research report (see Chapter 35). The final chapter also applies to potential researchers in these areas who are considering a possible focus for their own research. Although each of these topics is dealt with individually, it is recognized that considerable overlap and similarity exists.

The ability to make use of completed studies, and to initiate or facilitate new ones, depends on a firm understanding of the research process generally. Equally important is the availability of a research report – a major responsibility of the researcher (see Chapter 35). For this reason, this part, which deals with the production of a research report and the subsequent use of research, has been placed at the end of the book.

CHAPTER 35

Reporting and disseminating research

Desmond F. S. Cormack

The creation of a written report ('writing up') is required to complete all pieces of research, whether or not the report is to be published in full or in part(s). The research report is *the* major means by which the research is made known to, and can be considered for use by, others. Although report writing is only one part of the research process, it is a particularly important and challenging one. Throughout this text, it has been emphasized that there is no *blueprint* for a piece of research, and the same is true for a research report. The shape of a report will be determined by the variation of the research process used and the research design selected. Although an example structure will be used in this chapter to illustrate aspects of reporting research and to illustrate some general principles, many other variations and structures are possible.

The preparation of a written report will be necessary irrespective of the purpose for which the research was undertaken, and the same principles apply to an informal small-scale study, or to a doctor of philosophy thesis, or to a large-scale project undertaken by a team of researchers. Although this chapter will discuss the production of an entire report, many such reports are subsequently published, in parts, as articles in one or more than one journal. It would not be unusual for a number of discrete articles to be extracted from a doctoral thesis and published as individual papers. These might relate to the literature review, data collection, data analysis, part or all of the research findings, or to any other topic which is of sufficient interest on a stand-alone basis. A published article may be (rather unusually) a full report in miniature, in which case this chapter will apply. More commonly, an article will describe part of a report – in which case this chapter, although of some value, will be much less applicable. When preparing part(s) of a full research report for publication as one article, or more, some of the references at the end of this chapter may be of value.

It is often said that health care research is rarely read and less frequently implemented. This criticism may, in part, result from those reports which are badly written. Indeed, it may be argued that unless reports are written in a readable and meaningful form, their potential effectiveness is much reduced. However, it is more probable that difficulties are experienced by readers because of unfamiliarity with the research process, and with what reports are intended to achieve.

Many researchers experience some difficulty in preparing a written description of their work, a problem which relates as much to structure as to content. While the question of content can only be dealt with by the researcher and supervisors, some help can be offered with structure. This discussion is intended to minimize these difficulties and should be used *in addition* to any instructions offered by the institution which has commissioned the research, or with the requirements of the institution awarding the research degree. If the report is to be published, it is then written (or more usually rewritten) to comply with the requirements of the publisher.

An essential guide to structure is that no blueprint exists for all pieces of research and that, to a considerable extent, a structure already exists prior to 'writing up' in that the variation of the research process, and the design used, inform the researcher or the structure.

Structure

To a great extent the writing-up phase of the research can run parallel with all other phases of the process – an approach which is strongly commended, rather than only writing-up at the end of the research. However, it is known that some researchers will do almost all their writing at the end of earlier parts of the research. In either case it is widely accepted that a specific part of the 'time budget' should be set aside for this purpose. A useful starting point is to consider the structure of the research process generally, and the research design in particular, which in turn constitutes the structure of the report. Although there is no blueprint for the structure of the research process, that being influenced by the research design used, the report will reflect whichever process and design are used. The remainder of this chapter is based on one frequently used variation of the research process, and design, while acknowledging that there are others.

Introduction

A general introduction to the subject of the research will include a discussion of its importance, and of the need for it to be researched. The research problem is clearly identified, as will be the thinking process which prompted initiation of the research. Invariably, this section will contain references to previous research. These will be used to support all aspects of the introduction, and particularly the assertion by the researcher that the subject needs to be researched. Much research is an extention or continuation of previous work, seeking to answer questions raised by previous workers. Here, the references used will relate to those earlier works.

The relationship of the work to past, current and future projects is made clear. The background and experience of the researcher is often included here to place the work in a personal context. After reading the introduction the reader should be quite clear about the nature and purpose of the research.

At some point in the introduction will appear a series of words which will constitute the title of the work, accompanied by an 'operational definition' of all key words in the title. An operational definition differs from an accepted definition in that it is one which is created for the purpose of this particular study. For example, the study title may be *A study of the attitude of young expectant mothers to breast feeding*. Clearly 'young', 'expectant mothers' and 'breast feeding' need further explanation and definition. For example, 'young' might be defined as 'under the age of twenty years at the estimated date of conception'. Similarly, 'expectant mothers' might be defined as relating to women who are within an estimated one month of giving birth. Finally, 'breast feeding' might be defined as 'breast feeding in general, rather than *her* breast feeding'.

Aims of the research

The aims of the research are discussed in detail. The research question(s) which the study intends to answer are presented. Some, but by no means all, researchers state then test research hypotheses. The aims of the research are then listed in a concise form at the end of their more general discussion.

Literature review

A detailed presentation, review and evaluation of previously published relevant literature follows. This will demonstrate how the current research was influenced by, and will develop from, published literature, some of which will be research based, some of which will not. The purpose of the review is to inform the reader of relevant literature and of how it relates to the present study. Literature which is supportive of, *and* which disagrees with, the research being reported is included.

This part of the report will be much more easily prepared if all references previously collected are recorded on alphabetically filed index cards or on a computing system. It is *absolutely essential* that a well-organized record be kept of all references. See Chapters 8 and 9 for a discussion of searching and reviewing the literature, and how to incorporate references into the text.

Research design

The term *research design* is used to describe the overall research approach to be used. A variety of designs are used either singly or, in some instances, in combination; examples include qualitative and quantitative designs, and grounded theory, experimental, action, historical and evaluation research designs. The design of a study, which is not to be confused with data-collection methods which are part of the design, is described in detail. The report should include a clear justification for the choice of design(s).

This section also includes a detailed description of, and justification for, the data-collection method(s) to be used; examples include interview, observation and questionnaire. It also describes, in detail, *every* step of the means by which data will be collected. This description will enable readers to understand the data-collection methods, judge their suitability, and be able to repeat (replicate) them if necessary. The validity and reliability of all data-collection instruments are discussed, as are anticipated problems.

The population and sample selection are described, as will any sampling techniques used. If experimental methods feature in the research, they are reported in considerable detail.

Ethical considerations

The length of this section will depend on whether or not the research is likely to raise any ethical issues. If no such issues were anticipated, and none emerged during the research, this part of the report will be short; otherwise they are fully discussed, as are the steps taken to deal with them.

Assurances regarding confidentiality and anonymity are a common feature of many research projects. The means by which these are made to actual or potential respondents are described, as should the methods employed to achieve these assurances.

Entry to the research site

Most research studies are dependent on obtaining permission from individuals, committees or managers to enter a site for the purpose of collecting research data. Details of how this was achieved, including correspondence with research and ethics committees should be covered, as will be any problems associated with gaining entry.

Data collection

This section describes how research data were actually obtained. Any difficulties experienced during this phase, particularly if they affected the study, are acknowledged and discussed.

If this phase constitutes or includes a pilot study, its outcome in terms of adequacy or otherwise is included, as are any resultant changes in the research method.

Data analysis

Collected data are described, analysed and presented in a clear and unambiguous form. If data are subjected to statistical analysis, the choice of statistical test is explained.

Conclusions and discussion

The major aim of the closing section is to draw conclusions from the study while bearing in mind any limitations. The inclusion of informed opinion is not only permissible, it is essential providing that the reader can distinguish it from research-based fact.

The discussion will enable speculation about the meaning of the findings, recognition of the limitations of the study and suggestions for future research in the subject area. No new material in the form of research data is introduced in this section.

Finally, a brief summary of the major findings of the study is presented.

In addition to the structure, other aspects of the report are considered before and during the actual research, and while the report is being written. The report does not develop haphazardly. During its construction the following two points are borne in mind:

- *Reason* (Why the report is being written.)
- *Readership and language* (Who will be reading the report and what form of language will be best understood?)

Reasons for a research report

Irrespective of how many, or how few, people have an interest in the findings of a piece of research, it is necessary to prepare a written report of it. Apart from providing a permanent record of the work, the actual task of 'writing-up' the work adds much to the researcher's understanding of it and helps to avoid the use of generalities which are often a feature of verbal description. Many reports are written as a condition of the commissioning institution or by a grant-awarding body for example. Similarly, if the research is undertaken for a higher degree, producing a report in the form of a thesis will be necessary.

In terms of a more general readership, the report has two major purposes; to make the findings available, and to give details of the research design, including the data-collection methods, used.

To make findings available

The full details of the findings of a research report include those which supported any hypotheses or expectations, those which contradicted them, and those which were inconclusive. When possible raw data, or liberal samples of them, are included in addition to the more frequently used summaries of data.

Following the presentation of data (facts) there is a full discussion of the meaning and interpretation of the research findings which includes an important input which draws on personal experience and knowledge of the subject (opinion). In this concluding section the data will be interpreted, used to increase knowledge of the subject, and give direction to further related research.

Research methods used

In some instances only part of a report may be published – for example, an article might contain a summary of the findings. However, the full report will contain a detailed description of the methods used in the study. The reasons for including this section are to enable the reader to evaluate the quality of the methods used, to avoid similar mistakes if any were made, and to use similar or identical methods in future projects.

Evaluate the quality of the methods

The quality of a research study and its findings is only as good as the validity and reliability of the research methods used to collect data. It is necessary, therefore, that readers be given the opportunity to make a critical appraisal of the methods by being able to study them in the report. When a part of the research is published and does not include a detailed description of the methods used, the readers must be referred to the complete report to provide them with an opportunity to judge for themselves the quality of the methods used.

Avoid similar mistakes

An important function of a literature review as part of every piece of research is to learn from the problems experienced and mistakes made by other researchers. The methods section will therefore discuss all problems, solutions, shortcomings and strengths of the methods used.

Use similar or identical methods

Another reason for reviewing the literature before undertaking a study is to identify previously used methods which can be used, or adapted, in the planned study. Unless these are included in considerable detail in reports, the readers will be unable to judge the value, or otherwise, in completed studies.

Readership and language of the report

When writing a report, the needs of its readership are a major consideration: it is essential to use a 'language' which readers will understand. Although the formal language may be English, for example, decisions are made as to the use of technical terms, mathematical language and illustrative material such as photographs, tables and figures.

Readership of the report

The report may be written in different ways depending on its intended readership in the knowledge that, for example, a reader with a background in research will have needs which are different from the general public, most of whom have no such experience.

The general public

Because many readers in the general public may have limited professional or research background and skills, they require a jargon-free and relatively non-technical report. A report of this type may say very little about the reviewed literature or research design, with emphasis being placed on presenting, interpreting and discussing the findings.

An examiner

If the report – a dissertation or thesis, for example – is being submitted for examination it must comply with the marking and examination criteria set by the institution concerned. Such a work may focus on the theoretical and philosophical aspects of the research, in addition to the more practical issues.

Dissertations and theses deliberately deal with a number of issues which are not part of that particular study, but an understanding of these being indicative of an understanding of the research process generally. For example, the researcher may discuss a range of *potential* ethical issues and their possible solution, although these were not actually experienced. By doing so the writer indicates an understanding of an important aspect of research, although it did not actually arise.

A commissioning institution

If the research has been commissioned by an institution or organization, it is prudent to agree on the probable length and general structure of the final report as early as possible. It would clearly be problematical if a 50 000 word report in the style and level of a Ph.D. thesis was produced, when the commissioning body hoped for a 10 000 word report which could be read and understood by a wide readership with limited research knowledge.

It may be necessary to prepare and circulate a summary to a large number of people for information or comment. In this instance, a summarized version of the entire work may have to be prepared and reducing its 50 000 words to 1000 words would not be uncommon. If such a summary is required, this needs to be made known in advance, as should its specifications, including length. Although the readership of the summary will be varied, a limited knowledge of research language and a general understanding of the subject of the research may be assumed, unless informed otherwise.

Other researchers

Other researchers will be particularly interested in the research methods used, Indeed, an article extracted from the whole report may deal only with the research method. Similarly, full details of the statistical analyses, if used, would be included in a report prepared for other researchers. A knowledge of research, technical and statistical language may be assumed of this readership.

Specialists in the subject of the research

Specialists, such as others in the same discipline, may require a report, or report summary, in which the application of the findings to clinical practice are fully discussed. A knowledge of technical language and the subject of the research would be assumed of this readership.

Language of the report

The language of the report is, to a large extent, dependent on its readership and will include the use of words and possibly mathematical language and pictorial elements in the form of graphs and figures. It is unlikely that the report language will be exclusively of one kind, a combination of two or three types being more common.

Word language

Words are carefully chosen and written in a clear and understandable way. Reports which are badly written are difficult to read and are frequently not implemented for this reason. Readers are entitled to be critical of a work which is difficult to read. They are justified in assuming that an ambiguous, unclear and otherwise badly written report reflects muddled thinking by its writer. It is sad that an otherwise good piece of research has less impact than it deserves because it is badly written.

Mathematical language

Although not all research uses numbers and other mathematical symbols, they form an important, perhaps crucial, part of many studies. They may be used in tables, figures, in the text or to describe statistical concepts or findings. The range and complexity of use may vary from the simple 'Five per cent of the sample was female', to more complex statistical tests.

A proportion of health care professionals have some difficulty with mathematical language. If it is used in the report for anything other than basic descriptive statistics (percentages and averages, for example), consider whether some explanation is needed. This decision will obviously depend on the readership, researchers requiring less explanation than others with no research background.

Pictorial language (illustrations)

It is a truism that a picture can paint a thousand words, this being of considerable importance when writing a research report. The types of pictures used include tables, graphs, line drawings, sociograms, photographs and blueprints. These are sufficiently significant to the subject of writing to justify a chapter being devoted to the subject (see Chapter 34).

General hints for writing research reports

These hints are directed in particular at those writing a report for the first time. The list is not exhaustive, the hallmark of good report writing being innovation, imagination and experimentation with a variety of approaches. The points made are in addition to those raised in the earlier part of the text.

Time

A common error made by beginners is to underestimate the time needed to write a report. In general, it is prudent to allocate one-third of the time available to the entire project to writing the report. This writing-up time will not necessarily all be used at the end of the time allocated to the research. Perhaps one-half of the writing-up time, one-sixth of the total research time, will be used as the work is proceeding, the other half being used at the end of the project.

Starting to write

Writing the report begins as soon as possible, when ideas about the work first begin to develop. Written work is produced, however sketchy and disorganized, at every stage of the study. These first draft notes will form an important basis for the final report.

Experience will show that ideas are rarely fully developed and clarified until they are placed on paper. While it is easy to be vague and ambiguous in terms of thinking, and even in verbal discussions, these faults will be more easily identified and rectified when the material is placed on paper.

Write down the reasons for being interested in this particular research topic, why the research is felt to be necessary and include as much background information as possible.

References

All references consulted in relation to the study should be recorded and stored in an alphabetical card or computer system. The record will contain full bibliographical details of the reference, a summary of its contents, and a note of where it can be found. If the reference was consulted and found to be of no value to the study, this fact is noted. This important aspect of undertaking a research study is initiated as soon as the decision is taken to start the work. It is essential to the successful completion of the research report. (See Chapters 8 and 9 for a full discussion of this subject.)

Documents

All documents relating to the study, those collected as data and those used to collect data, are clearly labelled and stored for later use. Many will be presented in the body of the report or as appendices. If there is serious doubt as to whether a document needs to be included, err on the side of inclusion.

Structure

Draft a provisional structure of the final report during the planning stage of the research. As far as possible, this draft should contain as much detail as can be anticipated; chapters/major sections, headings, subheadings, and titles of figures, tables, line drawings and appendices for example.

The initial draft structure will, of course, be modified and remodified as the research progresses, with each subsequent draft structure adding considerably to the ease with which the report is written.

Shape

The grouping of material into chapters and sections of chapters, and the sequence of these parts is referred to as *shape*. The shape of the the report both in terms of chapters and their sequence, and in terms of the arrangement of material within chapters, requires careful consideration.

The size of each part of the report, and its size as a proportion of the work as a whole, is deliberate rather than left to chance. This decision will be influenced by the purpose of the report and its intended readership.

Title

A tentative title for the report is decided at the beginning of the study to provide both a focus for the work and a 'label' by which it becomes known to others. The title is re-examined as the work progresses and can be changed if it fails to encapsulate and accurately reflect the subject of the research. However, it is probable that such a change will be in emphasis only, rather than a completely new title. 'Gimmicky' titles are best avoided as they often fail to indicate the content of the report to potential readers.

Detail

Good research and good reports greatly depend on attention to detail. The content of the report will be exact, specific, unambiguous and sufficiently detailed as to leave readers in no doubt about its meaning. Although some professionals regard the detail required of a research report to be pedantic and unnecessary, these are essential features of successful research.

Accuracy

As in all forms of writing, a research report demands a high level of accuracy in presenting factual material which has emerged from the research. Although this accuracy is an important feature of the presentation of numerical data, it is by no means confined to that application. Whether qualitative or quantitative data are being described, the material is checked and rechecked for accuracy. This checking includes the data, research findings, and to the means used to describe them. It is essential that an otherwise excellent piece of research should not be regarded as 'suspect' because of inattention to accuracy in the report.

Drafts

Allow for making a number of drafts of the report, which will be expensive in time *and* finance if a typist is used, and should be taken into account when budgeting for time and money. In earlier drafts allow for making changes and additions; this will be made easier if wide margins are left and if pencil is used on one side of the page only. Better still, type all drafts on a word processor which will cope easily with all manner of corrections, changes, additions, movement of text and so on.

Earlier drafts are shown to, and discussed with, colleagues or those for whom the work is being prepared. If the research is being formally supervised, all drafts will be read and commented on by supervisors.

The final report should be attractively produced (in typescript), easy to read, and professionally presented. With minimal effort and relatively little expense, a research report of poor quality in terms of appearance can be transformed into a visually attractive item. This is not to suggest that high-quality presentation can ever be a substitute for high-quality content. However, poor-quality presentation detracts considerably from good content. Finally, readers expect and deserve reports which are carefully prepared in order to make them visually appealing and readable.

Summary (Abstract)

Whether or not a short summary (abstract) is requested by those for whom the report is being prepared, it is as well to prepare one. Summaries (abstracts) may typically be approximately 1000 words long. It needs considerable skill to write and summarize the entire content of the report. However, this skill will be developed by writing many drafts, by sharing them with colleagues, and by reading successful summaries/abstracts in other reports, particularly those which have been published in article form.

Confidentiality and anonymity

Unless those institutions, groups and individuals taking part in the study – by providing data, for example – have agreed to be identified, readers of the report should be unable to identify them. Confidentiality and anonymity can be maintained by stating generally thus;

> 'A 400 bed district general hospital...'
> or 'A sample of patients in a rural location...'
> or 'A midwife said...'
> or 'A consultant physician reported that...'
> or 'The view of the majority of health visitors was that...'.

Publishing research reports

Research reports may be published in the form of the written word or by other means such as papers read at conferences or on study days. It is necessary that the report be made available to those who commissioned the research and possibly, either in complete or summary form, to those who participated in it – this being particularly so if data were collected from fellow professionals. Unless there was any prior agreement to restrict circulation of the report, an effort is made to make it available to as wide an appropriate readership as possible. This is often most effectively achieved by publishing a series of articles or by converting the report into 'book form' for publication.

Conclusions

The preparation of a research report involves a number of steps in addition to those required for other types of writing for a professional readership. Although the writer has the advantage of working from a pre-existing 'blueprint' in the form of the structure of the research process and of the selected research design, the accuracy, detail and objectivity required in writing a research report call for careful attention, as is the case in all good writing.

Further reading

Bryer, R. (1994) The world of referencing. *Nursing Times* 90 (36): 38–41.

Burnard, P. (1993) The standard guide to making sense on paper. *Nursing Standard* 7 (29): 45–7.

Cormack, D.F.S. (1994) *Writing for Health Care Professions*. Oxford: Blackwell Scientific Publications. [In particular, see Chapter 4, 'Writing style and structure'; Chapter 5, 'References'; and Chapter 14, 'Dissertations and theses'.]

Hall, G.M. (1994) *How to Write a Paper*. London: BMJ Publishing Group.

Hicks, C. (1995) The shortfall in published research; a study of nurses' research and publication activities. *Journal of Advanced Nursing* 21: 594–604.

Kirk-Smith, M. (1996) Winning ways with research proposals and reports. *Nursing Times* 92 (11): 36–8.

Mander, R. (1995) Midwife researchers need to get their work published. *British Journal of Midwifery* 3 (2): 107–10.

Robinson, D., Collins, M. & Monkman, J. (1997) A practical guide to writing for publication. *Nurse Researcher* 5 (1): 53–64.

Sandelowski, M. (1994) The use of quotes in qualitative research. *Research in Nursing and Health* 17 (6): 479–82.

Weldman, S. (1998) Publishing your work in nursing journals. *Professional Nurse* 13 (7): 419–22.

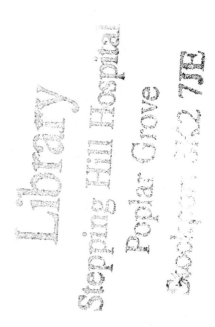

CHAPTER 36

The research, education, management and practice interface

Jennifer E. Clark

If nursing and midwifery care is to be effective, it must essentially be based on current research findings. Before this can become a reality an effective interface between nursing practice and nursing research needs to be established. It is the purpose of this chapter to present a dynamic model of this interface (Fig. 36.1). The essence of this model is the interaction that occurs between managers, educationalists and practitioners to create a research culture that not only initiates and facilitates some means to conduct research but also generates enthusiasm in every nurse and midwife to implement relevant findings into their practice.

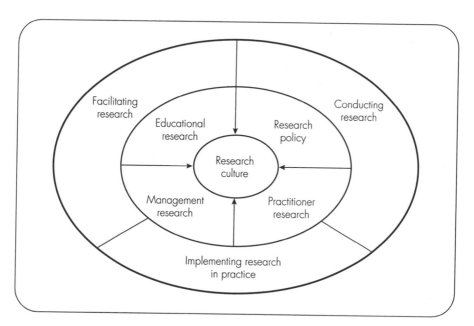

Fig. 36.1 The research, education, management and practice interface.

In Britain positive steps are being taken to underpin the National Health Service (NHS) with a strong research base, and the need for clinical practice to be based on scientific evidence is being strongly emphasized. In the past research has been generally the concern of academics in higher education institutions and research organizations with health care delivery remaining largely on the fringes. The government over recent years has introduced policies that reinforce the premise that research should be everybody's concern. It is essential today that all clinicians and managers understand research and are committed to implementing the findings to the best advantage of their patients. Indeed it would also be true to say that the need for research awareness stretches also to the patients, the consumers of health care, if they are to exercise informed choice and to take their rightful place as meaningful contributors to health care policy.

The NHS research and development strategy

The response of the NHS Management Executive to the House of Lords Report *Priorities in Medical Research* (House of Lords Select Committee on Science and Technology, 1988) was to appoint a director of research and development with a seat on the board of the NHS Executive. The remit of this post was to spearhead the research and development strategy for the NHS in England. The first edition of the strategy *Research for Health* (DoH, 1991) outlined the crucial role to be played by regions in the setting of their own regional research priorities and in the management of their own research agendas. As a result of this initiative, regional R&D committees were established under the directorship of regional R&D directors. *The Report on the NHS R&D Information Systems Strategy Study* (DoH, 1992a) was published to complement the implementation of the government's R&D strategy which was further enhanced by the publication of a report *Assessing the Effects of Health Technologies* (DoH, 1992b). This report stressed the importance of evaluating care and laid down guidelines for health technology assessment within the NHS.

Two further reports were published in 1993, namely *Research for Health* (DoH, 1993a) which built on the 1991 strategy (DoH, 1991) and the *Report of the Taskforce on the Strategy for Research in Nursing, Midwifery and Health Visiting* (DoH, 1993b). This strategy set a new agenda for nursing research and it emphasized two key objectives:

- To promote more and better research into nursing.
- To enhance the research skills of nursing staff, so as to increase their involvement in research in their own fields and in health services research generally.

The Culyer report

In order to support the R&D strategy the government instigated a task force under the chairmanship of Anthony Culyer. The report of the task force findings was published in 1994, and was entitled *Supporting Research and Development in the NHS* (Culyer, 1994). The task force in its consultation exercise identified five major areas of concern relating to R&D in the NHS:

- The system of support for R&D within the NHS was unco-ordinated, with little evidence that the NHS needs for R&D were being met and that the resources were being appropriately prioritized and targeted.
- There was conflict between the NHS internal market and the R&D agenda.
- There was poor quality control and accountability.
- There was confusion over the allocation of funds in terms of what funding went where.
- There was evidence of inadequate funding to community and primary care based R&D and for non-medical health service research, which includes nursing research and that conducted by the professions allied to medicine.

The premise that underpinned the Culyer report recommendations can be summarized in one word: 'enabling'. The recommendations were formulated with the intention of facilitating research individuals, groups and organizations to flourish providing they met the required quality conditions. The recommendations included:

- The instigation of a single source of funding for R&D in the NHS through the co-ordination and combination of previous sources of funding.
- The construction of a national register of all research activity in every NHS Trust which would ultimately inform the level of R&D funding to be allocated to each institution.
- The determination of means to measure the quality of research.

A more detailed implementation plan (DoH, 1995) and information relating to the new funding system (DoH, 1996) followed the Culyer report. The R&D strategy and especially the Culyer recommendations have been responsible for the creation of a new ethos in health services research in England which, in turn, has been responsible for generating a wave of activity within NHS Trusts. Most Trusts have now appointed directors of R&D who are responsible for co-ordinating and leading the Trust's R&D activity and their applications for funding.

Clinical effectiveness

It is necessary at this point to emphasize that the government in its R&D strategy is placing as great an importance on practice development as it is upon research. It is at great pains to stress that the dissemination of research findings into practice is an essential part of the research process, and that funding for research will depend heavily upon this criterion. It is acknowledged that not all practitioners will be researchers as this would be impracticable; however, it is expected that all practitioners will base their practice upon research findings.

This ethos of research-based practice is fundamental to the government's drive towards clinical effectiveness within the NHS. Clinical effectiveness has been defined by the Department of Health as:

> 'The extent to which specific clinical interventions when deployed in the field for a particular patient or population do what they are intended to do, i.e. maintain and improve health and secure the greatest possible health gain.'
> (DoH, 1998: 19)

Clinical governance

In its policy document *A First Class Service: Quality in the New NHS* (DoH, 1998) the government outlines a framework of accountability for NHS organizations for improving the quality of their services to patients. The Department of Health entitles this framework clinical governance and defines it as follows:

> 'Clinical governance can be defined as a framework through which NHS organisations are accountable for continuously improving the quality of their services and safeguarding high standards of care by creating an environment in which excellence in clinical care will flourish.' (DoH, 1998: 33)

Clinical governance is an all-embracing term given to a range of activities adopted by NHS organizations to promote and monitor excellence in clinical care. These activities are succinctly portrayed as the 10 Cs of clinical governance (Fig. 36.2).

- Clinical performance
- Clinical leadership
- Clinical audit
- Clinical risk management
- Complaints

- Continuing health needs assessment
- Changing practice through research evidence
- Continuing education
- Culture of excellence
- Clear accountability

Fig. 36.2 The 10 Cs of clinical governance (Heard, 1998).

Clinical governance is currently a top priority for all trusts who are required to establish systems for ensuring and improving the quality of the services they provide. To that end they are required to nominate a person to lead on the development of clinical governance and to publish an annual report on the steps they are taking to ensure and improve quality and the measures they are taking to implement clinical governance. All NHS Trusts are required to produce their first clinical governance reports in spring 2000.

A new impetus is evident within the NHS. The practice of basing health care largely upon opinion is no longer acceptable in the new NHS and the drive is towards research evidence of clinical effectiveness. The responsibility for achieving this goal within the nursing profession rests equally with nursing management, nursing education and nursing practice. The remainder of this chapter will address these three interdependent aspects, with special reference to how research in all these areas is conducted, facilitated and implemented.

Management research

Management activities are in many aspects similar to the research process. This is particularly evident in a manager's approach to problem-solving and decision-making when systematic enquiry is essential for the collection of data and the cognitive abilities of assessment and analysis are used to process those data. The crucial role played by nurse managers in supporting and facilitating the nursing research agenda is a strongly emergent theme from the literature (Champion & Leach, 1989; Camiah, 1997; Kenrick & Luker, 1997).

The role of the manager relating to research has three aspects:

- Conducting research into management issues
- Facilitating staff to undertake research
- Implementing research findings into their own management practices

Conducting research into management issues

There is no particular approach to management research that can be claimed as being 'the best'. Management research uses a wide spectrum of approaches. Gill & Johnson (1991) categorize these approaches as follows:

- The experiential deductive approach, which involves a structured and controlled environment, hypothesis testing, quantitative data and generalizable findings. The use of the true experiment in management research is relatively rare; however, one well-recognized example involves the Hawthorne studies, which have been described by Roethlisberger & Dickson (1939).
- The ethnographic approach, which involves subjective accounts generated by the researcher 'getting inside' situations and viewing phenomena through the eyes of the subject.

   'Emphasis within this approach is on theory grounded in empirical observation which takes account of the subject's meaning and interpretational systems in order to explain understanding.' (Gill & Johnson, 1991: 9)

This approach generates mainly qualitative data and it has been used within management research to investigate issues relating to role and to study the specific characteristics of managers and management practices.

- The survey approach involves the generation of both quantitative and qualitative data. In terms of methodological rigour, survey research adopts an intermediate position in between experiential research and ethnography. Survey approaches have been used extensively within management research. In recent years survey research has been used to determine the level of customer satisfaction towards the care received. Alternatively it has been used to ascertain the opinions of staff towards specific approaches to care.
- The action research approach, which involves the solving of a management problem whilst simultaneously adding to the body of knowledge of change processes. The approach is cyclical in nature and involves fact finding, action and evaluation at every level. The process is participative and collaborative in nature and involves the researcher working in tandem with the action organization to solve organizational problems. This approach has become increasingly popular over recent years as it is seen to offer a means of narrowing the gap between theory and practice and of empowering nurses to instigate change. Examples of action research studies include Christine Webb's study in which action research was utilized to develop nursing and management skills (Webb, 1989) and an action research study conducted by Titchen & Binnie (1997) to develop patient-centred nursing in an acute medical unit.

Facilitating research activity in staff

While only a few nurse managers will be actively involved in conducting research, all nurse managers have the responsibility of facilitating their staff to participate in research activity. Nurse managers, when addressing this aspect of their role, could consider two specific areas of development – namely, the development of their organization to support research and the development of the individual to participate in research activity.

Development of a positive research culture

Gloss & Cheater (1994) postulated that the effective utilization of research findings and the effective facilitation of research activity within an organization could only take place if a positive research culture existed. They also recognized that the creation of such an environment involved willingness on the part of all the salient players – that is, managers and individual practitioners. The Inter-

- There is flexibility in teaching, administrative and/or clinical assignments so that time for research is possible.
- Time is used for such activities as thinking about researchable questions, conducting library searches and discussion with colleagues regarding designing and carrying out a study.
- A system of formal rewards and recognition exists for persons involved in research such as promotion, salary increases and opportunities for travel.
- An informal reward system exists within the organization, i.e. peers are supportive of active (nurse) researcher's involvement and productivity in research.
- Research productivity or recognition for achievement in research is demonstrated through the numbers of grants obtained, papers presented and manuscripts published.
- There are sufficient (nurse) researchers in the organization to act as a critical mass for the development of research.
- Nurse researchers participate in multi-disciplinary research projects.

Fig. 36.3   The characteristics of an organizational culture that is supportive of research (The International Congress of Nurses, 1985).

national Congress of Nurses (1985) identified the characteristics of an organization supportive of nursing research (Fig. 36.3).

Development of the practitioner

The professional bodies stipulate that all nurses have a responsibility to be aware of research findings and to seek ways of implementing those findings appropriately and evaluating their effects. Such activities are described as research awareness and involve a broad understanding of the research process and its application and relevance to practice. This should be integral to every nurse. Involvement in research projects, however, demands higher level abilities that often require the practitioner to undertake a specific educational programme. Wabschall (1987), cited by McGee (1996), identifies the personnel attributes required by research-oriented practitioners (Fig. 36.4).

The manager will be aware that only some of the personnel attributes in Fig. 36.4 can be taught or developed; the others are innate within the individual's personality.

- Creative thinking
- Critical and independent thinking skills
- Objectivity
- Clarity in the expression of ideas
- The ability to learn from mistakes
- The ability to live with uncertainty
- Self-discipline and self-organization
- Sense of humour

Fig. 36.4   Attributes of a researcher (Wabschall, 1987).

Implementing research findings into nursing management

Managers select between two alternatives in their approach to management practice. They may select to use the scientific approach whereby they utilize a problem-solving approach which draws on research findings to underpin their management practice, or they may select to use the alternative 'seat of the pants' management which evolves from following impulses and personal beliefs.

> 'The value of the scientific approach to management cannot be stressed more strongly as it forces the manager to plan, organise, motivate and control logically and analytically. It also allows the manager to build contingency plans for all possible outcomes rather than face problems unprepared.' (La Monica, 1994: x)

The scientific approach to management utilizes methodologically sound research derived from a variety of disciplines, including business studies, educational administration and psychology. The amount of research that is relevant and available to managers is extensive; however, the attention of the reader is drawn to two specific areas that are particularly pertinent to managers in contemporary organizations. These are: the management of change and problem-solving.

The management of change

There has been much research interest in the topic of change management with many prescriptions for managing the process effectively. The following is a synopsis of the most interesting:

- Lewin (1951), building on his research, described a three-stage model of change that involved unfreezing the *status quo*, moving towards change and refreezing the new situation and he proposed a method called force field analysis to assess the driving and resisting forces involved in the change process.

- Stewart (1983) suggests an incremental approach to change and postulates that change needs to be anticipated by manager. She also advocates that attitudes towards change can be altered more easily by creating circumstances whereby people are required to behave as if the attitude change has happened. In this way they gradually accept that the new situation is not so bad and they conform to the new behaviour.

- Kanter (1984), in *The Change Masters*, identifies relevant information, appropriate resources and expert support as essential factors in the management of change. She also recommends 'the don't do too much all at once' maxim and suggests that an accepted compromise is better than the best solution poorly accepted.

- Peters (1988) in *Thriving on Chaos* and Handy (1989) in *The Age of Unreason* describe similar approaches to the change process. They advocate that managers must accept that organizations are in an era of unprecedented change and must become flexible enough to respond quickly to the environment. Managers require to become obsessive about change. Predictability is a luxury of the past.

Problem-solving

Problem-solving and associated decision-making is a constant activity for managers; it is therefore not surprising that much research has been undertaken to assist managers to understand and manage problems and decisions more effectively. Hicks (1991) identifies three types of problem-solving approach:

- The rational approach
- The creative approach
- The soft systems approach

The rational approach

This is concerned with logical analytical and structured thinking. Stoner (1982) advocates a problem-solving cyclical model that involves recognition, definition and analysis of the problem, option generation, option choice implementation and evaluation. Buzan (1988) presents managers with a useful analytical tool for the solving of problems, which is called *mind mapping*.

The creative approach

Creativity is about thinking in a different and innovative way. It results in the generation of new and novel solutions to problems. De Bono (1981) introduced managers to the concept of lateral thinking – a process whereby the mind is stimulated to break free of its restricting mindset and think creatively.

The soft systems approach

The soft systems approach to problem-solving (Checkland & Scholes, 1991) is holistic in nature as opposed to the reductionist approach of rational problem-solving. At face value it appears complicated, however the underlying framework is relatively simple to understand. Checkland & Scholes (1991) advocate a two-stage approach to solving a problem. First, they suggest that managers paint a 'rich picture' of the problem situation. This rich picture should be holistic, in line with systems thinking and include all the structures and processes involved in the situation. Second, they encourage managers to construct a root definition of the systems they would wish to see in place. From this root definition a conceptual model emerges against which the rich picture or actual situation can be compared. From this analysis an appropriate action plan can be determined.

Research within nursing education has an enormous remit; however, for ease of presentation this section will consider its role and impact for nurse educationalists within the context of conducting educational research, facilitating research activity in students, and implementing educational research findings into their own teaching practices.

Conducting educational research

Educational research embraces the total spectrum of research methodologies. It would be inappropriate to single out any one approach as 'the best' for the educational setting. However, it would appear that, within the remit of their role, nurse educationalists have a particular responsibility to assess the educational needs of their students and to evaluate the outcomes of their teaching and learning strategies. It would therefore be pertinent to discuss the approaches of needs assessment and evaluation research in greater detail.

Needs assessment

Polit & Hungler (1991: 203) define needs assessment as: 'A study in which a researcher collects data for estimating the needs of a group, community or organisation. A needs assessment provides informational input in a planning process.' They also identify three key approaches: namely, the survey approach, the key informant approach and the indicators approach.

Survey approach

This is the most frequently used approach. All students or a representative sample are interviewed or respond by questionnaire to specific questions relating to their role and the education/training they require to carry out that role. Within the survey approach to needs assessment the technique of importance/performance analysis is often utilized. This technique requires respondents to rate, using a rating scale, both the importance that they place upon an item in terms of their educational development and their perceived current level of competence relating to that item. This technique allows the educational researcher to prioritize educational objectives, giving preference obviously to those items that have been rated as highly important, but with low levels of competence.

Key informant approach

This approach, as the name implies, involves collecting information concerning the needs of students from key individuals. These informants would be representative of different student groups. Within nurse education the collection of data from key informants is usually ongoing, with elected student representatives providing feedback to staff through a variety of staff/student liaison committees and course management teams.

Indicators approach

Information relating to student educational needs may be obtained from an analysis of student records and reports. Assessment results, student evaluation reports and reports from clinical assessors and tutorial staff would all be pertinent sources of information.

Evaluation research

Evaluation research investigates how well a programme, practice or policy is achieving its desired outcomes. Within the literature a variety of approaches are described, however it is beyond the remit of this chapter to discuss them all in detail. Two models with differing underlying philosophies are, however, presented.

The goal-oriented model (traditional approach)

Evaluation within this approach involves assessing progress against predetermined measures, which will ultimately determine the outcomes of the programme. The goal-oriented approach embraces four distinct phases:

- Determining the objectives of the programme
- Determining the indicators of achievement relating to the objectives
- Collecting appropriate data
- Interpreting the data against the objectives and the indicators of achievement

The greatest difficulty with this approach lies in phase one and in the determination of objectives that have measurable outcomes. Critics of this approach are keen to point out this problem and to emphasize that rigid adherence to measurable objectives within evaluation research invariably provides a very narrow perspective.

The goal-free model (untraditional approach)

In this model, evaluation attempts are made to assess the outcome of the programme without pre-agreed objectives and indicators. This approach is more holistic in its style and attempts to assess the impact of the programme on all the key components. For example, a goal-free evaluation of a nursing programme would attempt to assess the outcomes of the programme not only for the students, but also for the managers commissioning places. It would also attempt to assess the impact on patient care and on clinical staff who are both peers and fellow team members. The advantage of this approach is that it is more creative and provides a broader perspective; however, it is often not practical owing to the time and cost involved.

Facilitating research activity

Nurse educationalists play an important role in educating nurses both to implement research into their practice and to participate in research projects. The knowledge and skills required for research awareness and the development of research-based practice serve in many respects as a foundation upon which the more advanced skills of the nurse researcher may be built. A wealth of research literature is available identifying the knowledge and skills required by nurses both to implement research and to conduct research (Hunt, 1987; Walsh, 1997; McSherry, 1997). Figure 36.5 attempts to summarize the findings of this research by presenting a broad overview of the knowledge and skill required by nurses to implement research into practice and to participate meaningfully in research projects.

- Numeracy and literacy skills
- Information retrieval skills
- Knowledge and skills in comparative analysis
- Knowledge and skills in systematic review
- Knowledge of the research process
- Knowledge of available networks of information
- Knowledge of relevant research methodologies
- Data analysis and basic understanding of statistical tests
- An understanding of differing models of evidence-based practice
- Research proposal formulation
- Ethical issues and procedures
- Critical appraisal skills
- Problem-solving and decision-making strategies
- Assessing and managing change
- Differentiation between audit and research
- Clinical auditing processes
- Clinical protocol procedures and policies
- Research project report writing skills

Fig. 36.5 Inventory of nursing research knowledge and skills.

Implementing research into nurse education

Education, as a discipline, has been widely researched through the years, drawing particularly upon the work of educational psychologists. This in turn has resulted in the provision of a wealth of educational theories. These theories have significantly influenced many aspects of nurse education, however it is within the context of curriculum design and development and teaching and learning that these theories can be seen to have had their greatest impact. It would be pertinent to stress, however, that the degree to which these theories have been tested within nurse education is in fact questionable. The attention of the reader is, therefore, drawn to the need to evaluate the effectiveness of these theories within his own situation. A broad overview of the most pertinent developments are presented in Tables 36.1 and 36.2.

Table 36.1   Curriculum design and development

Theorist	Date	Title and underlying principles
Tyler, R.	1949	The Behavioural Objectives (Product) Model • Determination of objectives of achievement • Planning learning experiences to achieve these objectives • Evaluating the achievement of objectives
Stenhouse, L.	1975	The Process Model • Emphasis on the learning experience • Teaching is geared towards unpredictable outcomes • Emphasis on student self-appraisal of achievement
Lawton, D.	1983	The Cultural Analysis Model • Analysis of the society • Determination as to how members wish to see their society develop • Determination of values and principles needed to achieve the developments identified • Determination of the education means of achieving above

Over recent years nursing curricula have tended to steer away from the use of curriculum models and have moved towards the use of taxonomies of learning to underpin curriculum. Popular taxonomies include Bloom (1956 – a taxonomy for the cognitive domain), Steinaker & Bell (1979 – an experiential taxonomy) and Benner (1984 – a taxonomy of skill acquisition in clinical nursing).

Practitioner research

Practitioner research could be described as the new paradigm in nursing research. Fuller & Petch (1995) suggest that practitioner research is an idea whose time has

Table 36.2 Teaching and learning strategies

Theorist	Date	Title and underlying principles
Ausabel, D. *et al.*	1978	Meaningful learning • Students must adopt an appropriate learning set • The learning task must have logical meaning to the student • New concepts must interact with the student's existing cognitive structures
Bruner, J.	1960	Discovery learning • Learning achieved through active participation • Students should be exposed to simple concepts before being exposed to the more complex
Kolb, D.	1984	Experiential learning • Students experience new situations • Students reflect on those experiences • Students create concepts and construct logical themes • Students test the theories in new situations
Schon, D.	1983	Reflective learning • Theory and practice are inseparable • Reflection adds theory to action while it is occurring • Two types of reflection are described: – Reflection on action (after the event) – Reflection in action (during the event)
Knowles, M.	1990	Andragogical (adult) learning • Self-direction in learning • Use of past experiences in the learning process • Emphasis on problem-solving and task-centred learning approaches • Student motivation is driven by self-esteem and self-actualization

come. Before offering the reader a definition of practitioner research it would be wise to explain the underpinning rationale and to set it into context. This chapter began by reminding the reader of the government's drive towards research-based practice in the NHS and that, as a result, research was becoming everyone's business. To nurse practitioners this has presented something of a dilemma – a dilemma that centres around a concept that we have called the theory–practice gap. Rolfe (1998) identifies that the prime purpose of nursing research has been to generate knowledge and to extend the body of nursing theory available to the profession. This, he argues, presents a problem in that nursing is primarily a practice-based profession and the application of generalizable findings to individually unique person-centred practice, the very ethos of the government's research-based practice initiative, has resulted in the theory–practice gap.

From the wealth of literature available regarding getting research findings implemented into nursing practice (Lomas & Haynes, 1988; Kitson *et al.*, 1996; Kenrick & Luker, 1997) it is evident that one of the major barriers is that nurse practitioners are not aware of the research available and if they are aware they fail to organize its relevance to their individual practice situation. This gap between theory and practice can be partly explained by two factors. First, research in nursing has historically been an elitist activity conducted by academics in higher education institutions and geographically displaced from the practice setting. Second, great emphasis has been placed on the deductive positivist research methodologies that produce quantitative findings that are generalizable to the wider nursing profession. These two factors have created a hierarchical situation involving a select group, mainly of academics, that pass down their findings to practitioners to implement. This model may well be very relevant to the more theoretical disciplines such as the social sciences, however within nursing this hierarchical relationship has resulted in a lack of confidence and a growing scepticism that professional knowledge has little relevance to practice situations.

There is a strong drive, therefore, towards a paradigm of clinical nursing research. Clinical research works in partnership with, and indeed complements, theoretical research; it is involved with investigating individual nursing situations and is conducted by practitioners in the clinical situation. Rolfe (1998: 72) states that: 'Clinical research to be effective in practice must be practitioner based research.'

Conducting practitioner research

By its very nature practitioner research invariably involves very small samples and this has been the source of considerable criticism regarding its intellectual rigour and validity. However, Rolfe (1998) argues that single case research is well established in sociology and psychology and identifies the work of Piaget and Freud who both used small numbers and the single in-depth case study approach to their ground-breaking work. Within single case research the full range of research methodologies are available to the researcher. However, the ethnographic case study approach and the action research previously described are invariably the favoured approaches.

Facilitating practitioner research

It is pertinent that this section should serve as the conclusion to the chapter as it allows the reader to see how nurse managers, nurse educationalists and nurse practitioners are interdependent upon each other for the successful facilitation of practitioner research. Increasingly NHS organizations are working in liaison with higher education organizations to support research-based practice and promote practitioner research. The educators in health care play an important role in ensuring that practitioners have the appropriate level of knowledge necessary to underpin their research activity and they may also act as a catalyst by generating a spirit of enquiry and by encouraging practitioners to reflect upon and question practice. Many NHS Trusts are establishing a specific post at Trust level for nursing R&D facilitators. These posts have the remit of leading the nursing R&D agenda for the Trust and one emerging model for these posts is to negotiate a joint appointment or an honorary lecturership with a local higher education institution. The creation of such posts will lead eventually to the establishment of a supporting infrastructure between the Trust and the academic institution allowing researchers greater access to practice settings and practitioners better access to the research facilities and the expertise of higher education.

As previously discussed, nursing management also plays a crucial role in facilitating practitioner research, primarily by providing both support and resources. An example of how this has been achieved within some Trusts is the establishment of nursing development units. The purpose of such a unit is to provide a supportive environment that will initiate and co-ordinate practitioner-based research activity.

The essence of nursing is the unique relationship that exists between the patient and the nurse. It is important, therefore, that nursing research improves our understanding of this therapeutic interactive process. Only practitioners can effectively conduct such research but they require the support of management to generate the appropriate resources and educationalists to promote the appropriate knowledge and skill. Given optimum circumstances, this dynamic team has tremendous potential to influence practice and to achieve the ultimate aim of all health care research, which is to improve the care given to patients.

References

Ausabel, D., Novak, J. & Hanesian, H. (1978) *Educational Psychology: A Cognitive View*. New York: Holt, Rinehart & Winston.

Benner, P. (1984) *From Novice to Expert. Excellence and Power in Clinical Nursing Practice*. London: Addison-Wesley.

Bloom, B. (1956) *Taxonomy of Educational Objectives. The Classification of Educational Goals. Handbook One: Cognitive Domain*. New York: MacKay.

Bruner, J. (1960) *The Process of Education*. Cambridge, Mass.: Harvard University Press.

Buzan, T. (1988) *Making the Most of Your Mind*. London: Pan Books.

Camiah, S. (1997) Utilisation of nursing research in practice and application strategies to raise awareness amongst nurse practitioners. *Journal of Advanced Nursing* 26: 1193–1202.

Champion, V. & Leach, A. (1989) Variables related to research utilisation in nursing: an empirical investigation. *Journal of Advanced Nursing* 14: 705–10.

Checkland, P.B. & Scholes, J. (1991) *Soft Systems Methodology in Action*. Chichester: John Wiley.

Culyer, A.J. (1994) Taskforce on research and development in the NHS. *Supporting Research and Development in the NHS*. London: HMSO.

De Bono, E. (1981). *Lateral Thinking for Management*. Harmondsworth: Penguin.

DoH (1991) *Research for Health: An R&D Strategy for the NHS*. London: HMSO.

DoH. (1992a) *The NHS R&D Information Systems Strategy Study*. Department of Health for NHS ME Research and Development Directorate. London: HMSO.

DoH (1992b) *Assessing the Effects of Health Technologies*. Department of Health Advisory Group on Health Technology Assessment. London: HMSO.

DoH (1993a) *Research for Health*. London: HMSO.

DoH (1993b) *Report of the Taskforce on the Strategy for Research in Nursing, Midwifery and Health Visiting*. London: HMSO.

DoH (1995) *Supporting R&D in the NHS: Implementation Plan*. London: HMSO.

DoH (1996) *The New Funding System for R&D in the NHS: An Outline*. London: HMSO.

DoH (1998) *A First Class Service: Quality in the New NHS*. London: HMSO.

Fuller, R. & Petch, A. (1995) *Practitioner Research: The Reflexive Social Worker*. Buckingham: Open University Press.

Gill, J. & Johnson, P. (1991) *Research Methods for Managers*. London: Paul Chapman Publishing.

Gloss, S.J. & Cheater, F.M. (1994) Utilisation of nursing research: culture, interest and support. *Journal of Advanced Nursing* 14: 762–73.

Handy, C. (1989) *The Age of Unreason*. London: Business Books.

Heard, S. (1998) The risk of missing the point of the quest for continuous improvement. *British Journal of Health Care Management* 4 (12, Supplement).

Hicks, M.J. (1991) *Problem Solving in Business and Management: Hard, Soft and Creative Approaches*. London: Chapman & Hall.

House of Lords Select Committee on Science and Technology (1988) *Priorities in Medical Research*, vol. 1. London: HMSO.

Hunt, M. (1987) The process of translating research findings into nursing practice. *Journal of Advanced Nursing* 12: 101–10.

International Congress of Nurses (1985) *Proceedings of Assembly*. London: Royal College of Nursing.

Kanter, R.M. (1984). *The Change Masters*. London: Allen & Unwin.

Kenrick, M. & Luker, K. (1997) An exploration of the influence of managerial factors on research utilisation in district nursing practice. *Journal of Advanced Nursing* 23: 697–704.

Kitson, A., Ahmed, L., Harvey, G., Seers, K. & Thompson, R. (1996) From research to practice: one organisational model for promoting research-based practice. *Journal of Advanced Nursing* 23: 430–40.

Knowles, M. (1990) *The Adult Learner: A Neglected Species,* 4th edition. Houston: Gulf Publishing.

Kolb, D. (1984) *Experimental Learning*. London: Prentice Hall.

La Monica, E. (1994) *Management in Health Care: A Theoretical and Experiential Approach*. London: Macmillan.

Lawton, D. (1983) *Curriculum Studies and Educational Planning*. London: Hodder & Stoughton.

Lewin, K. (1951) *Field Theory in Social Science*. New York: Harper & Row.

Lomas, J. & Haynes, R.D. (1988) A taxonomy and critical review of tested strategies for the application of clinical practice. Recommendations from official to individual clinical policy. *American Journal of Preventative Medicine* (Supplement) 77–95.

McGee, P. (1996) The research role of the advanced nurse practitioner. *British Journal of Nursing* 5 (5): 290–1.

McSherry, R. (1997) What do registered nurses know and feel about research? *Journal of Advanced Nursing* 25: 985–98.

Peters, T. (1988) *Thriving on Chaos*. London: Macmillan.

Polit, D.F. & Hungler, B.P. (1991) *Nursing Research: Principles and Methods*, 4th edn. Philadelphia: Lippincott.

Roethlisberger, F.J. & Dickson, W.J. (1939) *Management and the Worker*. Cambridge. Mass.: Harvard University Press.

Rolfe, G. (1998) The theory practice gap in nursing: from research based practice to practitioner based research. *Journal of Advanced Nursing* 28: 672–9.

Schon, D. (1983) *The Reflective Practitioner: How Professionals Think in Action*. New York: Basic Books.

Steinaker, N. & Bell, M. (1979) *The Experiential Taxonomy: A New Approach to Teaching and Learning*. New York: Academic Press.

Stenhouse, L. (1975) *An Introduction to Curriculum Research and Development*. London: Heinemann.

Stewart, V. (1983) *Change the Challenge of Management*. London: McGraw-Hill.

Stoner, J.A.F. (1982) *Management*, 2nd edn. Englewood Cliffs; NJ: Prentice Hall International.

Titchen, A. & Binnie, A. (1997) *Freedom to Practice: A Study of the Development of Patient-Centred Nursing in an Acute Medical Unit*. Oxford: RCN Institute.

Tyler, R. (1949) *Basic Principles of Curriculum and Instruction*. Chicago: University of Chicago Press.

Wabschall, (1987) The clinical nurse specialist as researcher. In S. Menard, (ed.) *The Clinical Nurse Specialist. Perspectives in Practice*. New York: John Wiley & Sons, pp. 145–88.

Walsh, M. (1997) Perceptions of barriers to implementing research. *Nursing Standard* 29: 34–7.

Webb, C. (1989) Action research: philosophy methods and personal experiences. *Journal of Advanced Nursing* 14: 403–10.

Epilogue

As nursing, midwifery and associated groups become professions in the fullest meaning of the term, there can be no doubt that they are developing a firm research base. Without such a base, they would undoubtedly lack the support, academic and clinical credibility, and professionalism which they deserve and require. Although there continues to be a place for the use of some intuition, opinion and untested theory by these groups, this is being tempered with a much stronger research input than has been the case in the past. Although the change of emphasis which will result in a greater research-mindedness is perceived by some as threatening, it need not be so. Nurses, midwives and other professions are not being criticized for the approaches to care which they have developed thus far; indeed all are to be applauded for the developments that have been achieved. Rather, they are embarking on a process of self-analysis and self-criticism which is making full use of a scientific tool not previously available to all their members – *research*.

Now that the research process is becoming better understood by increasing numbers of professionals, the possibility of making it accessible to all is becoming much more real. Thus far, the majority who have developed research skills have been based in academic establishments such as colleges and universities – a historical fact which is easy to understand in the context of research having a strong academic component. However, now that a number of academically oriented educators, clinicians and managers have taken steps towards making nursing and midwifery research-based professions, the time is now right to introduce a greater degree of research-mindedness into the thinking of all groups and individuals.

The groups for whom this book was written are composed largely of clinicians who are supported by a number of subgroups such as managers and educators. As clinicians – the *raison d'être* for all groups – more fully understand and make use of the research process, nursing, midwifery and associated groups will become increasingly research based. This book has been prepared with all these groups in mind, particularly those who are concerned with the delivery of direct patient care, and who wish to do so with a full appreciation of the value, meaning, utility and process of research.

Desmond F.S. Cormack

Index